An Introduction to the
Physics of Diagnostic Radiology

An Introduction to the
Physics of Diagnostic Radiology

EDWARD E. CHRISTENSEN, M.D.

*Professor of Radiology, University of Texas
Health Science Center at Dallas
and Parkland Memorial Hospital*

THOMAS S. CURRY, III, M.D.

*Professor of Radiology, University of Texas
Health Science Center at Dallas
and Parkland Memorial Hospital*

JAMES E. DOWDEY, Ph.D.

*Associate Professor of Radiology (Physics),
University of Texas Health Science Center
at Dallas and Parkland Memorial Hospital*

2nd Edition

Lea & Febiger   *Philadelphia*

Library of Congress Cataloging in Publication Data

Christensen, Edward E
    An introduction to the physics of diagnostic radiology.

    Includes bibliographies and index.
    1. Diagnosis, Radioscopic. 2. Medical physics.
I. Curry, Thomas S., joint author. II. Dowdey, James E.,
joint author. III. Title.
RC78.C467   1978   616.07′572   78-5405
ISBN 0-8121-0636-9

1st Edition, 1972
    Reprinted 1973, 1975, 1976, 1977
2nd Edition, 1978

Published in Great Britain by Henry Kimpton Publishers, London

PRINTED IN THE UNITED STATES OF AMERICA

Print number: 6   5   4   3

DEDICATED TO:

Dolly
Miss Winn
Vauda

Preface

In the preface to the first edition of this text we spoke of the understandable apprehension with which the radiology resident approached the study of physics. We must now acknowledge the terrible apprehension with which two of us (E.E.C. and T.S.C.) approached the preparation of the second edition. Advances in technology threaten to overwhelm the clinical radiologist. Understanding how to apply this technology in rendering improved patient care is difficult, but also understanding the complex physics that provides these techniques is just about impossible. In this edition, we attempt to introduce the important equipment advances and changes which confront radiology. Ultrasound requires us to explore the physics involved in the generation, propagation and detection of sonic waves. Computerized tomography uses many physical principles familiar to radiologists, but adds the complex mathematics of image reconstruction with strange new words like pixel and voxel. And then there is xeroradiography which detours us into the exotic realm of solid state physics. Even our old friends, intensifying and fluoroscopic screens and x-ray film, now emerge with new colors and compositions that include rare earths and other elements that most of us had rarely, if ever, even been aware of. Radiation protection has been accorded the chapter it deserves; the absence of this chapter from the first edition was our most frequent criticism. The topics of cineradiography, television and magnification have been considerably amplified.

Our purpose remains to present this material in an understandable format not only to radiology residents, but also to students of radiologic technology. Unfortunately, some of the new topics demand a little more arithmetic, but we have insisted on keeping things as simple as possible. That we have succeeded for only a few readers will make the effort amply rewarding. The following comment which we received from two young radiologists in New York describes our wish for all our students.

". . . your book actually made the subject understandable and almost believable. It was the most readable book since *The Joy of Sex,* although the illustrations were not quite as interesting."

Thank you. And good luck.

Dallas, Texas

E. E. CHRISTENSEN, M.D.
T. S. CURRY III, M.D.
J. E. DOWDEY, Ph.D.

Preface to the First Edition

The resident in Radiology, in seeking to attain proficiency in his chosen specialty, finds himself confronted with the need to assimilate knowledge from a number of different disciplines. Having completed medical school, he is well prepared to deal with the biological aspects of the subject, but the realization that physics is also included in the curriculum of diagnostic radiology often comes as an unpleasant surprise. The facts learned in the physics course taken in undergraduate school have usually been dimmed by the passing years or lost in the confusion produced by the massive onslaught of the medical school curriculum. Therefore, most residents in diagnostic radiology, when they reencounter the study of physics, enter the field with understandable apprehension. For several years we sympathized with our residents as they mounted an inefficient, time consuming offensive against this traditionally formidable subject. It soon became apparent that physics, by demanding a disproportionate share of their time, had distracted them from their other academic pursuits.

In an effort to provide assistance, in addition to sympathy, we prepared a series of lectures dealing primarily with some of the applications of physics to the clinical practice of diagnostic radiology. These were well received, and it is upon these lectures that the text of this book is based. The book is intended to be used by radiology residents beginning their study of the physics of diagnostic radiology. Two of us (E.E.C. and T.S.C.) are diagnostic radiologists, singularly unschooled in higher mathematics or advanced physics. Thus, our understanding and presentation are based on the experience of a clinician.

Our purpose is to introduce the student of radiology to the tools of his trade and to describe some of the physical and chemical phenomena which make those tools work for him. The subjects of electricity, magnetism, atomic structure, circuitry, and x-ray protection are not discussed, except where such subjects are necessary for the understanding of a specific point. We have attempted to introduce those topics that are truly important and must be mastered if the maximum amount of diagnostic information is to be obtained from the radiographic examination, whether this information be recorded on film, a fluoroscopic screen, or a television monitor. We begin with the production of x-rays and the interactions between the patient and the x-ray beam. Such considerations lead to a discussion of collimators, grids, x-ray film and its proper exposure and processing, magnification, subtraction techniques, stereoscopy, and tomography. We feel that it is equally important to examine the use of devices which decrease the radiation dose to the patient, such as the x-ray image intensifier and intensifying screens, and to determine how the use of these devices affects the final radiographic image.

We have endeavored to present this material in such a way that it can be understood by a student with no mathematical training other than arithmetic and basic algebra. Therefore, presentations are necessarily simple, often superficial, and sometimes incomplete. We propose that it is better to understand a few fundamental principles than to be thoroughly confused by a plethora of data. This text is intended to be used in preparation for the study of the more complete textbooks of the physics of diagnostic radiology.

At some time during his period of intensive study the student of diagnostic radiology must decide to cross the Rubicon and learn physics. We hope that the following pages will make the journey a little easier.

Dallas, Texas

E.E. CHRISTENSEN, M.D.
T.S. CURRY, M.D.
J.E. NUNNALLY, M.A.

Acknowledgments

With the publication of the second edition, we acknowledge the absence of one of the original authors. Geographic separation from James Nunnally required that we acquire a new physicist who could share our offices and thoughts on a daily, and usually hourly, basis, so we welcome James E. Dowdey, Ph.D. as a co-author.

We must expand our indebtedness to many more people who helped in the preparation of this new edition.

We received valuable assistance from the E. I. duPont de Nemours and Company and the Eastman Kodak Company. We must especially thank R. E. Warynen of duPont for his continued help, and Al Allard of Kodak for joining our long list of helpers.

Nancy Sciscenti and Jan Dolph prepared all the new illustrations. Their suggestions and beautiful handiwork are much appreciated.

Three photographers, Dorothy Gutekunst, Katie Belle Wolf and Nancy Schreiber, shared the responsibility of preparing reproductions of the illustrations.

John Moore again assumed the role of coordinator and critic. In our department, John is known as "the man who built the book."

For typing the manuscript we are fortunate to have had Glenda Parkinson, Carolyn Tunnell and Linda Wooldridge.

The continued support we received from our friends and colleagues in the Radiology and Physics Departments remains one of the most rewarding aspects of this effort. Drs. Mike Landay and Harold Smitson assumed many of our clinical responsibilities, and Bob Murry and Mike Tipton occupied similar positions in the Physics Department. Other radiologists sharing the burden of our repeated absence from work include Drs. George Curry, Jan Diehl, Geral Dietz, Bob Epstein, Bill Kilman, Ken Maravilla and Bob Parkey. And our reliable and extraordinary friend, Dr. Jack Reynolds remained available to review and edit many pages of the manuscript.

Finally, we must confess that the entire project was undertaken only after we received permission from our patient wives. We are not sure why they let us do it, but we guess we are glad they did.

E.E.C.
T.S.C.
J.E.D.

Contents

CHAPTER 1

Radiation

Wilhelm Conrad Roentgen, a German physicist, discovered x rays on November 8, 1895. Several fortunate coincidences set the stage for the discovery. Roentgen was investigating the behavior of cathode rays (electrons) in high-energy cathode ray tubes. The tube consisted of a glass envelope from which as much air as possible had been evacuated. A short platinum electrode was fitted into each end, and when a high voltage discharge was passed through this tube, ionization of the remaining gas produced a faint light. Roentgen had enclosed his cathode ray tube in black cardboard to prevent this light from escaping in order to block any effect the light might have on experiments he was conducting. He then darkened his laboratory room to be sure there were no light leaks in the cardboard cover. Upon passing a high tension discharge through the tube, he noticed a faint light glowing on a work bench about 3 feet away. He discovered that the source of the light was the fluorescence of a small piece of paper coated with barium platinocyanide. Since electrons could not escape the glass envelope of the tube to produce fluorescence, and the cardboard permitted no light to escape from the tube, he concluded that some unknown type of ray was produced when the tube was energized. We can imagine his excitement as he investigated the mysterious new ray. He began placing objects between the tube and the fluorescent screen: a book, a block of wood, and a sheet of aluminum. The brightness of the fluorescence differed with each, indicating that the ray penetrated some objects more easily than others. Then he held his hand between the tube and the screen, and to his surprise, the outline of his skeleton appeared on the screen. By December 28, 1895, he had thoroughly investigated the properties of the rays and had prepared a manuscript describing his experiments. In recognition of his outstanding contribution to science, Wilhelm Conrad Roentgen was awarded the first Nobel Prize for Physics in 1901.

THE ELECTROMAGNETIC SPECTRUM

X rays belong to a group of radiations called electromagnetic radiation. **Electromagnetic radiation is the transport of energy through space as a combination of electric fields and magnetic fields** (hence the name electromagnetic). Familiar members of the family of electromagnetic radiation include radio waves, radiant heat, visible light, and gamma radiation.

The interactions of electromagnetic radiations are difficult to understand. Some interactions of electromagnetic radiations are explained only if they are assumed to be particles, while other interactions are explained only by theories of wave propagation. **It is necessary to discuss electromagnetic radiations as if they were both particles and waves.**

1

Wave Concept of Electromagnetic Radiation

Electromagnetic radiations are propagated through space in the form of waves. They may be compared to a wave traveling down a stretched rope when one end is moved up and down in a rhythmic motion. However, while the waves with which we are familiar must be propagated in a medium (such as the example of the rope, waves traveling in water, or sound waves traveling in air), electromagnetic waves need no such medium; i.e., they can be propagated through a vacuum. Waves of all kinds have an associated wavelength and a frequency. The distance between two successive crests, or troughs, is the wavelength of the wave, and is given the symbol λ (the Greek letter **lambda,** the initial for length). The number of waves passing a particular point in a unit of time is called the frequency, given the symbol ν (the Greek letter **nu,** the initial for number). If each wave has a length λ, and ν waves pass a given point in unit time, the velocity of the wave is given by:

$$V = \lambda \times \nu$$

For example, if the wavelength is 4 feet and the frequency is 60 waves per minute, then the velocity is:

Velocity = 4 ft. × 60/min
Velocity = 240 ft./min

Electromagnetic radiations always travel at the same velocity in a vacuum. This velocity is 186,000 miles per second (3×10^8 meters per second), which is usually referred to as the velocity of light and given the symbol c. Therefore, we may express the relationship between velocity, wavelength, and frequency as:

$$c = \lambda\nu$$

c = velocity of light (m/sec)
λ = wavelength (meters)
ν = frequency (per second)

Since all electromagnetic radiations have the same velocity, the frequency of the radiation must be inversely proportional to its wavelength. All the radiations in the electromagnetic spectrum differ basically only in wavelength. The wavelength of a radiowave may be 5 miles long, while a typical x ray is only 1 billionth of an inch. The wavelength of diagnostic x rays is extremely short and it is usually expressed in angstrom units (Å). An angstrom is 10^{-10} meters. The wavelength of most diagnostic x rays is between 1Å and 0.1Å. The wavelength of an electromagnetic wave determines how it interacts with matter. For example, an electromagnetic wave 7000 Å long can be seen by the human eye as red light, and a wavelength of 4000 Å is seen as blue light. The frequency of blue light may be calculated by knowing its wavelength (4000 Å = 4×10^{-7} meters):

$$c = \lambda\nu \text{ or } \nu = \frac{c}{\lambda}$$

$$\nu = \frac{3 \times 10^8 \text{ meters per sec}}{4 \times 10^{-7} \text{ meters}}$$

$$\nu = 7.5 \times 10^{14} \text{ per sec}$$

Blue light, with a wavelength of 4000 Å, has a frequency of 7.5×10^{14} vibrations per second. Similarly calculated, the frequency of an x ray of wavelength 0.1 Å is 3×10^{19} vibrations per second.

The complete spectrum of electromagnetic radiations covers a wide range of wavelengths and frequencies. The various parts of the spectrum are named according to the manner in which the radiations are generated or detected. Some of the members of the group, listed in order of decreasing wavelength, are:

Radio, television, radar:	3×10^5 cm to 1 cm
Infrared radiation:	0.01 cm to .00008 cm (8,000 Å)
Visible light:	7,500 Å (.000075 cm) to 3,900 Å
Ultraviolet radiation:	3,900 Å to 20 Å
Soft x rays:	100 Å to 1 Å
Diagnostic x rays:	1 Å to 0.1 Å
Therapy x ray & gamma rays:	0.1 Å to 10^{-4} Å

There is considerable overlap in the wavelengths of the various members of the electromagnetic spectrum; the numbers listed are rough guides. It is again stressed that the very great differences in properties of these radiations are attributable to their differences in wavelength (or frequency).

The wave concept of electromagnetic radiations explains why these radiations may be reflected, refracted, diffracted, and polarized. However, there are some phenomena that cannot be explained by the wave concept.

Particle Concept of Electromagnetic Radiation

Short electromagnetic waves, such as x rays, may react with matter as if they were particles, rather than waves. The particles of which we speak are actually discrete bundles of energy, and each of these bundles of energy is called a **quantum** or a **photon.** These photons travel at the speed of light. The amount of energy carried by each quantum, or photon, depends upon the frequency (ν) of the radiation. If the frequency (number of vibrations per sec) is doubled, the energy of the photon is doubled. The actual amount of energy of the photon may be calculated by multiplying its frequency times a constant. The constant has been determined experimentally to be 4.13×10^{-18} keV sec, and it is called Planck's constant. The mathematical expression is written as follows:

$$E = h\nu$$
$$E = \text{photon energy}$$
$$h = \text{Planck's constant}$$
$$\nu = \text{frequency}$$

The ability to visualize the dual characteristics of electromagnetic radiation presents a true challenge. But we must unavoidably reach the conclusion that electromagnetic radiation behaves sometimes as a wave and at other times as a particle. The particle concept is used to describe the interactions between radiation and matter. Since we will be concerned principally with interactions, such as the photoelectric effect and Compton scatter, we will use the photon (or quantum) concept in this text.

The unit that is used to measure the energy of photons is the electron volt (eV). An electron volt is the amount of energy that an electron gains as it is accelerated by a potential difference of 1 volt. Since the electron volt is a small unit, x-ray energies are usually measured in terms of the kiloelectron volt (keV), which is 1000 electron volts. We will usually discuss x rays in terms of their energy rather than their wavelengths, but the two are related as follows:

$$c = \lambda\nu \text{ or } \nu = \frac{c}{\lambda}$$

$$\text{And: } E = h\nu$$

$$\text{Substituting } \frac{c}{\lambda} \text{ for } \nu$$

$$E = \frac{hc}{\lambda}$$

The product of the velocity of light (c) and Planck's constant (h) is 12.4, when the unit of energy is keV and the wavelength is in angstroms. The final equation showing the relationship between energy and wavelength is:

$$E = \frac{12.4}{\lambda}$$

$$E = \text{energy in keV}$$
$$\lambda = \text{wavelengths in angstroms (Å)}$$

Table 1–1 shows the relationship between energy and wavelength for various photons.

If a photon has 15, or more, electron volts of energy, it is capable of ionizing atoms and molecules, and it is called ionizing radiation. An atom is ionized when it loses an electron. Gamma rays, x rays, and some ultraviolet rays are all ionizing radiations.

Table 1–1. Correlation Between Wavelength and Energy

WAVELENGTH (Å)	ENERGY (keV)
.0005	24,800
.08	155
.1	124
1.24	10

SUMMARY

Wilhelm Conrad Roentgen discovered x rays on November 8, 1895. X rays are members of a group of radiations known as electromagnetic radiations, of which light is the best-known member. They have a dualistic nature, behaving in some circumstances as waves and under different conditions as particles. Therefore, two concepts have been postulated to explain their characteristics. A single particle of radiation is called a photon, and we will discuss x rays in terms of photons.

REFERENCE

1. Glasser, O.: *Wilhelm Conrad Roentgen and the Early History of the Roentgen Rays.* Springfield, Charles C Thomas, 1934.

CHAPTER 2

Production of X rays

DIAGNOSTIC X-RAY TUBES

X rays are produced by **energy conversion** when a fast-moving stream of electrons is suddenly decelerated in the "target" anode of an x-ray tube. The x-ray tube is made of Pyrex glass which encloses a vacuum containing two electrodes (this is a diode tube). The electrodes are designed so that electrons produced at the cathode (negative electrode or filament) can be accelerated by a high potential difference toward the anode (positive electrode or target electrode). The basic elements of an x-ray tube are shown in Figure 2–1, which is a diagram of a stationary anode x-ray tube. Electrons are produced by the heated

tungsten filament and accelerated across the tube to hit the tungsten target, where x rays are produced. It will be the purpose of this section to describe the design of the x-ray tube and to review the way in which x rays are produced.

The Glass Enclosure

It is necessary to seal the two electrodes of the x-ray tube in a vacuum. If gas were present inside the tube, the electrons which were being accelerated toward the anode (target) would collide with the gas molecules, lose energy, and cause secondary electrons to be ejected from the electron orbits of the gas molecules. By this

Figure 2–1   The major components of a stationary anode x-ray tube

process (ionization) additional electrons would be available for acceleration toward the anode. Obviously, this production of secondary electrons could not be satisfactorily controlled. Their presence would result in variation in the number and, more strikingly, the reduced speed of the electrons impinging on the target. This would result in a wide variation in tube current and in the energy of the x rays produced. Actually, this principle was used in the design of the early, so-called "gas" x-ray tubes, which contained small amounts of gas to serve as a source of secondary electrons. The purpose of the vacuum in the modern x-ray tube is to allow the number and speed of the accelerated electrons to be controlled independently. The shape and size of these x-ray tubes are specifically designed to prevent electric discharge between the electrodes.

It is necessary to seal the connecting wires into the glass wall of the x-ray tube. During operation of the x-ray tube, both the glass and the connecting wires are heated to high temperatures. Because of differences in their coefficients of expansion, most metals expand more than glass when heated. This difference in expansion would cause the glass-metal seal to break and destroy the vacuum in the tube if special precautions were not taken. Because of this problem, special alloys, having approximately the same coefficients of linear expansion as borosilicate glass, are usually used in x-ray tubes.

The Cathode

The negative terminal of the x-ray tube is called the cathode. In referring to an x-ray tube, the terms **cathode** and **filament** may be used interchangeably, a statement which is not true for other types of diode tubes. In addition to **the filament, which is the source of electrons** for the x-ray tube, the cathode has two other elements. These are: (1) the connecting wires which supply the source of voltage (average about 10 volts) and amperage (average about 3 to 5

amperes) which heat the filament, and (2) a metallic focusing cup. The number (quantity) of x rays produced depends entirely on the number of electrons which flow from the filament to the target (anode) of the tube. **The x-ray tube current, measured in milliamperes** (1 mA = 1/1000 ampere), **refers to the number of electrons flowing per second.** It is important to understand where these electrons come from and that the number of electrons determines x-ray tube current. For example, in a given unit of time, a tube current of 200 mA is produced by twice as many electrons as a current of 100 mA, and 200 mA produces twice as many x rays as 100 mA.

The filament is made of tungsten wire, about 0.2 mm in diameter, which is coiled to form a vertical spiral about 0.2 cm in diameter and 1 cm or less in length. When current flows through this fine tungsten wire, it becomes heated. When a metal is heated, its atoms absorb thermal energy, and some of the electrons in the metal acquire enough energy to allow them to move a small distance from the surface of the metal (normally, electrons can move within a metal, but cannot escape from the metal). Their escape is referred to as the process of **thermionic emission,** which may be defined as the emission of electrons resulting from the absorption of thermal energy. A pure tungsten filament must be heated to a temperature of at least 2200°C to emit a useful number of electrons (thermions). Tungsten is not as efficient an emitting material as other materials (alloys of tungsten) used in some electron tubes. However, it is chosen for use in x-ray tubes because it can be drawn into a thin wire that is quite strong, has a high melting point (3370°C), and has little tendency to vaporize; thus such a filament has a reasonably long life expectancy.

Electrons emitted from the tungsten filament form a small cloud in the immediate vicinity of the filament. This collection of negatively charged electrons forms what is called the **space charge.** This cloud of negative charges tends to prevent other electrons from being emitted from the filament until they have acquired sufficient thermal energy to overcome the force caused by the space charge. The tendency of the space charge to limit the emission of more electrons from the filament is called the **space charge effect.** When electrons leave the filament, the loss of negative charges causes the filament to acquire a positive charge. The filament then attracts some emitted electrons back to itself. When a filament is heated to its emission temperature, a state of equilibrium is reached quickly. In equilibrium the number of electrons returning to the filament equals the number of electrons being emitted. As a result the number of electrons in the space charge remains constant, the actual number depending on filament temperature.

The high currents which can be produced by the use of thermionic emission are possible because of the fact that large numbers of electrons can be accelerated from the cathode (negative electrode) to the anode (positive electrode) of the x-ray tube. The number of electrons involved is enormous. The unit of electric current is the ampere, which may be defined as the rate of "flow" when 1 coulomb of electricity flows through a conductor in 1 second. The coulomb may be defined as the amount of electric charge carried by 6.25×10^{18} electrons. Therefore, an x-ray tube current of 100 milliamperes (0.1 ampere) may be considered as the "flow" of 6.25×10^{17} electrons from the cathode to the anode in 1 second. **Electron current across an x-ray tube is in one direction only** (always cathode to anode). Because of the forces of mutual repulsion and the large number of electrons, this electron stream would tend to spread itself out and result in bombardment of an unacceptably large area on the anode of the x-ray tube. This is prevented by a structure called the cathode **focusing cup** which

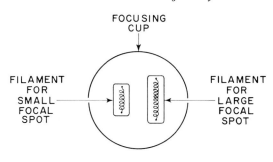

Figure 2–2   A double filament contained in the focusing cup

surrounds the filament (Figures 2–2 and 2–4). When the x-ray tube is conducting, the focusing cup is maintained at the same negative potential as the filament. The focusing cup is designed so that its electrical forces cause the electron stream to converge onto the target anode in the required size and shape. The focusing cup is usually made of molybdenum. Modern x-ray tubes may be supplied with a single or, more commonly, a double filament. Each filament consists of a spiral of wire, and they are mounted side by side or one above the other, one being longer than the other (Figure 2–2). It is important to understand that only one filament is used for any given x-ray exposure, the larger filament generally being used for larger exposures. The heated filament glows and can be easily observed by looking into the beam exit port of an x-ray tube housing (do not forget to remove the filter).

Vaporization of the filament when it is heated acts to shorten the life of an x-ray tube, because the filament will break if it becomes too thin. The filament should never be heated for longer periods than necessary. Many modern x-ray circuits contain an automatic filament-boosting circuit. When the x-ray circuit is turned on, but no exposure is being made, a "standby" current heats the filament to a value corresponding to low mA, commonly about 5 mA. This amount of filament heating is all that is required for fluoroscopy. When exposures requiring larger tube currents are desired, an automatic filament-boosting circuit will raise the filament current from the stand-by value to the required value before the exposure is made, and lower it to the stand-by value immediately after the exposure.

Tungsten which is vaporized from the filament (and occasionally the anode) is deposited as an extremely thin coating on the inner surface of the glass wall of the x-ray tube. It produces a color which becomes deeper as the tube ages. Old tubes acquire a bronze-colored "sunburn." This tungsten coat has two effects. It tends to filter the x-ray beam, gradually changing the quality of the beam. In addition, the presence of the metal on the glass increases the possibility of arcing between the glass and the electrodes at higher kVp values, and it may result in puncture of the tube.

Line Focus Principle

The focal spot is the area of the tungsten target (anode) which is bombarded by electrons from the cathode. **Most of the energy of the electrons is converted into heat,** less than 1% being converted into x rays. Since the heat is uniformly distributed over the focal spot, a large focal spot allows the accumulation of larger amounts of heat before damage to the tungsten target occurs. The melting point of tungsten is about 3370°C, but it is best to keep temperature below 3000°C. The problem posed by the need for a large focal spot to allow greater heat loading, and the conflicting need for a small focal area to produce good radiographic detail was resolved in 1918 with the development of the **line focus principle.** The theory of line focus is illustrated in Figure 2–3. The size and shape of the focal spot are determined by the size and shape of the electron stream when it hits the anode. The size and shape of the electron stream are determined by the dimensions of the filament tungsten wire coil, the construction of the focusing cup, and the position

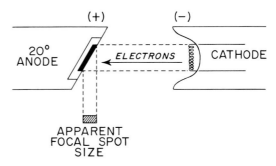

Figure 2–3   The line focus principle

of the filament in the focusing cup. The electron stream bombards the target, the surface of which is inclined so that it forms an angle with the plane perpendicular to the incident beam. The anode angle differs according to individual tube design and may vary between 6° and 20°. Because of this angulation, when the slanted surface of the focal spot is viewed from the direction in which x rays emerge from the x-ray tube, it is foreshortened and appears small. It is evident, therefore, that the size of the effective, or apparent, focal spot is considerably smaller than the actual focal spot. If the decrease in projected focal spot size is calculated, it is found that the size of the projected focal spot is directly related to the sine of the angle of the anode. Since sine 20° = 0.342 and sine 16.5° = 0.284, an anode angle of 16.5° will produce a smaller focal spot size than an angle of 20°. Thus, as the angle of the anode is made smaller, the apparent focal spot also becomes smaller. Some of the newer 0.3 mm focal spot tubes may use an anode angle of only 6°. Such small angles permit the use of larger areas of the target for electron bombardment (and heat dissipation), and yet achieve a small apparent focal spot size. For practical purposes, however, there is a limit to which the anode angle can be decreased as dictated by the heel effect (the point of anode cut-off). For general diagnostic radiography done at a 40-inch focus-film distance, the anode angle is usually no smaller than 15°.

Focal spot size is expressed in terms of the apparent or projected focal spot; sizes of 0.3 mm, 0.6 mm, 1.0 mm, 1.2 mm, and 2.0 mm are commonly employed.

The Anode

Anodes (positive electrodes) of x-ray tubes are of two types, **stationary** or **rotating.** The stationary anode will be discussed first as many of its basic principles also apply to the rotating anode.

The Stationary Anode

The anode of a stationary anode x-ray tube consists of a small plate of tungsten, 2 or 3 mm thick, which is embedded in a large mass of copper. The tungsten plate is square or rectangular in shape, each dimension usually being greater than 1 cm. The anode angle is usually 15° to 20°, as discussed above.

Tungsten is chosen as the target material for several reasons. It has a **high atomic number** (74), which makes it more efficient for the production of x rays. In addition, because of its **high melting point,** it is able to withstand the high temperature produced. Most metals melt between 300°C and 1500°C, while tungsten melts at 3370°C. Tungsten provides a reasonably good material for the absorption of heat and the rapid dissipation of the heat away from the target area.

The rather small tungsten target must be bonded to the much larger copper portion of the anode to facilitate heat dissipation. In spite of its rather good thermal characteristics, tungsten cannot withstand the heat of repeated exposures. Copper is a better conductor of heat than tungsten, thus the massive copper anode acts to increase the total thermal capacity of the anode and to speed its rate of cooling.

The actual size of the tungsten target is considerably larger than the area bombarded by the electron stream (Figure

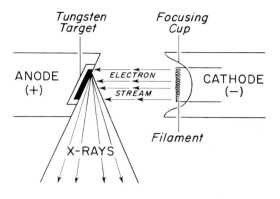

Figure 2–4 Lateral view of the cathode and anode of a stationary anode x-ray tube

2–4). This is necessary because of the relatively low melting point of copper (1070°C). A single x-ray exposure may raise the temperature of the bombarded area of the tungsten target by 1000°C or more. This high temperature is reached by any metal in the immediate vicinity of the focal spot. If the tungsten target were not sufficiently large to allow for some cooling around the edges of the focal spot, the heat produced would melt the copper in the immediate vicinity of the target.

All metals expand when heated, but they expand at different rates. The bonding between the tungsten target and the copper anode provides technical problems because tungsten and copper have different coefficients of expansion. If the bond between the tungsten and the copper were not satisfactorily produced, the tungsten target would tend to peel away from the copper anode.

The Rotating Anode

With the development of x-ray generators capable of delivering large amounts of power, the limiting factor in the output of an x-ray circuit became the x-ray tube itself. The ability of the x-ray tube to achieve high x-ray outputs is limited by the heat generated at the anode. The rotating anode principle is used to produce x-ray tubes capable of withstanding the heat generated by large exposures.

The anode of a rotating anode tube consists of a large disc of tungsten, or an alloy of tungsten, which theoretically rotates at a speed of about 3600 revolutions per minute when an exposure is being made. In practice, the anode never reaches a speed of 3600 rpm because of mechanical factors such as slipping between the rotor and bearings, so for purposes of calculating the ability of a tube to withstand high loads, a speed of 3000 rpm is usually assumed. While the actual speed of anode rotation varies even between new tubes of identical design, it is safe to assume that anode rotation of any functioning rotating anode will never drop below 3000 rpm, and will usually be greater than 3000 rpm, if 60 cycles per second current is used.

The tungsten disc has a beveled edge. The angle of the bevel may vary from 6° to 20°. The bevel is used to take advantage of the line focus principle previously described. **The purpose of the rotating anode is to spread the heat produced during an exposure over a large area of the anode.** Figure 2–5 presents a diagram illustrating this principle. (The dimensions are not drawn to scale.) If we assume that the filament and focusing cup of the x-ray tube produce an electron beam which covers an area of the anode 7 mm high and 2 mm wide, the area of the anode bombarded by electrons is represented by a 14 mm² rectangle. If the bevel of the target is 16.5°, the effective or apparent focal spot size in our illustration will be about 2 × 2 mm. If the anode were stationary, the entire heat load would be delivered to this one, small 14 mm² area of the target. However, if the target is made to rotate at a speed of 3600 rpm, the electrons will bombard a constantly changing area of the target. The total bombarded area of tungsten is represented by a track 7 mm wide which extends around the periphery of the beveled rotating tungsten disc. The effective focal spot will, of course, appear to remain stationary. At a speed of 3600 rpm, any given area on the tungsten disc comes opposite the electron stream only once every 1/60 second, and the remainder of the time heat generated during the exposure can be dissipated. During a 1/60 second exposure, the entire circumference of the tungsten disc will be exposed to the electron beam.

A comparison between the total and instantaneous target areas will illustrate the tremendous advantage offered by the rotating anode tube (Figure 2–5). At any instant, an area of 14 mm² is bombarded by the electron beam in our example. If we assume the average radius of the bombarded area of the tungsten disc to be 40 mm, which is a typical value, the circumference of the disc at a radius equal to 40 mm will be 251 mm. The total target area will then be represented by the height of the electron stream (7 mm) times the average circumference of the disc (251 mm) or a total of 1757 mm². Even though there has been an increase in the total loading area by a factor of about 125 (14 versus 1757 mm²), the apparent or effective focal spot size has remained the same.

The diameter of the tungsten disc determines the total length of the target track, and obviously affects the maximum permissible loading of the anode. Typical

$$C = 2\pi r$$
$$C = 2\pi\ 40\ \text{mm}.$$
$$C = 251\ \text{mm}.$$

$$7 \times 251 = 1757\ \text{mm}.^2$$

Figure 2–5 A rotating anode increases the total target area disc diameters will be found to vary between 75 and 100 mm (3 to 4 inches), although a tube with high capacity may have an anode 5 inches in diameter.

In order to make the anode rotate, some mechanical problems must be overcome, for the anode is contained within the vacuum of the glass tube. The power to effect rotation is provided by a magnetic field produced by stator coils which surround the neck of the x-ray tube outside the glass envelope (Figure 2–6). The magnetic field produced by the stator coils induces a current in the copper rotor of the induction motor, and this induced current provides the power to rotate the anode assembly. The clearance between the rotor and the glass neck of the tube is made as small as possible to insure maximum efficiency in utilization of the magnetic force supplied by the stator core and windings. Early in the development of rotating anode x-ray tubes, the life of the tube was quite short because of the lack of durable bearings on which the anode assembly could rotate. Because of the friction produced, it was necessary to lubricate the bearings, but ordinarily available lubricants could not be used. Lubricants such as oil would vaporize when heated and destroy the vacuum in the tube; dry lubricants such as graphite would wear off as a

powder and destroy the vacuum. This problem was solved by the use of metallic lubricants (especially silver), which are suitable for use in a high vacuum. In modern rotating anode tubes, bearing wear has become a negligible factor in overall tube life.

Heat dissipation in a rotating anode tube presents an additional problem. Heat generated in a solid tungsten disc is dissipated by radiation through the vacuum to the wall of the glass tube, then into the surrounding oil and tube housing. It will be recalled that heat is dissipated in a stationary anode by absorption and conductivity provided by the massive copper anode. In the rotating anode tube, absorption of heat by the anode assembly is undesirable because heat absorbed by the bearings of the anode assembly would cause them to expand and bind. It is because of this problem that the stem (Figure 2–6) which connects the tungsten target to the remainder of the anode assembly is made of molybdenum. Molybdenum has a high melting point (2600°C) and is a poor heat conductor. Thus, the molybdenum stem provides a partial heat barrier between the tungsten disc and the bearings of the anode assembly.

The length of the molybdenum stem is another important consideration. As the length of the stem is increased, the inertia of the tungsten disc increases; this increases the load on the bearings of the anode assembly. It is desirable to keep the stem as short as possible.

Even if all the factors which affect rotation of the relatively heavy anode assembly are optimally controlled, inertia still poses a problem. Because of this inertia, there is a short delay between application of force to the anode assembly and the time when the rotor reaches its full angular velocity. This period usually varies between ½ to 1 second, and can be several seconds when large (5-inch) anodes are used. A safety circuit is incorporated into the x-ray circuit which prevents an x-ray exposure from

Figure 2–6 The major components of a rotating anode x-ray tube

being made until the rotor has reached its full speed.

The life of a rotating anode x-ray tube is usually limited by roughening and pitting of the surface of the anode exposed to the electron beam. These physical changes are the result of thermal stress, and they act to diminish the x-ray output of the tube. The decreased output of x radiation from a rough target surface results from excessive scattering of the x rays (more radiation is directed away from the exit window of the tube) and increased absorption of x rays by the target itself. The combination of short exposure time and fast anode rotation causes very rapid heating and cooling of the surface of the anode disc. The loss of heat by radiation from the disc surface occurs before there is time for any significant amount of heat to be conducted into the main mass of the tungsten disc. Therefore, thermal expansion of the metal on the surface is much greater than expansion of metal immediately beneath the surface. This condition causes stresses to develop which distort the target surface of the anode disc. It has been found that an alloy of about **90% tungsten and 10% rhenium** (a heavy metal with good thermal capacity) produces an anode which is more resistant to surface roughening and has a higher thermal capacity than an anode of pure tungsten.

The usual speed of anode rotation using 60-cycle current varies between 3000 and 3600 rpm. If the speed of rotation is increased, the ability of the anode to withstand heat will become greater because any given area of the target is exposed to the electron beam for a shorter period of time during each revolution of the anode. By use of proper circuits, the speed of anode rotation can be increased to about 10,000 rpm. Three modifications of the tube help to overcome the problems associated with this increased velocity. (1) The length of the anode stem is made as short as possible to decrease the inertia of the anode. (2) The anode assembly rotates on two sets of bearings, which are placed as far apart as is possible. (3) Finally, the inertia of the anode is reduced by decreasing the weight of the anode itself. This is achieved by employing a compound anode disc in which the largest part of the disc is made of molybdenum (specific gravity 10.2) which is considerably lighter than tungsten (specific gravity 19.3). A relatively thin layer of tungsten-rhenium alloy which is attached to the molybdenum disc serves as the actual target for the electron beam. A high-speed anode should be used whenever large tube currents must be used, as during serial exposures in angiography.

Grid-Controlled X-ray Tubes

Conventional x-ray tubes contain two electrodes (cathode and anode). The switches used to initiate and stop an exposure with these tubes must be able to withstand the large changes in voltage applied between the cathode and anode. The rather involved topic dealing with the timers and switches used in the x-ray circuit will be considered in the next chapter. A grid-controlled x-ray tube contains its own "switch" which allows the x-ray tube to be turned on and off rapidly, as is required with cinefluorography (discussed in Chapter 16).

A third electrode is used in the grid-controlled tube to control the flow of electrons from the filament to the target. **The third electrode is the focusing cup which surrounds the filament.** In conventional x-ray tubes there is a focusing cup which is electrically connected to the filament. This focusing cup helps focus the electrons on the target. Since each electron is negatively charged, the electrons repel one other as they travel to the target. As a result, the electron beam (tube current) spreads out. The focusing cup is designed to counteract the spread of the electron beam which can be accomplished even with the cup and filament electrically connected.

In the grid-controlled tube, the focusing cup can be electrically negative relative to the filament. The voltage across the filament-grid produces an electric field along the path of the electron beam that pushes the electrons even closer together. If the voltage is made large enough, the tube current may be completely pinched off, a condition where no electrons go from the filament to the target. The voltage applied between the focusing cup and filament may therefore act like a switch to turn the tube current on and off. Since the cup and filament are close together, the voltage necessary to cut off the tube current is not extremely large. For example, to pulse (turn the tube current on and off with the focusing cup) a 0.3 mm focal spot tube operating at 150 kVp requires about -1500 volts between the filament and the cup.

Rotating Segmented Anode Tubes

A cup-shaped segmented anode has been developed by Machlett Laboratories and incorporated into their Dynamax "100" tube. Figure 2–7 shows a cross section of the tube. The cup-shaped anode is

GRAPHITE
ANODE

TUNGSTEN
SEGMENTS

CATHODE

X-RAY
BEAM

Figure 2–7 Segmented rotating anode tube. (Courtesy of Machlett Laboratories, Inc.)

made of graphite. Several hundred independent tungsten-rhenium segments line the inside of the cup. With a conventional anode, thermal stress weakens the tungsten-molybdenum bond and centrifugal force tends to tear the tungsten free. When a segmented anode rotates, the tungsten segments are forced against the graphite cup by centrifugal force. Rather than being stressed, the bond is strengthened by rotation.

Segmented anodes tolerate the heat of instantaneous exposures better than conventional anodes. The breaks between segments behave like expansion joints in a concrete sidewalk. They are controlled breaks that protect the anode from thermal stress. Segmented anode tubes also tolerate greater cumulative heat loads. Graphite has a larger heat storage capacity than molybdenum on a per gram basis. Compared to a conventional 4-inch diameter target of the same weight, anode heat storage is increased by more than a factor of 2 (approximately 700,000 heat unit storage capacity).

Field Emission Tubes

The electric field about a conductor is determined by its radius of curvature. A needle point has the smallest radius of curvature of any geometric shape; therefore, for a given impressed voltage and cathode-anode separation, a needle point cathode will have the maximum electric field that can be established. Figure 2–8 compares the electric fields of a wire coil, like the filament in a conventional x-ray tube, and a needle point. The force lines are spread out over the surface of the coil but concentrated at the point of the needle. If a voltage is applied to a conventional x-ray tube before the filament is heated, no current flows because the electric field is too weak to pull electrons free of the coil. When a voltage is applied to a needle point cathode, an extremely high electric field is established at the point of the needle, and electrons are pulled free to

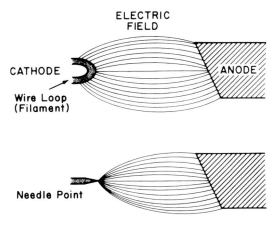

ELECTRIC
FIELD

CATHODE

Wire Loop
(Filament)

ANODE

Needle Point

Figure 2–8   Comparison of the electric field for a wire loop (filament) and a needle point

CATHODE
(Needles)

ANODE

X-RAY BEAM

Figure 2–9   Field emission tube

establish a current in the tube. **The process of removing electrons from a metal by an electric field is called field emission.** Since no heated element is used to liberate electrons, the process is also called cold cathode emission.

Field emission units are used clinically for high (350) kVp chest and some neonatal radiography. The design of commercially available tubes is shown in cross section in Figure 2–9. A conical anode is surrounded by a cylindrical cathode containing facing rows of needle points (only two shown). The x-ray beam passes through a window in the end of the tube. The focal spot is doughnut shaped on pin-hole radiographs and the intensity of the beam is somewhat decreased in the center of the field. The generators for field emission units are usually of the capacitor discharge type. A series of capacitors are charged to a preset voltage, then discharged quickly through the field emission tube.

Saturation Voltage

When the filament of an x-ray tube is heated, a space charge is produced, as previously discussed. When a potential difference is applied between the cathode and anode, electrons flow from the filament to the anode to produce the tube current. If the potential applied across the tube is insufficient to cause almost all electrons to be pulled away from the filament the in-

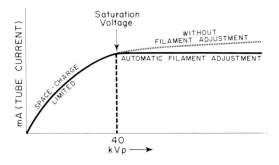

Figure 2–10   Saturation voltage

stant they are emitted, a **residual space charge** will exist about the filament. As we described earlier in this chapter, this residual space charge acts to limit the number of electrons available, and thus it limits the current flowing in the x-ray tube. From the accompanying chart (Figure 2–10) it can be seen that, up to about 40 kVp, an increase in kilovoltage produces a significant increase in x-ray tube current even though filament heating remains the same. Above 40 kVp, however, further increases in kilovoltage produce very little change in tube current. In our example, 40 kVp defines the location of the saturation point of this x-ray tube. Below 40 kVp, the current flowing in the tube is limited by the space charge effect (space charge limited). Above 40 kVp (the **saturation voltage**) the space charge effect, theoretically, has no influence on current flowing in the x-ray tube. In this region the current is determined by the number of electrons made available by the heated filament and is said to be emission limited or temperature limited. Reference to Figure 2-10 will show that in actual practice, a continued increase of kilovoltage above 40 will produce a slight increase in tube current. This is because of a small residual space charge effect. In modern x-ray circuits this slight increase in milliamperes accompanying increased kilovoltage is undesirable for, because of it, the tube current could not be precisely controlled. By the use of resistors, the circuit automatically compensates for this change by producing a slight decrease in filament heating as kilovoltage is increased.

The Heel Effect

The intensity of the x-ray beam which leaves the x-ray tube is not uniform throughout all portions of the beam. The intensity of the beam depends on the angle at which the x rays are emitted from the focal spot. This variation is termed the heel effect.

Reference to Figure 2–11 will show that

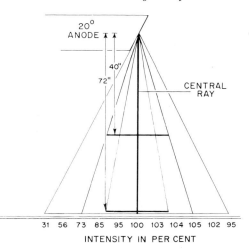

Figure 2–11   The heel effect

the intensity of the beam toward the anode side of the tube is less than that which angles toward the cathode. The lessened intensity of the x-ray beam which is emitted more nearly parallel to the surface of the angled target is caused by the absorption of some of the x-ray photons by the target itself. Beam intensity, as related to the angle of emission, varies depending on the physical characteristics of individual x-ray tubes. Figure 2–11 contains average values taken from charts published in several textbooks and is used for purposes of illustration only. If, for example, a 14 × 17 inch film is oriented so that its long axis corresponds with that of the tube, the heel effect can be studied. At a 40-inch target-film distance, the anode end of the film will receive a relative exposure of 73% and the cathode end will receive a relative exposure of 105%. Thus, there is about 30% difference in the intensity of exposure between the two ends of the film. If the target-film distance is increased to 72 inches, it can be determined from the chart that the difference in exposure intensities will be considerably less, roughly 87 to 104%. Three clinically important aspects of the heel effect are illustrated with this example. First, **the intensity of film exposure on the anode side of the x-ray tube is significantly less than that on the cathode side of the tube.** This factor can be used in obtaining balanced densities in radiographs of body parts of different thicknesses. The thicker parts should be placed toward the cathode (filament) side of the x-ray tube. This is usually illustrated by pointing out that an AP film of the thoracic spine should be made with the tube oriented so that its anode end is over the upper thoracic spine where the body is less thick; the cathode end of the tube is over the lower thoracic spine where thicker body structures will receive the increased exposure, which they require. Second, it can be seen that **the heel effect is less noticeable when larger focus-film distances are used.** Third, for equal target film distances, the **heel effect will be less for smaller films.** This is because the intensity of the x-ray beam nearest the central ray is more uniform than that toward the periphery of the beam.

Tube Shielding and High-Voltage Cables

Although we usually think of x rays as being confined to the beam emerging from the tube, they are, in fact, emitted with more or less equal intensity in every direction from the target. In addition, the x rays are scattered in all directions following collisions with various structures in and around the tube. The tube housing serves to absorb primary and secondary x rays which would otherwise produce a high intensity of radiation around the tube, resulting in needless exposure of patients and personnel and excessive film fogging. The effectiveness of the tube housing in limiting leakage radiation must meet the specifications listed in the National Council on Radiation Protection and Measurements Report #33 which states: "The leakage radiation measured at a distance of 1 meter from the source shall not exceed 100 mR (milliroentgens) in 1 hour when the tube is operated at its maximum continuous rated current for the maximum rated tube potential."

Another function of the tube housing is to provide shielding from the high voltages required to produce x rays. The high voltage cables, which are connected to the tube through appropriate receptacles in the tube housing, contain a grounding sheath of wires to provide proper grounding of the tube to earth. To prevent short circuiting between the grounding wires and the tube, the space between them is filled with very thin mineral oil. Thus, the x-ray tube is contained within the tube housing, and oil, inside the housing, surrounds the tube. The housing is then carefully sealed to exclude all air, since air would expand excessively when heated and rupture the housing. This oil has good electrical insulating and thermal cooling properties. Because of its insulating properties, the use of oil allows more compact tubes and shields to be used as it permits points of high potential difference to be placed closer to each other. In addition, convection currents, which are set up in the oil, help to carry heat away from the tube. Heat from the oil is absorbed through the metal of the tube shield to be dissipated into the atmosphere.

As the oil in the tube housing is heated it will, of course, expand. A metal bellows within the tube shield allows the oil to expand without increasing pressures upon the tube and shield, thus averting possible damage. In addition, the expanded bellows can be made to operate a microswitch, which will automatically prevent further exposures if maximum heating of the oil has occurred.

Tube Rating Charts

It is customary to speak of the total load which can be applied to an x-ray tube in terms of kilovoltage, milliamperes, and exposure time. The limit on the load which can be safely accepted by an x-ray tube is a function of the heat that is generated during the exposure. The maximum temperature to which tungsten can be safely raised is generally considered to be 3000°C. Above this level, considerable vaporization of the tungsten target occurs. The rate at which heat is generated by an electric current is proportional to the product of the voltage and the current (kV and mA). Thus, the total heat produced is a product of voltage and current and exposure time. This total energy is expressed in terms of heat units. **The heat unit (HU) is defined as the product of mA × kVp × seconds.** For example, the heat units developed in an x-ray tube during an exposure of 75 kVp, 100 mA, and 2 seconds would be 75 × 100 × 2 = 15,000 heat units.

The amount of heat which can be applied to an x-ray tube is primarily determined by three factors: (1) the type of rectification (to be discussed in Chapter 3), (2) the surface area of tungsten bombarded by electrons (focal spot size), and (3) the length of the exposure. The ability of the tube to withstand heating when it is used with a single phase generator is expressed in terms of heat units per second. When a tube is used with high speed anode rotation and a three phase generator, it is common to speak of its power rating, or the kilowatt (kW) rating. By convention, **the kW rating of an x-ray tube is 1/1000 of the (kVp x mA) maximum for a 0.1 second exposure.** For example, a tube capable of withstanding an exposure of 125 kVp at 800 mA for 0.1 second would be rated at 100 kW $\left(\frac{125 \times 800}{1000} = 100\right)$. When reference is made to the kW rating of an x-ray tube, it is assumed that it is the high speed, three phase rating unless otherwise specified.

The basic principles controlling permissible heat loads for stationary and rotating anode tubes are the same, but it is obvious that the rating of the stationary anode tube will be much lower. It should be recalled that the means of heat dissipation are different in stationary and rotating anode tubes. The stationary anode tube depends on the ability of a large copper anode to transfer heat. The rotating anode tube dissipates heat by radiation from the tungsten disc through the vacuum to the glass enclosure and the surrounding oil, and, eventually, to the tube housing.

In considering tube rating, three characteristics are encountered: (1) the ability of the tube to withstand a single exposure, (2) the ability of the tube to function despite multiple rapid exposures (as in angiography), and (3) the ability of the tube to withstand multiple exposures during several hours of heavy use.

The safe limit within which an x-ray tube can be operated for a single exposure can be easily determined by the tube rating chart which is supplied with all x-ray tubes. An example of such a chart is given in Figure 2–12. For example, if it is determined that an exposure will require 50 mAs (500 mA at 1/10 second), reference to the rating chart will show that the lines signifying 500 mA and 1/10 second cross at a point which limits maximum kilovoltage to about 100 kVp. In similar fashion, the safe loading for any combination of exposure factors can be determined from the tube rating chart. This chart is used as an

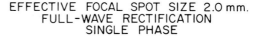

EFFECTIVE FOCAL SPOT SIZE 2.0 mm.
FULL-WAVE RECTIFICATION
SINGLE PHASE

Figure 2–12 An x-ray tube rating chart

example only. The manufacturer of the x-ray tube used in any diagnostic installation always supplies tube rating charts for the specific circumstances under which the tube will be used. Tube rating charts contain information for many different kilovoltages, usually ranging from 50 kVp to the maximum operating kilovoltage of the tube in steps of 10 kVp.

Angiographic techniques requiring multiple exposures during a short period of time produce large amounts of heat. For any tube used for angiography, appropriate ratings will be made available in the form of graphs or charts. Several special considerations must be kept in mind when a tube is subjected to the stresses of rapid-sequence radiography. (1) The surface of the target can be overheated by repeating exposures before the surface heat has had time to dissipate into the body of the anode. (2) The entire anode can be overheated by repeating exposures before the heat in the anode has had time to radiate into the surrounding oil and tube housing. (3) The tube housing can be overheated by making too many exposures before the housing has had time to lose its heat to the surrounding

air. (4) The total heat units of a series of exposures made in rapid-sequence must not exceed the heat units permissible for a single exposure of a duration equal to the total elapsed time required to complete the series of exposures.

The chart used to calculate the maximum loading of the x-ray tube for a single exposure (Figure 2–12) can also be used to determine the ability of the tube to withstand multiple rapid exposures. For example, assume exposure factors of 500 mA, 1/10 second, 100 kVp, with 10 exposures to be made in 10 seconds. Incidentally, this technique would not produce good quality films, but it will provide easy figures to use for calculating this example. First, reference to the chart will show that the single exposure is within the capability of the tube. Each exposure will produce $500 \times 100 \times 1/10 = 5000$ HU. Ten exposures will produce 50,000 HU in the 10-second interval. The maximum number of heat units the x-ray tube can accept during a 10-second period can be calculated from the chart. Actually, for an exposure time as long as 10 seconds, the number of heat units produced is relatively

Table 2–1. Dynamax 69 Angiographic Rating Chart (Used with Permission of the Machlett Laboratories, Inc., Stamford, Conn. 06907)

EFFECTIVE FOCAL SPOT SIZE   1.20 MM
STATOR FREQUENCY   180 HERTZ

TOTAL NUMBER OF EXPOSURES

EXPOS. PER SEC	2	5	10	20	30	40	50	60
	MAXIMUM LOAD IN PKV X MA X SEC PER EXPOSURE (*)							
1	45000	27000	17500	10800	7400	5500	4400	3700
2	30000	20000	13600	8800	6600	5400	4400	3700
3	24000	16500	11600	7600	5800	4700	4100	3600
4	19500	14000	10000	6800	5200	4300	3700	3300
5	17000	12200	9000	6200	4800	4000	3400	3000
6	14800	11000	8200	5700	4500	3700	3200	2900
8	11800	9200	7000	5000	4000	3400	2950	2650
10	10000	7800	6200	4500	3600	3100	2700	2400
12	8600	7000	5500	4000	3300	2900	2550	2250

independent of the kilovoltage used, and the permissible loading of the tube during the 10-second period can be calculated from any convenient kilovoltage curve. On our chart, this calculation could be made using 50 kVp or 100 kVp. For example, 50 kVp applied for 10 seconds could be used with a maximum milliamperage of 200, and 50 × 200 × 10 would allow 100,000 heat units input in 10 seconds. The same calculation for 100 kVp for 10 seconds at approximately 125 mA would allow 125,000 heat units input. In our example, the input of 50,000 heat units in 10 seconds is well within the capability of the tube.

Angiographic rating charts are now frequently available. Such a chart is illustrated in Table 2–1 (this is the angiographic rating chart of a Machlett Dynamax 69 tube used with three-phase rectification, high speed anode rotation and 1.2 mm focal spot). Notice the asterisk which reminds you to correlate this chart with the graph for single exposure ratings. Let us assume we wish to make 20 exposures at a rate of 2 exposures per second; the chart indicates we can use 8,800 HU per exposure. This results in heat input of 176,000 HU in 10 seconds. Reference to the single exposure graph for this tube (not illustrated) would show that the tube could accept a 10 second continuous exposure at 70 kVp and 250 mA, or an input of 175,000 heat units (10 × 70 × 250) in 10 seconds. One would also check the single exposure graph to insure that the tube could accept each individual exposure in the series. Both the angiographic rating chart and the single exposure rating graph must be used to insure that planned exposure factors will not damage the tube.

The ability of an x-ray tube to withstand heat loading over a period of several hours depends upon the anode heat storage characteristics. Figure 2–13 illustrates an anode capable of storing 110,000 HU. It will be noted that anode cooling is much more rapid when the anode has accumulated large amounts of heat. This is a practical application of the physical law stating that **heat loss by radiation is proportional to the fourth power of the**

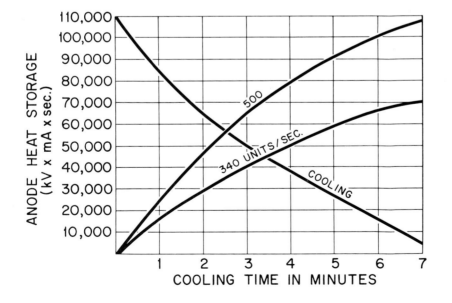

Figure 2–13 A chart of the anode heat storage capacity of an x-ray tube

temperature. The rate at which an anode heats during a period of constant exposure is of importance in fluoroscopy. For example, reference to Figure 2–13 shows that a continuous heat input of 500 units per second will produce an accumulation of the maximum number of heat units in the anode in about 7 minutes. Therefore, if the tube is used during fluoroscopy at 100 kVp and 5 mA (100 × 5 × 1 = 500 HU/second), continuous fluoroscopy beginning with a cold tube will be limited to 7 minutes. On the other hand, if fluoroscopy is carried out at 90 kVp and 3.8 mA (about 340 HU/second), fluoroscopy can be continued indefinitely without causing excessive anode heating.

One of the most important uses of this anode heat storage chart is to determine the length of time the tube must be allowed to cool before additional exposures can be made. For example, assume that an angiographic procedure produces 5000 HU per exposure. If a rapid filming procedure required 20 exposures, the total anode heating would be 100,000 HU. If Figure 2–13 represented the anode heat storage chart for the tube in question, it could be determined from the chart that it would require approximately 6 minutes for the tube to cool from 100,000 to 10,000 HU. Thus, if repeat rapid filming were necessary, a delay of 6 minutes would be needed because of the limitation imposed by the ability of the anode to store heat.

Additional consideration must be given to the ability of the entire tube housing to withstand heat. The tube housing can absorb an enormous amount of heat (a figure of 1,500,000 HU is not unreasonable). While the tube housing can absorb large amounts of heat, it also requires considerable time for cooling. Reference to some typical charts will show that it takes, in general, about 30 minutes for a tube housing to dissipate 600,000 HU. If more rapid cooling of a tube housing is required, the use of air circulators will usually double the cooling rate. Cooling rates exceeding 96,000 heat units per minute are possible.

INTERACTION OF THE ELECTRON BEAM WITH THE TARGET OF THE X-RAY TUBE

Atomic Structure

Before attempting to describe the phenomena which occur when fast-moving electrons encounter the tungsten target in an x-ray tube, we must briefly examine the structure of an atom. In 1897, J. J. Thomson discovered a negatively charged particle much smaller than any atom, which came to be called the electron. Based on the work of Rutherford and Bohr, a simple model of an atom may be visualized as a massive positively charged nucleus surrounded by electrons in orbits of specific diameters. The solar system is organized in similar fashion.

The Nucleus

The nucleus of an atom is made up of several types of elementary particles, which are termed **nucleons.** Of the nucleons, only **protons** and **neutrons** will be considered in this discussion, since they are the only ones of importance outside the field of nuclear physics. The proton has a positive electrical charge numerically equal to the charge of the electron, while the neutron has zero electrical charge. The neutron and proton have about the same mass (1.66×10^{-24} gm), which is approximately 1836 times greater than the mass of an electron. The number of protons in the nucleus is called the **atomic number** of the atom, and is given the symbol **Z.** The total number of protons and neutrons in the nucleus of an atom is called the **mass number** and is symbolized by the letter **A.** For example, stable gold (Au) has a nucleus with 79 protons (Z = 79) and 118 neutrons (A = 197). All atoms of an element have the same atomic number (Z), but an element may have several isotopes. All the isotopes of an element have the same number of protons in the nucleus, i.e., the same atomic number, but they have different numbers of neutrons and therefore different atomic masses.

In summary: the nucleus of an atom contains protons and neutrons, has a positive electrical charge, and contains almost all the mass of an atom.

Electron Orbits and Energy Levels

The electrons are negative charges revolving around the nucleus. Since an atom is always electrically neutral in its normal state, it must contain an equal number of protons and electrons. The simplest picture of an atom is to visualize a central positive nucleus with electrons in circular orbits about the nucleus. In this description, the atom resembles a tiny planetary system, with the nucleus as the sun and the electrons as the orbiting planets. Unlike the Solar System with one planet in each orbit, the atomic system allows 2 electrons in the first orbit, up to 8 in the second, up to 18 in the third, up to 32 in the fourth, and up to 50 in the fifth. The electron orbits are designated by letters: K, L, M, N, O, and so on.

The planets of the Solar System are all nearly in the same plane, whereas the electrons move about the nucleus in spherical shells. An electron in the shell closest to the nucleus is in the K-shell and the electron is called a K-electron. L-electrons are in the L-shell, the second nearest shell to the nucleus. As in the planets, the diameters of the electronic shells are determined by the nuclear force on the electron, and the angular momentum and energy of the electron. Angular momentum simply indicates that the electron is moving in a curved path. The attractive force between the positively charged nucleus and the negatively charged electron is the force that keeps the electrons in the atom. This force is called the binding force of the electron and it is inversely proportional to the square of the distance between the nucleus and electron. Therefore, a K-electron has a larger binding force than an L-electron. Of course, the binding force of the electron is directed towards the nucleus, and the electron would move towards the nucleus were it not moving in a

curved path. The attractive force due to the nucleus keeps the electrons moving in a circular path. The earth has a gravitational force towards the sun, but it continues to move around the sun in a stable orbit. Similarly, electrons are in stable orbital shells.

The earth has energy which is the sum of its potential energy and kinetic energy. The earth's potential energy is due to the gravitational effect of the sun; its kinetic energy is due to its motion. By definition, kinetic energy must be positive, but potential energy may be either positive or negative. Thus, the total energy may be positive or negative. **Bound particles always have negative energy.** The earth is in a negative energy state, and electrons in an atom are also in negative energy states. To free an electron from an atom, it must be raised to zero or a positive value. The energy that an electron in a shell must be given to raise the energy value to zero is called the binding energy of the electron. This is also the energy value designated for the atomic shell that houses the electron. The atomic shells are also called **energy shells.** Tungsten has a K-shell energy of 70 keV and an L-shell energy of 11 keV. Remember, these are negative energy values. To free a K-electron from tungsten, the electron must be given 70 keV of energy, while only 11 keV are required to free an L-electron. The L-electron has 59 keV more energy than the K-electron. The binding energy of the electron shells varies from one element to another. For example, tungsten, with an atomic number of 74, has a K-shell binding energy of 70 keV, while copper, with an atomic number of 29, has a K-shell binding energy of only 9 keV.

If a small amount of energy were taken from the earth, it would move a bit closer to the sun. However, atomic structural laws prohibit small additions or subtractions of energy from the bound electrons. An electron cannot have any more, or less, energy than that associated with its energy shell. However, an electron may jump from one energy shell to another, if the shell to which it jumps is not already filled. An electron can move to either a higher or lower energy shell. Electron movement to a lower energy shell, for example from an L to a K-shell, results in the emission of energy. The amount of energy is equal to the difference in the binding energy between the two shells. The energy takes the form of a photon. If the quantity of energy is sufficient, the photon may be called an x ray. Electron movement to a higher energy shell, for example from a K to an L-shell, requires the addition of energy to the electron. One of the sources of this addition may be the absorption of an x-ray photon.

Each of the atomic energy shells, except the K-shell, has subshells of slightly different energies. For example, the L-shell has 3 subshells and an electron in the L-shell may have one of 3 energy values. Of course, a single electron will have only one energy value, but the 8 electrons needed to fill the L-shell will be divided with 2 electrons in the lowest, 3 in the middle, and 3 in the highest subshells. In a transition from the L-shell to the K-shell, an electron will emit energy precisely equal to the difference in the energy of the shells. If an L-electron leaves the highest subshell and goes to the K-shell, it will emit some value of energy. However, if it leaves the middle shell and goes to the K-shell, it will emit a slightly different value. An L-electron in the lowest subshell may not go to the K-shell. This transition is called a Forbidden Transition.

There are more elaborate models of atomic structure which suggest that the orbits are elliptical (so are the orbits of the Solar System) or that the electron is just a standing wave about the nucleus. However, for diagnostic radiology the circular orbit model is sufficiently accurate.

The diameter of the nucleus of an atom is about 5×10^{-15} meters, and the diameter of the entire atom is about 5×10^{-10} meters. This means that the diameter of the atom is about 100,000 times larger

than the diameter of its nucleus. Most of an atom is an empty space, and this explains why a high-speed electron may go through many atoms before colliding with any of the components of an atom. It is interesting to visualize the hydrogen atom in terms of balls. Suppose the hydrogen nucleus (a proton) were a ball 3 inches in diameter. The electron (assuming the electron density to be equal to proton density) would be a ball ¼ inch in diameter. The K-shell would have a diameter of 1.5 miles. A normal hydrogen atom would be visualized as a 3-inch ball with a ¼-inch ball moving on a spherical shell ¾ of a mile away. Further, if all the electrons in the atoms of the world could be removed and the nuclei packed together (a condition that exists in the white dwarf stars), the diameter of the earth would be reduced to about one-tenth mile.

The production of x rays makes use of three properties of the tungsten atoms in the target of the x-ray tube: (1) the electric field of the nucleus, (2) the binding energy of orbital electrons, and (3) the need of the atom to exist in its lowest energy state.

Production of X rays

X rays are produced by **energy conversion** when fast-moving electrons from the filament of the x-ray tube interact with the tungsten anode (target). The kinetic energy (E) of the electron in passing across a voltage (V) is increased by

$$E = eV$$

where e is the electronic charge. Since the electric charge (e) of the electron does not change (e = 1.60×10^{-19} coulombs), it is apparent that increasing the voltage (V) across the x-ray tube will increase the kinetic energy of the electron. Voltage is expressed as the peak kilovoltage (kVp) applied across the x-ray tube (100 kVp = 100,000 peak volts). We must clearly distinguish between **kVp** and **keV** (kiloelectron volts). The expression 100 kVp means that the maximum voltage across the tube causing acceleration of the electrons is 100,000 volts. The expression keV denotes the energy of any individual electron in the beam (100 keV = 100,000 electron volts). When the x-ray tube is operated at 100 kVp, few electrons acquire a kinetic energy of 100 keV because the applied voltage pulsates between some lower value and the maximum value (kVp) selected. It takes the electrons something like 10^{-10} seconds to go from the cathode to the anode, separated by 1 inch, when the applied voltage is 100 kilovolts (kV). Each electron will acquire a kinetic energy (eV) where V is the instantaneous voltage across the tube. In a single-phase, full-wave rectified circuit, the voltage varies from 0 to the maximum (kVp) value selected, at a rate of 120 times per second. This will be discussed in more detail in Chapter 3. For the present discussion, it is adequate to state that the voltage (V) providing the potential to accelerate the electrons is pulsating, so that the energy (eV) of electrons that encounter the target (anode of the x-ray tube) covers a broad range. In other words, **the high-speed electrons striking the target do not have the same energy.**

X rays are generated by two different processes when the high-speed electrons lose energy in the target of the x-ray tube. One involves reaction of the electrons with the nucleus of the tungsten atoms, producing x rays that are termed **general radiation,** or **bremsstrahlung.** The second involves collision between the high-speed electrons and the electrons in the shell of the target tungsten atoms, producing x rays that are called **characteristic radiation.** To repeat, when high-speed electrons lose energy in the target of an x-ray tube, x rays are produced by two different processes: (1) general radiation (bremsstrahlung), and (2) characteristic radiation.

General Radiation (Bremsstrahlung)

When an electron passes near the nucleus of a tungsten atom, the positive charge of the nucleus acts on the negative charge of the electron. The electron is attracted toward the nucleus and is thus deflected from its original direction. The electron loses energy and is slowed down when its direction changes. The kinetic energy lost by the electron is emitted directly in the form of a photon of radiation. The radiation produced by this process is called general radiation or bremsstrahlung ("braking radiation" as translated from the German). Figure 2–14 is a schematic representation of the production of bremsstrahlung.

Most of the electrons which strike the target give up their energy by interactions with a number of atoms. The electron gives up only part of its energy in the form of radiation each time it is "braked." Electrons penetrate through many atomic layers before giving up all their energy, therefore, not all x rays are produced on the surface of the target. Occasionally, the electron will collide "head-on" with a nucleus. In this type of collision all the energy of the electron appears as a single x-ray photon.

Usually, an electron will undergo many reactions before coming to rest, and the energy it loses with each reaction is small. In addition, the electrons in the beam striking the target have widely different

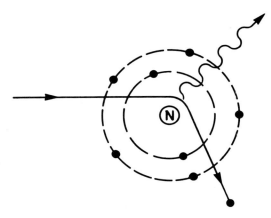

Figure 2–14 The production of general radiation (bremsstrahlung)

energies. These two factors cause a wide distribution in the energy of the radiation produced by this braking phenomenon. Most of the radiation will have little energy, and will appear as heat. Few x rays will appear, because over 99% of all reactions produce heat. The energy of the radiation is the amount of energy lost by the electrons. As we discussed in Chapter 1, the energy of a photon of radiation is inversely related to its wavelength. The wavelength of x-ray photons produced when the electron is braked by the tungsten nuclei in the target is related to the energy (keV) of the electron. The energy of the electron is related to the potential difference (kVp) across the x-ray tube. Consider the case of a head-on collision between the electron and nucleus. All the energy of the electron is given to the resulting x-ray photon. The minimum wavelength (in angstroms) of this x-ray photon can be calculated:

$$\lambda_{min} = \frac{12.4}{kVp}$$

For example, using 100 kVp x-ray tube potential, the maximum energy (eV) an electron can acquire is 100 keV. An electron with this energy can produce an x-ray photon with a minimum wavelength of 0.124 Å.

$$\lambda_{min} = \frac{12.4}{100} = 0.124 \text{ Å}$$

Remember, 0.124 Å is the shortest wavelength (highest energy) x-ray photon that can be produced with an x-ray tube potential of 100 kVp. Most of the x rays produced will have wavelengths longer than 0.124 Å. In fact, the wavelength of over 99% of the radiations will be so long that the radiation will produce only heat. The energy of the emitted x-ray photon resulting from deceleration of electrons in the electric field of a nucleus depends on: (1) how close the electron passes to the nucleus; (2) the energy of the electron; and (3) the charge of the nucleus. Figure 2–15 is a graph of the distribution, or "continu-

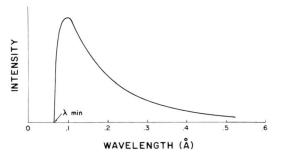

Figure 2–15   The continuous spectrum of x rays produced by bremsstrahlung

ous spectrum," of the wavelengths of x rays resulting from bombardment of the x-ray tube target by electrons. Notice that there will be a well-defined minimum wavelength (λ_{min}) of x rays produced; this λ_{min} will, of course, depend on the kVp used. The x-ray beam will also contain all wavelengths of x rays longer than the minimum wavelength. Filters (Chapter 6) are used to remove the very long wavelength, low-energy x rays, from the beam. Therefore, the highest energy x-ray photon leaving the x-ray tube depends on the kVp used; the lowest energy x-ray photon leaving the x-ray tube does not depend on kVp, but is determined by the filter used (or absorption of low-energy x rays by the glass envelope of the tube if no filter is used).

To review, **the wavelength of x rays in the continuous spectrum varies. The variation is produced by the different energies with which the electrons reach the target and by the fact that most electrons give up their energy in stages.** The minimum wavelength x-ray photon is dictated by the x-ray tube voltage (kVp). The maximum wavelength (lowest-energy) x rays escaping the tube will depend on the filtering action of the glass enclosure of the x-ray tube and any added filtration.

Characteristic Radiation

Characteristic radiation results when the electrons bombarding the target eject

electrons from the inner orbits of the target atoms. Removal of an electron from a tungsten atom causes the atom to have an excess positive charge, and the atom thus becomes a positive ion. In the process of returning to its normal state, the ionized atom of tungsten emits radiation which has wavelengths within the x-ray range. X rays produced in this manner are called characteristic x rays because the wavelengths of the x rays produced are characteristic of the atom which has been ionized. For the purposes of illustration, we will discuss ejection of an electron from the K-shell of tungsten, then apply the principles to electrons in other shells of the tungsten atom.

The binding energy of an electron in the K-shell of tungsten is about 70 keV. Therefore, a cathode electron must have energy of more than 70 keV to eject the K-shell electron from its orbit. A 60 kVp electron beam will not contain any electrons with enough energy to eject a K-shell electron from tungsten. After an impinging electron uses 70 keV of its energy to eject the K-shell electron, the remaining energy is shared between the initial electron and the ejected electron. Both these electrons leave the atom (Figure 2–16). The ionized tungsten atom is unstable, and the K-shell electron is rapidly replaced, usually with an electron from the L-shell. However, the replacement electron may come from other shells in the atom. The electron in the L-shell has more energy than the K-shell electron, as we discussed earlier. In its transition from the L- to the K-shell, the electron must give up its excess energy. The energy lost by the L-shell electron is radiated as a single x-ray photon. In tungsten, the energy of this x-ray photon is approximately 59 keV, which is the difference between the binding energy in the K-shell (about 70 keV) and the L-shell (about 11 keV). For tungsten, the energy of this x-ray photon will always be the same, regardless of the energy of the electron which ejected the K-shell electron. Thus, the x-ray photon

energy is a "characteristic" of the K-shell of a tungsten atom. This process is illustrated in Figure 2–16.

When the L-shell electron moves into the K-shell, a vacancy is created. This vacancy may be filled from the M-shell, and another x-ray photon will be produced.

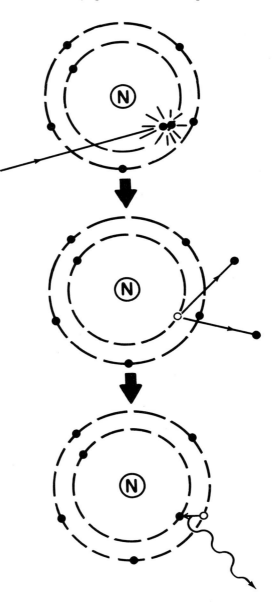

Figure 2–16 The production of characteristic radiation

However, the energy of the L-characteristic radiation will be much less than that of the K-characteristic radiation. In tungsten, L-characteristic x-ray photons have an energy of about 9 keV (L-shell binding energy is about 11 keV, that of the M-shell about 2 keV). Characteristic radiations will also be generated from transitions involving the outer electron shells of tungsten. The energy of this radiation is small, and ionization in these outer shells produces mostly heat or x rays which are absorbed by the glass walls of the x-ray tube.

Figure 2–17 diagrams the energy of the K-characteristic x rays of tungsten, superimposed on the continuous spectrum (bremsstrahlung). There is actually more than one binding energy for each inner shell in the tungsten atom except the K-shell, and this causes the appearance of several different energies of characteristic radiation. In Figure 2–17 the α_1 (59.3 keV) and α_2 (57.9 keV) characteristic x rays arise from transition of L-shell electrons to the K-shell. The β_1 (67.2 keV) results from an M-shell to K-shell transition, and the β_2 (69 keV) from an N-shell to K-shell transition. The dashed line in Figure 2–17 represents the low energy x rays, produced by bremsstrahlung, which are removed from the x-ray beam by the glass enclosure of the x-ray tube and the added filtration.

What contribution does the characteristic radiation make to the total production of x-rays by a standard x-ray tube? Below 70 kVp there is no K-shell characteristic radiation. Between 80 and 150 kVp characteristic radiation (K-shell characteristic) contributes about 10% (80 kVp) to 28% (150 kVp) of the useful x-ray beam. Above 150 kVp the contribution of characteristic radiation decreases, and it becomes negligible above 300 kVp.

Intensity of X-ray Beams

The intensity of an x-ray beam is defined as the number of photons in the beam multiplied by the energy of each photon.

Figure 2–17   The spectrum of bremsstrahlung and K-characteristic radiation

The intensity is commonly measured in roentgens per minute (defined on page 396. See Chapter 27). The intensity of the x-ray beam varies with the kilovoltage, the x-ray tube current, the target material, and the filtration.

Target Material

The target material used determines how much radiation (the quantity) will be produced by a given applied voltage (the next section will define the effect of this voltage on the radiation). **The higher the atomic number of the target atoms the greater will be the efficiency of the production of x rays.** For example, tungsten (Z = 74) would produce much more bremsstrahlung than tin (Z = 50) if both were used as the target of an x-ray tube and compared at identical tube potential (kVp) and current (mA). Earlier in this chapter we pointed out that tungsten is used as the target material because of its relatively high atomic number (74) and its high melting point (3370°C). Platinum, with a more favorable atomic number of 78, has a melting point of 1770°C, and stable gold (Z = 79) melts at 1063°C. Thus, **for the continuous spectrum, the atomic number of the target material determines the quantity of x rays produced.**

The relationship between atomic number and the production of characteristic radiation is quite different. **The atomic number of the target material determines the energy,** or quality, **of characteristic x rays produced.** For example, the K-shell characteristic x rays for tungsten (Z = 74) vary from 57 to 69 keV; those of tin (Z = 50) vary from 25 to 29 keV; and those of lead (Z = 82) have energies between 72 and 88 keV.

Molybdenum Target. With a high atomic number anode like tungsten, the x-ray beam consists almost entirely of bremsstrahlung radiation. The contribution from characteristic radiation varies somewhat with tube voltage, but it never makes up a large percentage of the total beam. With lower atomic number anodes, bremsstrahlung production is less efficient. Efficiency also diminishes as the tube voltage is decreased. The combination of a low atomic number anode and low tube voltage reduces the efficiency of bremsstrahlung production to the point where characteristic radiation assumes a greater importance. Molybdenum anode tubes are designed to take advantage of this principle for breast radiography. Maximum tube voltages for mammography are approximately 40 kVp. At this voltage, the K-characteristic radiation of molybdenum forms an intense band between 17.9 and 19.5 keV, which is about optimum for mammography.

To summarize, the atomic number of the target material determines the quantity (number) of bremsstrahlung produced and determines the quality (energy) of the characteristic radiation.

Voltage (kVp) Applied

We have reviewed how the energy of the photons emitted from the x-ray tube depends on the energy of the electrons in the electron stream which bombards the target of the x-ray tube. The energy of the electrons is, in turn, determined by the peak kilovoltage (kVp) used. Therefore, **the kVp determines the maximum energy (quality) of the x rays produced.** In addition, higher kVp techniques will also increase the quantity of x-rays produced. The amount of radiation produced increases as the square of the kilovoltage:

Intensity is proportional to $(kVp)^2$

The wavelength of the characteristic radiations produced by the target is not changed by the kVp used. Of course, the applied kilovoltage must be high enough to excite the characteristic radiation. For example, using a tungsten target, at least 70 kVp must be used to cause the K-characteristic x rays to appear.

X-ray Tube Current

The number of x rays produced obviously depends on the number of electrons which strike the target of the x-ray tube.

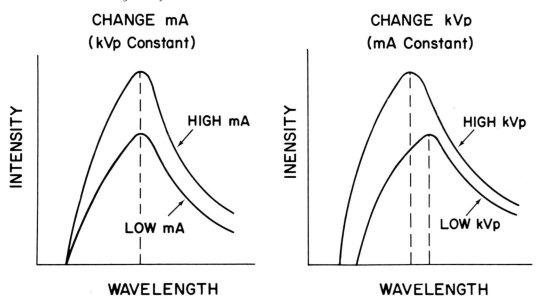

Figure 2–18   The effect of kVp and mA on the quality and intensity of the x-ray beam

The number of electrons depends directly on the tube current (mA) used. The greater the mA, the more electrons produced; consequently, more x rays will be produced. This principle was reviewed earlier in this chapter.

The effect of kVp (x-ray tube potential) and mA (x-ray tube current) on the wavelength (quality) and intensity of the x-ray beam is illustrated in Figure 2–18.

SUMMARY

X rays are produced by energy conversion when a fast-moving stream of electrons is suddenly decelerated in the target of an x-ray tube. An x-ray tube is a specially designed vacuum diode tube. The target of an x-ray tube is tungsten or an alloy of tungsten. Heat production in the x-ray tube is minimized by using the line focus principle and a rotating anode.

X rays are generated by two different processes, resulting in (1) the production of a continuous spectrum of x rays (bremsstrahlung), and (2) characteristic x rays. The quantity (number) of the x rays generated is proportional to the atomic number of the target material (Z), the square of the kilovoltage [$(kVp)^2$], and the milliamperes of x-ray tube current (mA). The quality (energy) of the x rays generated depends almost entirely on the x-ray tube potential (kVp).

CHAPTER 3

X-ray Generators

An x-ray generator is the device that supplies electrical power to the x-ray tube. It is not a generator in the strict sense of the word, since by definition a generator converts mechanical energy into electrical energy. An x-ray generator begins with a source of electrical energy (usually 120- or 220-volt, 60-hertz alternating current) and then modifies this energy to meet the needs of the x-ray tube. The tube requires electrical energy for two purposes: (1) to boil electrons from the x-ray filament, and (2) to accelerate these electrons from the cathode to the anode. The x-ray generator has a circuit for each of these functions, and we will refer to them as the filament and high-voltage circuits. Also, the generator has a timer mechanism, a third circuit, which regulates the length of the x-ray exposure. These three circuits are all interrelated, but to simplify the discussion, we will describe them separately. We will not, however, discuss the overall design of the electrical system but we will leave the technical problems in the capable hands of the x-ray equipment manufacturer.

The mechanism of an x-ray generator is contained in two separate compartments: a control panel (box) and a transformer assembly. A representative control panel is shown in Figure 3–1. The panel contains a main switch to turn on the unit, three selector controls, two meters, and two exposure buttons. The controls allow the operator to select the appropriate kVp,

mA, and exposure time for a particular radiographic examination. The meters measure the actual mA and kVp during the exposure. One exposure button (stand-by) readies the x-ray tube for exposure by heating the filament and rotating the anode, and the other button starts the exposure. The timing mechanism terminates the exposure.

The second component of the x-ray generator, the transformer assembly, is a grounded metal box filled with oil. It contains a low-voltage transformer for the filament circuit and a high-voltage transformer and a group of rectifiers for the high-voltage circuit. The potential differences in these circuits may be as high as 150,000 volts, so the transformers and rectifiers are immersed in oil. The oil serves as an insulator and prevents spark-

CONTROL PANEL

Figure 3–1 An x-ray control panel

ing between the various components. By definition, **a transformer is a device that either increases or decreases the voltage in a circuit. A rectifier changes alternating current into direct current.**

TRANSFORMERS

As we mentioned earlier, the x-ray generator receives 120- or 220-volt, 60-hertz (cycles per second) alternating current. Filament heating requires a potential difference of approximately 10 volts, while electron acceleration requires a potential difference that can be varied between 40,000 and 150,000 volts. Transformers are used to change the potential difference of the incoming electrical energy to the appropriate level.

Before we describe transformers, we must pause briefly to discuss the meaning of potential and potential difference. Potential is a relative term. For a discussion of electrical circuits, the earth (ground state) is considered to be at zero potential. A point in a circuit with an excess of electrons has a negative potential, while a point with a deficiency of electrons has a positive potential. Both potential and potential difference are measured in volts. If one point has a negative potential of 10 volts, and another point has a positive potential of 10 volts, the potential difference between them is 20 volts, and electrons will tend to flow toward the positive potential. Now suppose one point has a negative potential of 30 volts and another point a negative potential of 10 volts; the potential difference is still 20 volts. Electrons will flow toward the point with a negative potential of 10 volts. This flow of electrons represents a current, and it is produced by a potential difference. A voltmeter is used to measure the potential difference between two points. The terms potential difference and voltage are synonyms and will be used interchangeably.

A transformer consists of two wire coils wound around the opposite sides of an iron ring as shown in Figure 3–2A. The

Figure 3–2 Current induction by a transformer

circuit containing the first coil is called the primary circuit, and that with the second coil the secondary circuit. **When current flows through the primary coil, it creates a magnetic field within the iron ring, and this magnetic field induces a current in the secondary coil.** However, current only flows through the secondary circuit when the magnetic field is changing (either increasing or decreasing), and no current flows while the magnetic field is in a steady state. We can demonstrate this principle with a simple experiment. In Figure 3–2A the primary circuit is connected to a battery and the secondary circuit to a voltmeter. When the switch in the primary circuit is closed, the battery drives current through the primary coil, which creates a magnetic field in the iron core. As the magnetic field increases, it induces a current through the secondary coil. This current builds up a potential difference between the two ends of the coil, and the voltmeter needle swings to one side. As soon as the magnetic field stabilizes, the potential across the secondary coil drops to zero and remains there until the switch in

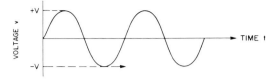

Figure 3-3   Alternating current wave form

the primary coil is opened. When the switch is opened, the magnetic field decreases, and again this changing field induces a potential difference across the secondary coil. However, the polarity of the potential is reversed, and the voltmeter needle moves in the opposite direction. The voltage across the primary coil is shown in Figure 3-2B, and that across the secondary coil in Figure 3-2C. The important fact to remember is that a current only flows in the secondary circuit when the magnetic field is increasing or decreasing. No current flows while the magnetic field is stable. For this reason, steady, direct current (like that from a battery) in the primary coil cannot be used to produce a continuous current through the secondary coil.

Alternating current is used for a transformer because it is produced by a potential difference (voltage) that changes continuously in magnitude and periodically in polarity (Figure 3-3). Current flows in one direction while the voltage is positive and in the opposite direction while the voltage is negative. The most important characteristic of alternating current is that its voltage changes continuously, so it produces a continuously changing magnetic field. Therefore, an alternating current in the primary coil of a transformer produces an alternating current in the secondary coil.

The Laws of Transformers

Two simple laws govern the behavior of a transformer:

1. **The voltage in the two circuits is proportional to the number of turns in the two coils.**

$$\frac{N_p}{N_s} = \frac{V_p}{V_s}$$

N_p = number of turns in primary coil
N_s = number of turns in secondary coil
V_p = voltage in primary circuit
V_s = voltage in secondary circuit

For example, suppose the primary coil has 100 turns and the secondary 30,000 turns. If the potential difference across the primary coil is 100 volts, the potential difference across the secondary coil will be:

$$\frac{100}{30,000} = \frac{100}{V_s}$$

$$V_s = 30,000 \text{ volts}$$

A transformer with more turns in the secondary coil than in the primary coil increases the voltage of the secondary circuit, and appropriately, it is called a "step-up" transformer. One with fewer turns in the secondary coil decreases the voltage and is called a "step-down" transformer.

2. The second law of transformers is simply a restatement of the law of the conservation of energy. A transformer cannot create energy. An increase in voltage must be accompanied by a correspondingly large decrease in current. **The product of the voltage and current in the two circuits must be equal.**

$$V_p \, I_p = V_s \, I_s$$

V_p = voltage in the primary coil
I_p = current in the primary coil
V_s = voltage in the secondary coil
I_s = current in the secondary coil

In our previous example the voltage across the primary coil was 100 volts and that across the secondary coil 30,000 volts. If the current in the primary coil is 30 amperes, then the current in the secondary coil will be:

$$100 \times 30 = 30,000 \times I_s$$
$$I_s = 0.1 \text{ amperes (100 mA)}$$

The product of voltage and current is power. If the potential difference is in volts and the current is in amperes, then power will be in watts.

$$W = V \times I$$
W = watts
V = volts
I = amperes

In the last example, the power in the transformer is 3000 watts; it is the same on both the high voltage (100 V × 30 A) and low voltage (30,000 V × 0.1 A) sides of the transformer. The wire in the transformer must be large enough to carry the current without overheating. As a result, high voltage transformers are both large and heavy, which also makes them very expensive.

In summary, a step-up transformer increases the voltage and decreases the current, while a step-down transformer decreases the voltage and increases the current. These laws assume 100% transformer efficiency, which cannot be achieved, but they are sufficiently accurate for our purposes.

THE FILAMENT CIRCUIT

The filament circuit regulates current flow through the filament of the x-ray tube. The circuit contains a variable resistor and a step-down transformer as shown in Figure 3–4. The filament is a coiled tungsten wire. A potential difference of approximately 10 volts produces a current of 3 to 5 amperes through the filament. This current merely heats the filament, and it does not represent the current across the x-ray tube. The potential difference of the incoming electrical supply (120

or 220 volts) is considerably higher than the voltage required across the filament. The step-down transformer in the filament circuit has approximately ten times as many turns of wire in the primary coil as in the secondary coil, and it reduces the potential to the appropriate level of about 10 volts.

The variable resistor in the primary circuit of the step-down transformer (Figure 3–4) is the mA selector for the x-ray exposure. It regulates the amount of current that flows through the x-ray filament. Decreasing the resistance increases the current flow and thus increases the temperature of the filament. A hotter filament emits more electrons. Remember that the voltage across the x-ray tube is usually sufficient to accelerate all available electrons to the anode. Since these electrons represent the current (mA) through the tube, increasing the filament temperature actually increases the x-ray (cathode-anode) current.

THE HIGH-VOLTAGE CIRCUIT

A simplified schematic of the high-voltage (cathode-anode) circuit is shown in Figure 3–5. The circuit has two transformers: an autotransformer and a step-up transformer. The autotransformer is actually the kVp selector and it is located in the control panel. The voltage across the primary coil of the step-up transformer can be varied by changing the number of turns in the autotransformer. Only five selections are shown in the illustration, but actually the kVp can be adjusted in steps from approximately 40 to 150 kVp.

The step-up transformer, which is sometimes called the high-voltage transformer, has many more turns in the secondary coil than in the primary coil, and it increases the voltage by a factor of approximately 600. The potential difference across the secondary coil may be as high as 150,000 volts, so the step-up transformer is immersed in oil in the transformer assembly for maximum insulation.

Figure 3–4 Filament circuit

Figure 3–5 High-voltage (cathode-anode) circuit

Two meters are incorporated into the high-voltage circuit: one to measure kVp and the other to measure mA. The meters themselves are located on the control panel, but their connections are in the high-voltage circuit as shown in Figure 3–5. They indicate the potential across the x-ray tube and the actual current flowing through the tube during an x-ray exposure. A voltmeter measures the difference in electrical potential (kVp) between two points. Electrons moving through the difference in potential constitute an electric current. In a closed circuit, the same number of electrons flows through all points. An ammeter (mA meter) merely counts the number of electrons flowing past a point per unit time, and it can be placed in the circuit wherever it is most convenient.

The ratio of the voltage across the primary and secondary coils in a transformer is proportional to the number of turns in the two coils. Some voltage is lost in the rectifier circuit, but with the appropriate calibrations, the potential difference in the high voltage side of the circuit, i.e. across the x-ray tube, can be measured indirectly on the low voltage side of the transformer. Therefore, the kVp meter can be placed in the circuit between the autotransformer and step-up transformer as shown in

Figure 3–5. The voltage in this circuit is relatively small and the meter can be located on the control panel with a minimum of insulation, and without serious risk of electrical shock.

The connections for the mA meter must be in the secondary coil of the high-voltage transformer to record current flow accurately. Transformers are not 100% efficient, so the current through the primary coil is not an accurate representation of the current in the secondary coil. The mA meter is in a circuit with a potential difference of up to 150 kVp, and to minimize the risk of an electric shock, the connections are at the place where the transformer is grounded, which is the center of the coil. With a voltage across the coil of 150 kVp, the potential on one side is +75 kVp and on the other side −75 kVp. The center of the coil is at zero potential, and if the meter is connected at this point, it may be placed on the control panel without risk of shock to the operator. Remember, even though the meter is remote from the x-ray tube, it measures the actual current flow across the tube, since the same number of electrons flows through all portions of a closed circuit.

The switch (Figure 3–5) that opens and closes the high-voltage circuit is located between the autotransformer and high-voltage transformer. This switch begins and terminates the x-ray exposure. It is operated by a timer mechanism which we will discuss later in this chapter.

Rectification

Rectification is the process of changing alternating current into direct current, and the device that produces the change is called a rectifier. The circuits that we have described to this point are entirely capable of producing x rays. The current is still alternating, so the potential difference between the cathode and anode changes back and forth from positive to negative 60 times each second. When the cathode is negative with respect to the anode, electrons are propelled between the two, which of course produces x rays. During the next half of the electrical cycle, the target of the x-ray tube is negative and the filament positive, so electrons would tend to flow away from the target. However, no electron cloud exists about the target, so no electrons are available to produce a current through the tube. By blocking current flow in the inverse half of the electrical cycle, the x-ray tube changes an alternating current into a direct current, so in effect it is a rectifier. Since only half of the electrical wave is used to produce x rays, the wave form is called **half-wave rectification.** Figure 3–6 shows the wave form of the incoming electrical supply (A) and that of half-wave rectification (B) for comparison. Only the upper half of each electrical cycle is used to produce x rays. When the x-ray tube itself serves as a rectifier, the circuit is called self-rectified.

Self-rectification has two disadvantages. First, half of the available electrical cycle is not utilized to produce x rays, so exposure times need to be twice as long as they would if the whole cycle were utilized. Second, as repeated or prolonged exposures heat the anode, it may become hot enough to emit electrons and to produce a current during the inverse half cycle. The electrons in this current will bombard the

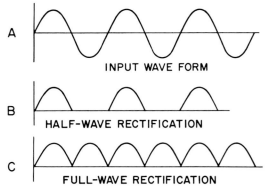

Figure 3–6   Electrical wave forms for full-wave and half-wave rectification

filament and eventually destroy it. Therefore, to protect the x-ray tube and improve the efficiency of x-ray production, special rectifiers, called valve tubes, are incorporated into the high-voltage circuit. Of course, the current must be rectified in the secondary circuit of the step-up transformer, since a transformer will not function with direct current in the primary circuit.

Rectifier Tubes

Rectifier tubes, also called valve tubes, have the same effect on an alternating electric current as heart valves have on blood flow; i.e., they permit flow in only one direction. Rectifier tubes, like x-ray tubes, are thermionic diodes. They have a heated filament and an anode (plate), both enclosed in an evacuated glass envelope. The filament is heated by a secondary circuit, and it serves a dual function as both a filament and a cathode. The structural design of a rectifier tube is different from an x-ray tube in two respects: the plate of a valve tube is much larger than the x-ray target and the rectifier filament has no focusing cup. We will discuss the importance of these differences as we describe the function of valves.

The current across the rectifier tube is a flow of electrons through a vacuum. Two things are required to produce a current, a source of electrons and a force (potential difference) to move them. The heated filament produces a source of electrons for current flow from the cathode to the plate. However, no source is available for current flow in the reverse direction, so the valve stops current flow in the inverse half of the electric cycle, thus protecting the x-ray tube. It is imperative that the plate be kept below the temperature at which it would emit electrons. The plate is large and the tube has no focusing device, so the electron stream is disbursed over a sizable area, which prevents any point from becoming hot enough to emit electrons. Plate heating is further limited by the relatively low potential across the valve (approximately 0.5 kV). The electrons do not have enough energy to heat the anode to any significant degree.

Valve tubes are always incorporated into the x-ray circuit in series with the x-ray tube as shown in Figure 3-7. Exactly the same number of electrons (current) flows through the x-ray tube and valve tubes. However, the valve filament is heated to a very high temperature, and it produces an overabundance of electrons, many more than are needed for the current. Because of this difference in filament heating between the valve tubes and the x-ray tube, most of the potential difference from the

high-voltage transformer appears across the x-ray tube. In Figure 3–7, the potential difference between the input leads of the high-voltage transformer is 100 kV (−50 to +50 kV). The voltage across each valve tube is only 0.5 kV, while the voltage across the x-ray tube is 99 kV. Since the voltage across the valve tube is relatively small, the electrons flowing through the valve do not have sufficient energy to produce x rays. If a valve tube produces x rays, the voltage across the valve is too high. It can be lowered by heating the filament to a higher temperature, which increases the number of electrons in the electron cloud, and decreases the voltage required to move a current.

In recent years, solid-state silicon rectifiers have completely replaced vacuum valve tubes. Solid-state rectifiers have the same electrical characteristics, but they have several advantages. They are physically smaller than vacuum tubes, and they do not require a heated filament, so they have a longer life expectancy.

Half-wave Rectification

We have already described one form of half-wave rectification, self-rectification by the x-ray tube. The same wave form is produced by two rectifiers connected in series with the x-ray tube as shown in Figure 3–7. With the voltage shown in the illustration, current flows through the x-ray tube from the cathode to the anode. When the voltage reverses during the inverse half of the alternating cycle, the rectifier stops current flow. When rectifiers are used in this manner, they produce half-wave rectification. The only advantage of the rectifiers is that they protect the x-ray tube from the full potential of the inverse cycle.

Full-wave Rectification

Almost all modern x-ray generators employ full-wave rectification, which utilizes the full potential of the electrical supply. Figure 3–6C shows the wave form

Figure 3–7   The circuit for half-wave rectification

that is produced by full-wave rectification. Both halves of the alternating voltage are used to produce x rays, so the x-ray output per unit time is twice as large as it is with half-wave rectification.

Figure 3–8 is a schematic presentation of the high-voltage circuit for full-wave rectification. The voltage across the circuit is supplied by the step-up transformer. Current flows along the solid lines and in the direction of the arrows. The valve tubes prevent flow along the dotted lines, since no current can flow from the plate to the filament of a valve. The polarity is in one direction in (A) and in the opposite direction in (B). In both cases, current flows from the cathode to the anode of the x-ray tube. Thus, the current through the x-ray tube is a direct current (unidirectional) even though the input current is alternat-

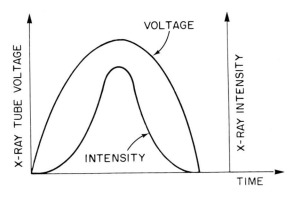

Figure 3–9 X-ray intensity superimposed upon the electrical voltage

ing. However, the voltage across the tube still fluctuates from zero to its maximum level, and x rays are generated in 120 short bursts each second. Figure 3–9 shows the intensity of the x-ray beam superimposed on the electrical voltage of the x-ray tube during one-half cycle. As you can see, most of the x rays are generated during the central, high-voltage portion of the cycle.

The principal disadvantage of pulsed radiation is that a considerable portion of the exposure time is lost while the voltage is in the valley between two pulses. This disadvantage is not shared by three-phase generators, which we will discuss next.

THREE-PHASE GENERATORS

Three-phase generators produce an almost constant potential difference across the x-ray tube, and in recent years they have become more popular for both angiography and routine radiography.

Commercial electrical power is usually produced and delivered by three-phase alternating current generators. It is easier to understand three-phase current if we think of each phase in terms of degrees rather than in time. Figure 3–10 shows all three phases separately and superimposed upon one another (bottom). Phase two lags 120° behind phase one, and phase three 120° behind phase two. Thus a three-phase

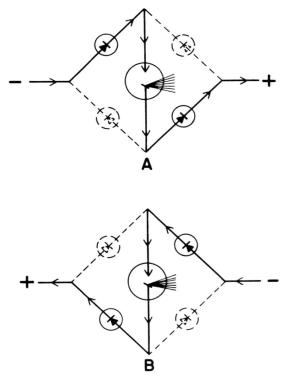

Figure 3–8 The circuit for full-wave rectification

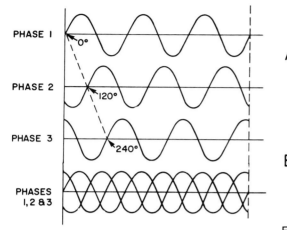

Figure 3–10 Three-phase alternating current wave forms

Figure 3–11 Wave forms from three-phase generators

generator produces an almost constant voltage as there are no deep valleys between pulses.

Three-phase generators are extremely complex, and we will not attempt to outline their circuits. Two wave forms can be produced by three-phase generators, depending upon the manner in which the circuits are connected. These are shown in Figure 3–11. In one (A), the wave form has 6 pulses per cycle (1/60 sec), and in the other, 12 pulses per cycle. As you can see, the voltage is more nearly constant with the 12-pulse generator.

The "ripple factor" is the variation in the voltage across the x-ray tube expressed as a percentage of the maximum value. The theoretical ripple factor for a 6-pulse generator is 13%, while for a 12-pulse generator, the ripple factor is only 3%. In actual practice, the ripple is somewhat larger, but compared to the 100% ripple factor of a single-phase system, three-phase generators produce a nearly constant potential.

The major advantage of three-phase generators is a much higher tube rating for extremely short x-ray exposures. This is due to the fact that near maximum loading is applied to the tube throughout the exposure, so that the electron beam is spread across a sizable area of the rotating anode. Three-phase generators are now being built to deliver a tube current of up to 2000 mA. They make it possible to produce radiographs with extremely short exposure times and high repetition rates, so they are excellent for angiography.

BATTERY POWERED GENERATORS

Some portable x-ray machines employ a series of batteries to generate the high voltage and filament currents. These units are designed to operate in areas where the electrical supply is inadequate for conventional generators. Figure 3–12 shows a schematic outline of a battery powered unit. Each cell in the battery pack supplies a potential difference of approximately 1.5 volts, about the same as a standard flashlight battery, so thousands of cells are required to produce the high voltages that are used in diagnostic radiology.

The controls on a battery generator are similar to those of a conventional generator. The kV selector in the high voltage circuit regulates the potential difference across the x-ray tube by adding or subtracting batteries from the series. Note that the high voltage selector is a kV, and

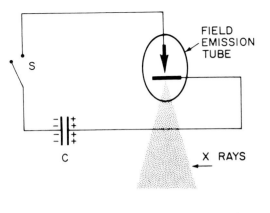

Figure 3-13 Circuit for a capacitor-discharge generator

Figure 3-12 Circuit for a battery powered generator

not a kVp selector, because the batteries supply a constant potential. The filament current (mA selector) is adjusted by a variable resistor in the filament circuit. An amp meter (A) on the low voltage side of the x-ray tube (near ground potential) measures the current in the circuit. A timing device simply breaks a connection (S) on the grounded side of the circuit, so no high voltage timer is required. The batteries must be recharged periodically, but they carry enough energy so that they can be used for numerous radiographic exposures.

CAPACITOR DISCHARGE GENERATORS

Another type of generator, a capacitor discharge unit, is now being used in clinical radiology with cold cathode field emission x-ray tubes. These tubes have no filament. Electrons are drawn off the points of multiple needle-like cathodes by a strong electric field. The electric field is supplied by an array of capacitors, wired together in both series and parallel, in a complex circuit that we have represented in Figure 3-13 with a single capacitor (C). A capacitor is an electrical device for storing

charge, or electrons. It consists of two metal plates separated by a space. The space is filled with a dialectric material, but for our purposes, we can picture the space as filled with air. When a number of electrons are forced onto one plate of the capacitor, for instance from a storage battery, a like number is forced off the other plate. No current flows across the capacitor. In a capacitor discharge generator, the capacitors are discharged through the field emission x-ray tube. If the capacitor is sufficiently charged, closing the switch (S) in Figure 3-13 will produce x rays.

The capacitors are charged to a high voltage, 350 kilovolts in one commercial field emission unit,* by a step-up transformer-rectifier circuit like the one shown in Figure 3-14. This circuit is exactly the same as the one shown earlier in our discussion of rectification, except that the x-ray tube has been replaced with a capacitor. The rectifiers (valve tubes) change the alternating current from the transformer to a direct current through the capacitor limb of the circuit. Note that the current always flows in the direction of the arrows shown on either side of the capacitor in the illustration. A relatively

*Manufactured by Hewlett-Packard Co.

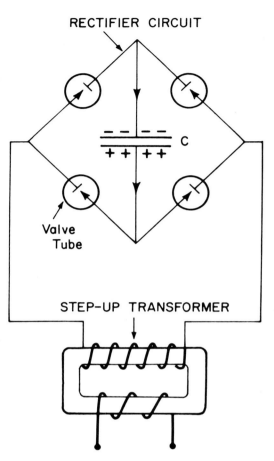

RECTIFIER CIRCUIT

C

Valve
Tube

STEP-UP TRANSFORMER

Figure 3–14   Transformer-rectifier circuit for a capacitor-discharge generator

small transformer-rectifier assembly can be used in the charging circuit, because the charge on the capacitor builds up gradually over a period of time. In a conventional x-ray generator, the transformer and rectifiers must build up to full power (voltage times current) in a few milliseconds (thousandths of a second) and then maintain this power throughout the exposure. A capacitor discharge circuit may take up to 2 minutes to reach full charge, and then discharge in a few nanoseconds (10^{-9} sec or 1 millionth of a millisecond).

The principal advantage of capacitor discharge generators is that they deliver a

relatively large amount of power in an extremely short burst. Exposure times are so short that they can freeze the motion of a bullet in flight. Unfortunately, a single relatively large burst of power is not enough for most clinical situations. Multiple bursts are required. This is accomplished by incorporating many capacitors into the circuit, and firing them sequentially in pulses 1 millisecond apart.

The voltage across the x-ray tube is maximum the instant the switch is closed. At this time the full charge of the capacitors is released and a large current flows across the x-ray tube. As the current flows, the charge on the capacitors decreases and the voltage drops. The drop continues until the voltage is inadequate to pull electrons free of the needle-like cathodes. At this time, the flow of the current and production of x rays ceases. The exact voltage at which x-ray production ceases will depend upon the design of the x-ray tube. The shape of the electrical pulse is shown in Figure 3–15. The voltage builds up rapidly, almost instantaneously, and then falls off in two phases. In the first phase, the voltage drops precipitously in a brief period of time, while in the second phase, the voltage drops less precipitously and over a more prolonged period of time. Compared to a conventional single-phase generator, the pulse from a capacitor discharge unit is exceedingly short, i.e. 1/120 second compared to a few billionths of a second. Nevertheless, these two generator types both produce a pulsed voltage, and consequently more relatively low energy radiation than either battery powered or three phase generators, both of which produce a constant, or nearly constant voltage.

TIMING THE X-RAY EXPOSURE

The length of an x-ray exposure is regulated by an exposure timer. The timer controls are located in the x-ray control panel, but the timer itself may be located in either the control panel or transformer

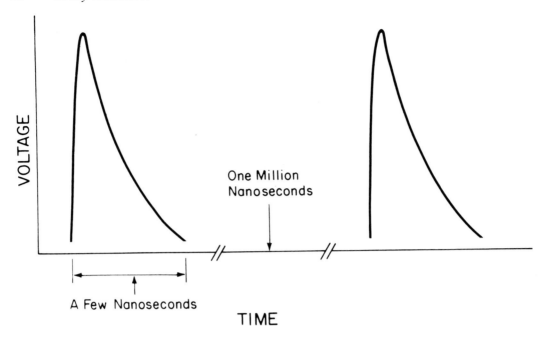

Figure 3–15 Voltage pulses from a capacitor-discharge generator

assembly depending upon the design of the generator. The timer controls include a timer selector and two exposure buttons. Pushing the first button causes the filament to heat and the anode to rotate in preparation for an exposure. Pushing the second button activates the timer and closes a switch in the high-voltage circuit to begin the exposure. The timer automatically opens the switch and terminates the exposure at the preselected time. Timer switches are always located in the high-voltage circuit, i.e., the circuit supplying current between the cathode and anode of the x-ray tube. The filament circuit cannot be used to regulate exposure times. The filament heats and cools gradually, so its response time is relatively long. The high-voltage circuit has an almost instantaneous response time, so it is more practical to regulate the length of the exposure in the high-voltage circuit.

X-ray exposure timers and switches have separate but interdependent functions. Timers are thinkers, and switches are workers. A timer tells a switch to close or open a circuit, and the switch responds to the best of its ability. However, a switch is not always capable of following the timer's instructions, and the actual exposure time may be considerably different than the anticipated time. For optimal results at the lowest possible cost, both the timer and switches should be designed for the same level of performance. Three factors must be considered in the design of a timer mechanism: (1) the minimum exposure time; (2) the current load of the circuit; and (3) the recycle time (the amount of time between exposures).

Early x-ray tubes had a low heat-storage capacity, so they had to be operated with small tube currents (low mA). Exposure times were long, and a relatively simple timing mechanism was entirely adequate. With larger tubes came a need for faster, more accurate timers and switches. When serial filming and cinefluorography were developed, the timer was confronted with a new problem, that of recycling to make ready for the next exposure. Each stage in the development of x-ray tubes and generators has demanded a more sophisticated timing system, and the circuitry of the newer timers is extremely complex.

Switches

An x-ray switch functions like the switch on a reading lamp; it turns the current in the x-ray tube on or off. When an electric current is started or stopped abruptly in an inductive (transformer) circuit, a sudden surge of current results. These abnormally high currents may damage the electrical components in the circuit. They also produce an unpredictably large x-ray output which results in radiographs that are not uniform from one exposure to the next. This problem is not difficult to solve with a single-phase generator. The circuit can be opened and closed when the alternating current is at zero voltage. At this time there is no potential difference, and no current, so of course there is no inductive surge.

The problem of inductance is much more difficult to solve in a three-phase system. When one phase is at zero, the other two phases are 87% of their maximum level. One approach to the problem is to "sequence switch," to switch each of the three phases individually as their voltages pass through zero. This does not work well with very short exposure times, and usually three-phase generators are used to produce short exposures. Manufacturers have overcome the problem of inductive surges in three-phase circuits by a variety of complex means, mostly employing capacitors to store the surge. With newer timers and switches, it is possible to obtain exposure times as short as 1/1000 of a second (1 millisecond).

Mechanical Switches

The simplest x-ray switches are mechanical contactors. They are usually opened and closed by solenoids (electromagnets) which are activated by the exposure timer. They are always connected into the low voltage (primary) side of the high voltage circuit and perform satisfactorily with small currents and relatively long exposure times. The size of the contactor must be proportional to the amount of current it will carry. Large contactors have considerable inertia and require powerful electromagnets. They are noisy and tend to arc with large voltages. The maximum accuracy of mechanical contactors is one-half cycle of a full-wave rectified circuit (1/120 sec). They have a relatively slow recycle time which limits them to 2 or 3 exposures per second.

Mechanical contactors may be used singly or in pairs. When they are used in pairs, one contactor closes the x-ray circuit and starts the exposure, and the second contactor opens the circuit and terminates the exposure.

Electronic Switches (Thyratrons)

The most important advance in the evolution of x-ray switches was the development of the thyratron tube. **A thyratron is a gas-filled triode that functions as an electronic switch.** The tube is filled with a small amount of inert gas (argon, neon, or mercury vapor). Thyratrons have three

Figure 3–16   Thyratron tube

electrodes (Figure 3–16): an anode, a cathode, and a grid. A heating element boils electrons from the cathode (thermionic emissions), and these electrons eventually form the current through the tube. Electron emission is similar to that of an x-ray tube, except that the cathode is heated indirectly. The electron cloud around the cathode is repelled by the third electrode, a grid, with a small negative potential (−3 volts) relative to the cathode. The grid behaves like a fine wire screen. Its negative potential creates an electrostatic field which blocks the flow of electrons, but it does not physically impede their flow. Even though the grid has a relatively small negative potential, it is able to hold back the electron stream because of its close proximity to the cathode. While the grid is sufficiently negative, no current flows through the tube.

To start a current flowing through a thyratron tube, the grid voltage must be reduced (made less negative) below a critical level. This permits a few electrons to escape the grid's electrostatic field. These electrons are accelerated toward the anode and, as they move through the tube, they ionize gas molecules forming ion pairs—electrons (negative ions) and atoms with an electron deficiency (positive ions). These ions in turn ionize other atoms and create an avalanche effect. The positive ions migrate back to the grid and further diminish its negative potential. The grid loses control of the electron cloud as soon as ionization begins. If an outside force increases the grid's negative potential, it merely attracts more positive ions, which increases the efficiency and current flow through the tube. The only way that the current can be stopped is by removing the potential difference between the anode and cathode. Thus, a thyratron is like a trigger that can start, but cannot stop, a current flow.

Thyratrons are controlled by electronic timers. Since they are strictly one-way switches, they are always used in combination with either another thyratron or a mechanical switch. Frequently, the current from a thyratron is used to operate an electromagnet, in which case the current from an electronic switch (thyratron) operates a mechanical switch. Thyratrons are capable of conducting a large current with only a negligible drop in voltage. They have two obvious advantages over mechanical timers: (1) an almost instantaneous response time, because they have no inertia, and (2) an almost instantaneous recycling time. For this reason, they are capable of utilizing only a portion of an x-ray pulse, the intense central portion, so they can produce a nearly square wave form and exposure times as short as 1 millisecond.

In recent years, solid-state thyratrons have almost completely replaced gas-filled tubes. They are called either silicon-controlled switches or silicon-controlled rectifiers. Their characteristics are identical to gas-filled thyratrons, but they are smaller and do not require a heater. Even more recently, high-voltage thyratrons have been developed, and they are occasionally incorporated into the secondary circuit of the high-voltage transformer with good results.

Grid-controlled X-ray Tubes

A grid-controlled x-ray tube is a triode tube (see page 12). The focusing cup functions as the grid, and behaves like a switch much like the grid in the thyratron tube that we just discussed. The grid has a relatively small negative potential, but it is close to the cathode, so it exerts a strong influence on the electron cloud. Grid-controlled tubes have the same advantages as thyratron switches, but in general, they cannot control as large a current flow. For this reason, they are seldom used for routine radiography, but they are used for cineradiography.

Exposure Timers

X-ray exposure timers have developed through several stages beginning with simple mechanical timers and ending with highly sophisticated automatic electronic timers. All of the various stages are still in use, and we will discuss them in the order of their appearance.

Mechanical Timers

The simplest exposure timer is a mechanical device that functions much like a spring-driven clock. The timer is set by turning a dial to the appropriate time. Turning the dial winds a spring and opens a mechanical contactor to prepare for the exposure. When the timer button is pushed, the exposure begins and the spring drives the dial back to its starting position terminating the exposure. A mechanical timer activates a solenoid (electromagnet) in the x-ray circuit, and the solenoid opens and closes a single mechanical switch.

Mechanical timers are usually used in low-power dental and portable radiographic units. They are only accurate to approximately 0.25 seconds, so they cannot be used to regulate the short exposures of high-power equipment.

Synchronous Timers

A synchronous timer is driven by a small synchronous motor. The speed of the motor is controlled by the frequency of the alternating current supplied by the electric power company, so it is fairly accurate. The motor drives a cam that activates an electromagnet to open and close a single contactor switch. Synchronous timers are accurate to 0.1 second. They have a fairly long recycle time and cannot be used for rapid serial exposures.

Electronic Timers

As the power of x-ray generators increased, exposure times became too short to control with synchronous timers. Something better was needed, and the electronic timer was developed to meet this need. Electronic timers are far superior to any other timer, and they are incorporated into almost all modern x-ray generators.

All electronic timers operate on the same general principle. **The length of the x-ray exposure is determined by the time required to charge a capacitor** to a predetermined level. Electronic timers have two essential components, a variable resistor and a capacitor. The capacitor is always connected to the grid of a thyratron-type switch. Since all electronic timers have a resistor and a capacitor, they are frequently called **resistance-capacitor (RC) circuits.** Figure 3–17 shows the basic RC circuit. The switch (S) is closed between exposures. This short circuits the capacitor so that it does not accumulate a charge. At the beginning of an exposure, the switch is opened. At the same time that the timer switch is opened, another switch closes the main x-ray circuit and begins the exposure. In the RC circuit, electrons migrate toward the lower plate and away from the upper plate of the capacitor. Electrons flowing away from the upper plate are impeded by the resistor, and the greater the resistance, the slower their flow. The upper plate is connected to the grid (third electrode) of a thyratron. While the thyratron grid remains negative, it can contain the electron cloud about the cathode, and no current flows through the thyratron tube. As a positive charge accumulates on the upper plate of the capacitor, it lowers the negative potential of the thyratron grid. Eventually the grid reaches its critical level, and suddenly, a current flows through the thyratron. This current opens a switch in the x-ray circuit and terminates the exposure.

The amount of time required to reach the critical voltage of the thyratron depends upon the resistance in the capacitor circuit. When we select an x-ray exposure

Figure 3–17 Electronic timer circuit

time, we change the resistance in the capacitor circuit. Increasing the resistance increases the exposure time, and decreasing the resistance shortens the exposure time.

The basic resistor-capacitor circuit and thyratron tube produce an accurately timed electric current. This current can be used in a variety of ways. It may be used to activate an electromagnet and thus open a mechanical contactor to terminate the x-ray exposure (impulse timer). When used in this manner, a second mechanical switch is employed to close the circuit at the beginning of the x-ray exposure.

Electronic timers may also be used entirely with electronic (usually silicon-controlled) switches in which case they have a shorter activation time and an almost instantaneous recycling time. They are capable of delivering an x-ray pulse as short as 1 millisecond with an activation time (the time delay between the command to make an exposure and the beginning of execution) of 1 millisecond. They can control more than 60 exposures per second. Electronic timers can be incorporated into either the primary or the secondary circuit of the high-voltage transformer.

Phototimers

All of the exposure timers that we have discussed to this point are subject to human error. The operator selects the exposure time that he believes will produce a film of the desired density. He can measure the patient's thickness, but he must estimate the density of the tissues that will be included in the radiographic field. If his estimate is incorrect, the resultant radiograph will be improperly exposed. Phototimers have been developed to eliminate human error. They measure the amount of radiation that is transmitted through the patient and terminate the exposure when the transmitted radiation reaches a predetermined level. Several types of radiation detectors could be used in phototimers, but only two are in common usage—

photomultiplier tubes and ionization chambers. We will describe them separately.

Photomultiplier Tubes. Figure 3–18 shows the essential components of a photomultiplier tube-timer circuit. The tube is radiopaque so it must be positioned beneath the film to prevent its image from appearing on the radiograph. The timing circuit consists of a photomultiplier tube, capacitor (C), switch (S) and thyratron. After x rays pass through both the patient and film, they strike the photomultiplier tube, which produces a small electric current. This current is used to charge the capacitor in the phototimer in a manner similar to that described for electronic timers. In fact, the only difference between a phototimer and an electronic timer is in the resistor. A phototimer does not require a resistor. The patient serves this function. In an electronic timer, the amount of resistance determines the time that is required to charge the capacitor. In a phototimer, the density of the patient determines the capacitor charge time. With a thick anatomic part, only a small amount of radiation is transmitted through the patient. A comparably small amount of current flows from the photomultiplier tube, the capacitor charges slowly, and the radiographic exposure is prolonged. The

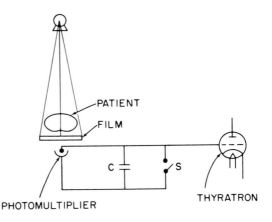

Figure 3–18 Photomultiplier timing circuit

Figure 3–19   Photomultiplier tube

anode of the photomultiplier tube is connected to the grid of a thyratron tube which serves as the switch for a photo-timer.

Figure 3–19 is a schematic diagram of a photomultiplier tube. It consists of a small fluorescent screen, a photocathode, several intermediate electrodes (called dynodes), and an anode. The photocathode is coated with a photoemissive surface. When it is struck by light, it emits electrons in numbers proportional to the intensity of the light. The intermediate electrodes are coated with a material that emits secondary electrons when struck by another electron. The photocathode is at a more negative potential than any of the dynodes, and the potential difference between the electrodes diminishes in steps down to the anode. Only three dynodes are shown in Figure 3–19 but there may be as many as ten. When x rays strike the fluoroscopic screen, the screen emits light. The light strikes the photocathode, and it in turn emits electrons. These electrons are accelerated toward the next electrode, and they acquire additional energy en route. When they strike the electrode, they emit a specific number of secondary electrons, and the process is repeated over and over down to the anode. At each step the number of electrons increases by a specific amount. It is important to realize that this is not an avalanche effect. **The output current is proportional to the amount of irradiation striking the fluorescent screen.** The electrical signal is amplified as it passes through the photomultiplier tube, and this signal supplies the current to charge the capacitor.

Ionization Chambers. The ionization chambers for phototimers are designed to be as radiolucent as possible so that they can be positioned in front of the x-ray film as shown in Figure 3–20. The chamber casts its image on a film, but the image is so faint that it is lost in the stronger superimposed images of anatomic parts. This radiolucency gives ionization chambers a definite advantage over photomultiplier tubes which must be placed behind the film because of their radiopacity. For example, an ionization chamber can be permanently mounted in the center of a fluoroscopic screen. In this position, it is ideally positioned for spot film radiography (discussed in Chapter 14), and yet does not interfere with routine fluoroscopy. A photomultiplier tube must be moved out of the radiographic field for fluoroscopy, and brought back for spot films. Even then its image obstructs the fluoroscopist's view of the spot film image. With the phototimer between the patient and the film, any type of cassette, regardless of the nature of

Figure 3–20   Ionization chamber timing circuit

its back, can be used to hold the film. Special cassettes must be used with photomultiplier tubes, cassettes with a translucent back, since the detector measures the transmitted radiation. If a lead back cassette is inadvertently used with a photomultiplier tube, the film will be overexposed.

Ionization chambers are filled with air, so they do not have to be enclosed in a glass envelope. The glass envelope around photomultiplier tubes is required to maintain a vacuum.

An ionization chamber consists of two electrodes, one a thin sheet of metal folded on itself to form two parallel plates, and the other a fine wire grid positioned equidistant between the plates, as shown in Figure 3–20. Before the x-ray exposure, the chamber is charged by applying a direct current voltage across the electrodes. As radiation passes through the chamber, air molecules are ionized. Each molecule produces an ion pair. The negative ions (electrons) move to the grid, which is the positive electrode, while the positive ions migrate to the negative plates. These moving electrons form an electric current. The current decreases the negative voltage on the grid of a thyratron tube, i.e. makes it more positive, and thus terminates the x-ray exposure.

Phototimer detectors (photomultiplier tubes and ionization chambers) are frequently used in pairs or triplets to sample several areas of the radiographic field. For example, paired detectors are used for PA chest films. The detectors are positioned on either side of the mid-line, hopefully in the upper lung fields. If the patient has a left upper lobe pneumonia, the detectors will average the readings from the two sides and expose the film accordingly. In this case, the right lung will be a little overexposed, but not as much as it would have been with only a single detector positioned on the left side. For the lateral chest film, the paired detectors are turned off and the exposure is regulated with a third detector placed near the center of the film.

The sensitivity of phototimers is adjusted empirically. Multiple radiographs are made on a test phantom until the desired density is achieved. The sensitivity of the phototimer is changed with a small variable resistor. Once adjusted, it should produce radiographs of uniform average density, regardless of the thickness of the patient. Phototimers usually have an automatic safety timer that controls the maximum exposure time. Safety timers are incorporated into the circuit to protect the x-ray tube, and they will terminate an exposure prematurely to prevent the anode from being overheated.

A   B   C

Figure 3–21   Spinning top (A); Radiographs from a single-phase (B) and from three-phase (C) generator

Testing the Accuracy of X-ray Timers

With a pulsating x-ray beam, the accuracy of an x-ray exposure timer can be measured with the aid of a **spinning top.** A photograph of a spinning top is shown in Figure 3–21A. It consists of a 3- to 4-inch metal disc attached to a stem and mounted on a base-plate for support. The disc has a narrow slit (or hole) near its edge and it must be free to rotate either on the stem or base-plate. The disc may be made of lead, steel, brass, or any other rigid radiopaque material.

Spinning tops function best with pulsating radiation; i.e., circuits with either half-wave or full-wave rectification. To test a timer, the spinning top is placed on an x-ray film (usually enclosed in a cassette). The top is manually rotated, and the film is exposed by radiation that passes through the narrow slit. As the disc rotates, the x-ray pulses are recorded as a series of broad dashes (or dots). Each dash represents an exposure time of 1/120 sec with full-wave and 1/60 sec with half-wave rectification, so the number of dashes measures the length of the exposure. The speed of disc rotation is not important provided it is fast enough to separate the individual pulses on the radiograph, and not so fast that the disc makes a complete revolution during the exposure.

Figure 3–21B shows a test film made with the exposure timer set for 1/10 sec in a circuit with full-wave rectification. The 12 broad dashes on the film represent an exposure time of 12 × 1/120 sec, or 1/10 sec. Since both the anticipated and measured exposure times are the same, the timer is functioning properly.

Figure 3–21C shows a radiograph of a spinning top taken with a 12-pulse three-phase generator. The exposure is recorded as a broad, continuous arc consisting of bands of varying density. These density variations represent ripple pulsations. The exposure timer was set for 1/30 sec, which is two cycles of alternating current. Since there are 12 pulses per cycle, 24 pulsations should be visible on the radiograph. However, the generator was not operating at full potential during the first portion of the exposure, so it is difficult to count the ripples. This points out another use for the spinning top; i.e., it provides a method of recording the intensity of an x-ray exposure at various instances in time.

A timer can also be evaluated with a photoconductor coupled to an oscilloscope. A photoconductor is a material which conducts a current when exposed to either light or x rays. This current can be displayed on an oscilloscope in exactly the same way that electricity from the heart is displayed for an electrocardiogram. Figure 3–22 shows the x-ray output of a three phase, 12-pulse generator for an exposure set at 1/60 of a second. The exposure time can be calculated either by counting the pulses or measuring the distances between the ascending and descending limbs of the exposure. Twelve pulses are shown on the oscilloscope, which is the correct number for a 1/60 sec exposure. The vertical lines on the oscilloscope are 5 milliseconds (msec) apart. A 1/60 sec exposure lasts 16.7

Figure 3–22 Oscilloscopic display of an x-ray exposure (12-pulse three phase generator)

msec (1000 ÷ 60), so the ascending and descending limbs of the exposure should be 16.7 msec apart. The limbs are not perfectly vertical, so an exact measurement is impossible, but the timer is certainly functioning at an acceptable level of accuracy.

The height of the exposure on the oscilloscope is a measure of relative x-ray intensity. With careful calibration, this height could be used as an exact measure of the x-ray exposure in roentgens. However, it is much easier to measure x-ray output with an ionization chamber, or some similar device designed specifically for this purpose. In general, the height of the exposure on the oscilloscope is used only to compare the various parts of the exposure, which in this case is almost perfectly uniform except for ripple pulsations.

SUMMARY

An x-ray generator supplies electrical energy to the x-ray tube and regulates the length of the radiographic exposure. The x-ray tube requires two sources of energy: one to heat the filament and the other to accelerate electrons between the cathode and anode. The filament circuit contains a variable resistor, which is the mA selector, and a step-down transformer. The cathode-anode circuit, which is called the high-voltage circuit, contains an autotransformer and a step-up transformer. The autotransformer is the kVp selector.

The incoming electrical supply to the x-ray generator has an alternating potential, which tends to move current from the anode to the cathode during half of each electric cycle. Rectifiers are electronic valves that transmit a current in only one direction. They are incorporated into the high-voltage circuit between the step-up transformer and the x-ray tube to prevent a reverse current. Half-wave rectification produces 60 x-ray pulses per second, while full-wave rectification produces 120 pulses.

Radiographic exposure timers open and close switches in the high-voltage circuit. These switches may be either mechanical (usually operated by an electromagnet) or electronic. Electronic switches, which are called thyratrons, have an almost instantaneous response and recycling time. Most modern x-ray generators have electronic timers. An electronic timer contains a variable resistor and a capacitor. The exposure time is determined by the amount of time required to charge the capacitor to a predetermined level. The variable resistor is the time selector. Phototimers are a special type of electronic timer in which the patient replaces the electrical resistor. The capacitor is charged by a current from a photomultiplier tube which measures the radiation transmitted through the patient. Another type of detector, an ionization chamber, can be used in place of the photomultiplier tube. Ionization chambers are radiolucent, so they can be permanently mounted in front of the x-ray film. Because of their radiolucency, they have replaced photomultiplier tubes in most installations.

CHAPTER 4

Basic Interactions between X rays and Matter

Atoms are bonded into molecules by electrons in the outermost shell. X-ray photons may interact with either orbital electrons or the nucleus of atoms. In the diagnostic energy range, the interactions are always with orbital electrons. If these electrons happen to be the ones bonding atoms into molecules, the bonds may be disrupted and the molecular structure altered. However, the molecular bonding energies are too small to influence the type and number of interactions. A group of oxygen atoms will stop the same number of x-ray photons, regardless of their physical state. It does not matter if the oxygen is free as a gas or bound to hydrogen as water. The important factor is the atomic makeup of a tissue and not its molecular structure.

There are five basic ways that an x-ray photon can interact with matter. These are:

1. Coherent scattering
2. Photoelectric effect
3. Compton scattering
4. Pair production
5. Photodisintegration

As we go through a discussion of each of the interactions, you will see that at times x-ray photons are **absorbed,** while at other times they are merely **scattered.** When photons are absorbed, they are completely removed from the x-ray beam and cease to exist. When photons are scattered, they are deflected into a random course, and no longer carry useful information. Since their direction is random, they cannot portray an image, and the only thing they produce on a film is blackness. In the language of the information transfer theorist, scatter radiation adds **noise** to the system. You can gain some insight into the effect of noise with a simple analogy. Imagine yourself listening to music on your car radio as you drive past an airport. As a plane approaches, the music becomes more difficult to hear, until finally, when the plane is directly overhead, it becomes completely inaudible. Even though the music is still there, you cannot hear it. Radiation noise does exactly the same sort of thing. It destroys image quality. We refer to the noise created by scatter radiation as film fog. When an x-ray film is badly fogged, the image may be completely obscured. It is still there, but we cannot see it. An understanding of the production of scatter radiation is of vital importance, so pay particular attention to it as we discuss the basic interactions between x rays and matter.

COHERENT SCATTERING

The name coherent scattering is given to those interactions in which radiation undergoes a change in direction without a change in wavelength. For this reason, the name unmodified is sometimes used. There are two types of coherent scattering—Thomson scattering and Rayleigh scattering. In Thomson scattering a single electron is involved in the interaction. Rayleigh scattering results from a cooperative interaction with all of the electrons of an atom. Both types of coherent scattering may be described in terms of a wave-particle interaction, and are therefore sometimes called classical scattering. Rayleigh scattering is shown diagrammatically in Figure 4–1. Low energy radiation encounters the electrons of an atom and sets them into vibration at the frequency of the radiation. A vibrating electron, because it is a charged particle, emits radiation. The process may be envisioned as the absorption of radiation, vibration of the atom, and the emission of radiation as the atom returns to its undisturbed state. This is the only type of interaction between x rays and matter that does not cause ionization. In order to produce an ion pair, a photon must transfer energy to the atom. No energy is transferred, and no ionization occurs with coherent scattering. Its only effect is to change the direction of the incident radiation. The percentage of radiation that undergoes coherent scattering is small compared to the other basic interactions; in general, it is less than 5%. Some coherent scattering occurs throughout the diagnostic energy range, but it never plays a major role. Even though it produces scattered radiation, which contributes to film fog, the total quantity is too small to be important in diagnostic radiology.

PHOTOELECTRIC EFFECT

Before beginning a discussion of the photoelectric effect, we are going to digress a moment to review a few points about atomic physics. Atomic structure is extremely complex, but we can greatly simplify it and still have a fairly good idea of how these interactions occur. The atom consists of a central nucleus and orbital electrons. The nucleus is important in our present discussion only as a means of keeping the electrons in the atom. The positively charged nucleus holds the negatively charged electrons in specific orbits, or shells. The innermost shell is called the K-shell, and the more peripheral shells are named consecutively L, M, N, etc. These shells have a limited electron capacity. The K-shell can hold only two electrons. If more electrons are present in the atom, they must move out to the L-shell, which has a capacity of eight electrons. Each shell has a specific binding energy. The closer the shell is to the nucleus, the tighter the electrons in that shell are bound to the nucleus. The electrons in the outermost shell are loosely bound. They are essentially free, and appropriately, they are called free electrons. The energy value of electronic shells is also determined by the atomic number of the atom. K-shell electrons are more tightly bound in elements with high atomic numbers than they are in elements with low atomic numbers. In fact, the differences are sizable. For example, the K-shell binding energy for lead is 88

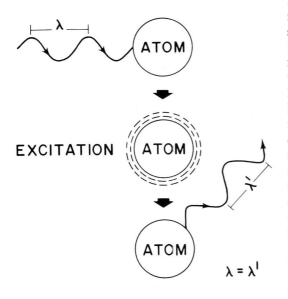

Figure 4–1   Coherent Rayleigh scattering

keV, while the K-shell binding energy for calcium is only 4 keV. Electrons in the K-shell are at a lower energy level than electrons in the L-shell. If we consider the outermost electrons as free, then inner-shell electrons are all in energy debt. Their energy debt is greatest when they are close to the nucleus in an element with a high atomic number.

The photoelectric effect is shown diagrammatically in Figure 4–2. We will quickly run through the whole interaction and then fill in some details later. An incident photon, with a little more energy than the binding energy of a K-shell electron, encounters one of these electrons and ejects it from its orbit. The photon disappears, giving up all of its energy to the electron. The majority of the photon's energy is needed to overcome the binding energy of the electron, and the excess gives

the electron kinetic energy. The electron, which is now free of its energy debt, flies off into space as a photoelectron. It becomes a negative ion, and it is absorbed almost immediately, since charged particles have little penetrating power. The atom is left with an electron void on the K-shell, but only for an instant. An electron immediately drops into the void to fill the K-shell. This electron usually comes from the adjacent L-shell, occasionally from the M-shell, and on rare occasions, from free electrons from the same, or another, atom. As an electron drops into the K-shell, it gives up energy in the form of an x-ray photon. The amount of energy is characteristic of each element, and the radiation produced by the movement of electrons within an atom is called characteristic radiation. When the K-shell void is filled by an outer-shell electron from the same atom, the atom is left with a deficiency of one electron, and it remains a positive ion. If a free electron from another atom fills the void, then the other atom becomes a positive ion, and the result is the same. The photoelectric effect always yields three end products: (1) characteristic radiation, (2) a negative ion (the photoelectron), and (3) a positive ion (an atom deficient one electron).

Probability of a Photoelectric Reaction

Three simple rules govern the probability of a photoelectric reaction.

1. **The incident photon must have sufficient energy to overcome the binding energy of the electron.** For example, the K-shell electrons of iodine have a binding energy of 33.2 keV. An x-ray photon with an energy of 33.0 keV absolutely cannot eject them from their shell. The photon may interact at the L- or M-shells, but not at the K-shell.

2. **A photoelectric reaction is most likely when the photon energy and electron binding energy are nearly the same,** provided of course that the photon's energy is greater. A 34 keV photon is

1. → • **Photoelectron**

2. **Characteristic Radiation**

3. **Positive Ion**

Figure 4–2   Photoelectric effect

much more likely to react with a K-shell electron of iodine than a 100 keV photon. In fact, the probability of a photoelectric reaction drops precipitously as photon energy increases. It is inversely proportional to approximately the third power of energy, or expressed in mathematical form:

$$\text{Photoelectric effect} \sim \frac{1}{(\text{Energy})^3}$$

3. **The tighter an electron is bound in its orbit, the more likely it is to be involved in a photoelectric reaction.** Electrons are more tightly bound in elements with high atomic numbers than in elements with low atomic numbers, as shown in Table 4–1. Most interactions occur at the K-shell in elements with low atomic numbers, since the K-shell contains the most tightly bound electrons. However, in elements with high atomic numbers, the energy of the incident photons is frequently insufficient to eject a K-shell electron, and many photoelectric reactions take place at the L- and M-shell levels. Since elements with high atomic numbers bind their electrons more tightly, they are more likely to undergo photoelectric reactions. The probability of the photoelectric effect increases sharply as the atomic number increases. In fact, it is roughly proportional to the third power of the atomic number:

$$\text{Photoelectric effect} \sim (\text{Atomic number})^3$$

In summary, photoelectric reactions are most likely to occur with low-energy photons and elements with high atomic numbers, provided the photons have sufficient energy to overcome the forces binding the electrons in their shells.

Characteristic Radiation

We first met characteristic radiation when we discussed the production of x rays in Chapter 2. Characteristic radiation generated by the photoelectric effect is exactly the same. The only difference is in the modality used to eject the inner-shell electron. In an x-ray tube, a high-speed electron is the moving force, while in a photoelectric reaction, the force is an x-ray photon. In both cases, the atom is left with an excess of energy equal to the binding energy of the ejected electron. All physical systems seek the lowest possible energy state. For example, water always runs downhill. An atom with an electron deficiency in the K-shell is in a higher energy state than an atom with an L-shell electron deficiency. The atom releases this excess energy in the form of photons. Usually, an electron from an adjacent shell drops into

Table 4–1. K-Shell Electron Binding Energies (keV) of Elements Important in Diagnostic Radiology

ATOMIC NUMBER	ATOM	K-SHELL BINDING ENERGY (keV)
6	Carbon	0.284
7	Nitrogen	0.400
8	Oxygen	0.532
13	Aluminum	1.56
20	Calcium	4.04
50	Tin	29.2
53	Iodine	33.2
56	Barium	37.4
74	Tungsten	69.5
82	Lead	88.0

Figure 4–3 Characteristic radiation from iodine

an inner-shell void as shown for an iodine atom in Figure 4–3. The K-shell binding energy for iodine is 33.2 keV, while the L-shell is 4.9 keV, and more peripheral shells have even lower binding energies. When an electron from an L-shell falls to the K-shell, a 28.3-keV (33.2 − 4.9 = 28.3) photon is released. The void in the L-shell is then filled with a photon from the M-shell with the production of a 4.3-keV photon. This process is continued until the whole 33.2 keV of energy has been converted into photons. Of course, the lower-energy photons are of no importance in diagnostic radiology, since they are absorbed immediately. Occasionally, an inner-shell void is filled by an electron from distant peripheral shells, or even free electrons. When a free electron moves into the K-shell void in iodine, a single photon of 33.2 keV is generated. This is the maximal energy characteristic radiation that iodine can produce.

The K-shell binding energies of some elements important in diagnostic radiology are shown in Table 4–1. Calcium, which has the highest atomic number of any element found in the body in significant quantity, emits a 4-keV maximal energy characteristic photon, which is little energy by x-ray standards. It is absorbed within a few millimeters of its site of origin. The contrast agents iodine and barium are the only elements encountered in diagnostic radiology that emit characteristic radiation energetic enough to leave the patient and fog an x-ray film.

Characteristic radiation is usually referred to as secondary radiation to differentiate it from scatter radiation, a distinction that hardly seems necessary since the end result is the same for both, a photon that is deflected from its original path.

The Photoelectric Effect in Diagnostic Radiology

As diagnostic radiologists we can look at the photoelectric effect in two ways, one good and the other bad. Starting with the good, it produces radiographic images of excellent quality. The quality is good for two reasons; first, the photoelectric effect does not produce scatter radiation; and second, it enhances natural tissue contrast. X-ray image contrast depends upon some tissues absorbing more x rays than other tissues. Contrast is greatest when the difference in absorption between adjacent tissues is large. Since the number of reactions depends upon the third power of the atomic number, the photoelectric effect magnifies the difference in tissues composed of different elements, such as bone and soft tissue. So from the point of view of film quality, the photoelectric effect is desirable. However, from the point of view of patient exposure, it is undesirable. Patients receive more radiation from photoelectric reactions than from any other type of interaction. All of the energy of the incident photon is absorbed by the patient in a photoelectric reaction. Only part of the incident photon's energy is absorbed in a Compton reaction, as you will see in the next section. Since one of our primary goals is to keep patient doses at a minimum, we must keep this point in mind at all times. The importance of the photoelectric effect can be minimized by using high-energy (kVp) techniques. In general, we should use radiation of the highest energy consistent with diagnostic-quality x-ray films in order to minimize patient exposure.

In summary, the likelihood of a photoelectric interaction depends upon two factors: first, the energy of the radiation, and second, the atomic number of the absorber. The reaction is most common with low-energy photons and absorbers with high atomic numbers. Photons usually strike tightly bound K-shell electrons, and they must have more energy than the electron binding energy. Photoelectric reactions are desirable from the point of view of the film quality, since they give excellent contrast without generating significant scatter radiation. Unfortunately, patient exposures are much higher than with any other type of interaction.

COMPTON SCATTERING

Almost all of the scatter radiation that we encounter in diagnostic radiology comes from Compton scattering. Figure 4–4 shows the reaction diagrammatically. An incident photon with relatively high energy strikes a free outer-shell electron, ejecting it from its orbit. The photon is deflected by the electron so that it travels in a new direction as scatter radiation. The photon always retains a part of its original energy. The reaction produces an ion pair, a positive atom and a negative electron, which is called a recoil electron.

The energy of the incident photon is distributed in two ways. Part of it goes to the recoil electron as kinetic energy, and the rest is retained by the deflected photon. Unlike a photoelectric reaction, where most of a photon's energy is expended freeing the photoelectron from its bond, in a Compton reaction no energy is needed for this purpose, since the recoil electron is already free. The incident photon always retains some of its original energy. Two factors determine the amount of energy the photon retains: first its initial energy, and second, its angle of deflection off the recoil electron. If you think of the Compton reaction as a collision between two billiard balls, the energy transfer is easier to understand. The cue ball is the incident photon, and the second ball is a free electron. When the cue ball strikes the second ball, they both deflect in a predictable manner. With a glancing blow, the angle of deflection of the cue ball is small, and only a small quantity of energy is transferred to the second ball. The cue ball retains almost all of its initial energy. With a more direct hit, the cue ball deflects at a greater angle and loses more energy. Finally, with a direct hit, maximal energy is transferred to the second ball, but unlike the cue ball in billiards, a Compton photon never gives up all its energy. The photon retains some energy and deflects back along its original path at an angle of 180°. Figure 4–5 shows the amount of energy a 75-keV photon retains as it is deflected through various angles. As you can see, more energy is lost with larger angles of deflection.

To make our comparison between a Compton reaction and billard balls complete, we must make one last adjustment in the analogy. Billiard balls all have the same mass. However, we want to compare them with photons whose energies vary. We can keep our analogy going by using cue balls of different masses. Thus, a light cue ball

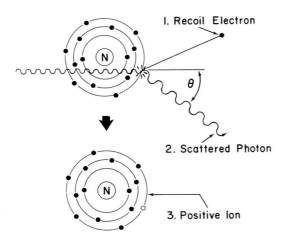

1. Recoil Electron

θ

2. Scattered Photon

3. Positive Ion

Figure 4–4   Compton scattering

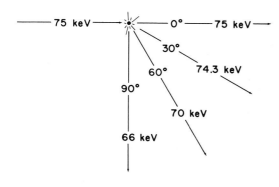

Figure 4-5 Energy of Compton-scattered photons

tion of events that are occurring in three dimensions. You can picture the three-dimensional distribution by rotating the pattern around its longitudinal axis. With lower-energy radiation, fewer photons scatter forward and more scatter back at an angle of 180°. This distribution is fairly constant throughout the diagnostic energy range.

The classic formula for calculating the change in wavelengths of a scattered photon is:

$$\Delta\lambda = 0.024 (1 - \cos\theta)$$
$$\Delta\lambda = \text{Change in wavelength (Å)}$$
$$\theta = \text{Angle of photon deflection}$$

simulates a low-energy photon, and a heavy cue ball simulates a high energy photon. Now, imagine both the light and the heavy cue balls striking a second ball a glancing blow at an angle of 45°. The light ball has little momentum, and it will deflect at a much greater angle than the heavy ball which has more momentum. Photons also have momentum, and the higher the energy of the photons, the more difficult they are to deflect. With x-ray energies of 1 MeV (million electron volts), most scattered photons deflect in a forward direction. However, in the diagnostic energy range the distribution is more symmetrical. Figure 4-6 shows the pattern of distribution of scattered photons from a 100-keV x-ray beam. The distance from the point of the interaction is used to express the percentage of scattered photons at various angles. Remember, this is a flat representa-

Most of us think in terms of kilovoltage and not wavelengths. We can change wavelengths from the above formula to kilovoltage with the following conversion factor:

$$kV = \frac{12.4}{\lambda}$$

$$\lambda = \text{Wavelengths (Å)}$$
$$kV = \text{Kilovoltage}$$

The amount of energy retained by scattered photons after a Compton reaction is shown in Table 4-2. In the diagnostic energy range up to 150 keV, the photon retains most of its original energy, and very little is transferred to the recoil electron. At narrow angles of deflection, scattered photons retain almost all of their original energy. This creates a serious problem in diagnostic radiology, because photons that are scattered at narrow angles have an excellent chance of reaching an x-ray film and producing fog. They are exceedingly difficult to remove from the x-ray beam. In fact, they cannot be removed by filters, because they are too energetic, and they cannot be removed by grids, because their angle of deflection is too small. Since we have no way of removing them from the useful beam, we must accept them and tolerate an image of diminished quality.

Scatter radiation from Compton reactions is also a major safety hazard. As you

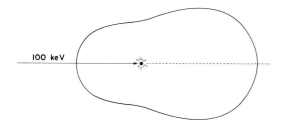

Figure 4-6 Distribution of Compton-scattered photons

Table 4–2.   Energy of Compton-Scattered Photons for Various Angles of Deflection

ENERGY OF INCIDENT PHOTON (keV)	ENERGY OF SCATTERED PHOTONS (keV)			
	Photon Deflection Angle			
	30°	60°	90°	180°
25	24.9	24.4	24	23
50	49.6	47.8	46	42
75	74.3	70	66	58
100	98.5	91	84	72
150	146	131	116	95

can see in Table 4–2, even after a photon has been deflected 90°, it still retains most of its original energy. This means that the scatter radiation that arises in the patient during a fluoroscopic examination is almost as energetic as the primary beam. It creates a real safety hazard for the fluoroscopist and other personnel who must be in exposure rooms.

Probability of a Compton Reaction

The probability of a Compton reaction depends upon the total number of electrons in an absorber, which in turn depends upon its density and the number of electrons per gram. In Chapter 5, we will show that all elements contain approximately the same number of electrons per gram, regardless of their atomic number. Therefore, the number of Compton reactions is independent of the atomic number of the absorber. However, the likelihood of a reaction does depend upon the energy of the radiation and density of the absorber. The number of reactions gradually diminishes as photon energy increases, so that a high-energy photon is more likely to pass through the body than a low-energy photon.

Since Compton reactions occur with free electrons, we must define this term a little more precisely. An electron can be considered free when its binding energy is a great deal less than the energy of the incident photon. With the photon energies used in diagnostic radiology (10 to 150 keV), only the outer-shell electrons are free in the elements with high atomic numbers. However, for the elements with low atomic numbers, those found in soft tissues, all electrons can be considered free, because even those on the K-shell are bound with an energy of less than 1 keV.

PAIR PRODUCTION AND PHOTODISINTEGRATION

The last two basic interactions, pair production and photodisintegration, do not occur in the diagnostic energy range. They have no importance in diagnostic radiology, and we will only discuss them briefly. In pair production, a high-energy photon interacts with the nucleus of an atom, the photon disappears, and its energy is converted into matter in the form of two particles. One is an ordinary electron. The other is a positron, a particle with the same mass as an electron, but with a positive charge. Since the mass of one electron is equal to 0.51 MeV, and pair production produces two electrons, the interaction cannot take place with photon energies less than 1.02 MeV.

In photodisintegration, a part of the nucleus of an atom is ejected by a high-energy photon. The ejected portion may be either a neutron, proton, alpha particle, or a cluster of particles. The photon must have sufficient energy to overcome nuclear binding energies of the order of 7 to 15 MeV.

Since pair production does not occur with photon energies less than 1.02 MeV, and photodisintegration with energies less than 7 MeV, neither of these interactions is of any importance in diagnostic radiology, where we rarely use energies above 150 keV.

RELATIVE FREQUENCY OF THE BASIC INTERACTIONS

Figure 4–7 shows the percentage of each type of interaction for water, compact bone, and sodium iodide with photon energies from 20 to 100 keV. The total number of reactions is always 100%. The contribution of each interaction is represented by an area in the illustration. Thus, if coherent scattering accounts for 5% of the interactions, Compton scattering for 20%, and the photoelectric effect for 75%, the total is 100%. Water is used to illustrate the behavior of tissues with low

atomic numbers, such as air, fat, and muscle. The total number of reactions is less for air than for water, but the percentage of each type is approximately the same. Compact bone contains a large amount of calcium, and it represents elements with intermediate atomic numbers. Iodine and barium are the elements with the highest atomic numbers that we encounter in diagnostic radiology, and they are represented by sodium iodide.

As you can see in the illustration, coherent scattering usually contributes around 5% to the total, and plays a minor role throughout the diagnostic energy range. In water, Compton scattering is the dominant interaction, except at very low photon energies (20 to 30 keV). The contrast agents, because of their high atomic numbers, are involved almost exclusively in photoelectric reactions. Bone is intermediate between water and the contrast agents. At low energies, photoelectric reactions are more common, while at high energies, Compton scattering is dominant.

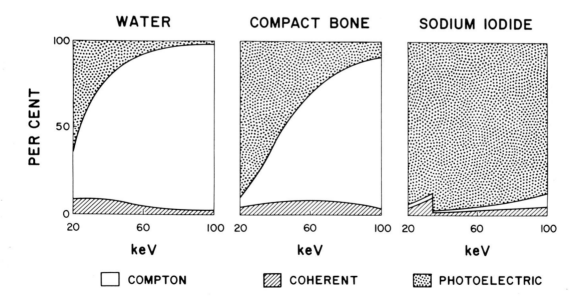

Figure 4–7 Percentage of coherent, photoelectric, and Compton reactions in water, compact bone, and sodium iodide

SUMMARY

Only two interactions are important in diagnostic radiology—the photoelectric effect and Compton scattering. Coherent scattering is numerically unimportant, and pair production and photodisintegration occur at energies above the useful energy range. The photoelectric effect is the predominant interaction with low-energy radiation and high atomic number absorbers. It generates no significant scatter radiation, produces high contrast in the x-ray image, but unfortunately, exposes the patient to a great deal of radiation. At higher diagnostic energies, Compton scattering is the most common interaction between x rays and body tissues, and it is responsible for almost all scatter radiation. Radiographic image contrast is less with Compton reactions than with the photoelectric effect.

CHAPTER 5

Attenuation

Quantity and quality are two terms used to express the characteristics of an x-ray beam. Quantity refers to the number of photons in the beam, and quality refers to their energies. The intensity of a beam is the product of the number and energy of the photons, so it is dependent upon both quantity and quality. A beam of 50-keV photons has a greater intensity than a beam made up of a comparable number of 20-keV photons. **Attenuation is the reduction in the intensity of an x-ray beam as it traverses matter by either the absorption or deflection of photons from the beam.** Because it is a measure of a change in x-ray intensity, attenuation depends upon both the quantity and quality of the photons in a beam. For our purpose, it would be simpler to think of attenuation only in terms of quantity. Then a reduction in intensity would be simply a reduction in the number of photons in the beam. We can do this if we limit our discussion to the attenuation of monochromatic radiation. Later in the text, we will clarify why quality does not change with monochromatic radiation. To further simplify our discussion, we will disregard the attenuation of secondary radiation resulting from coherent or Compton's scattering and the characteristic radiation of the photoelectric effect. Once a photon has undergone any of these reactions, it will be considered completely attenuated, i.e. totally removed from the beam.

ATTENUATION OF MONOCHROMATIC RADIATION

The attenuation of a beam of monochromatic radiation is shown schematically in Figure 5–1. A beam of 1000 photons is directed at a water phantom. The intensity of the beam is decreased to 800 photons by the first centimeter of water, which is an attenuation of 20%. The second centimeter of water decreases the intensity to 640 photons, which is 20% less than had passed through the first centimeter. With each succeeding centimeter of water, 20% of the remaining photons are removed from the beam.

The quality of monochromatic radiation does not change as it passes through an

Figure 5–1 Attenuation of monochromatic radiation

absorber. Remember, we are only discussing primary photons, i.e. the photons that do not undergo any kind of interaction. If we begin with a group of photons with an energy of 60 keV, then the transmitted photons will all have the same energy. Their numbers will be reduced, but their quality will not be changed. So when we talk about a change in the intensity of a monochromatic beam, we are really talking about a change in the number, or quantity, of photons in the beam. A 50% reduction in the number of photons is a 50% reduction in the intensity of the beam. The attenuation of polychromatic radiation is much more complicated, and we will not discuss it until near the end of the chapter.

When the number of transmitted photons and absorber thickness are plotted on linear graph paper, they plot a curved line as shown in Figure 5–2A. The initial portion of the curve is steep, since more photons are removed from the beam by the first few centimeters of absorber. After the beam has passed through many centimeters of water, only a few photons remain. While each centimeter continues to remove 20% of the photons, the total numbers are small, and the end of the curve is almost flat. The same numbers plot a straight line on semi-logarithmic graph paper as shown in Figure 5–2B. When the number of photons remaining in the beam decreases by the same percentage with each increment of absorber, as they do with monochromatic radiation, the attenuation is called exponential. Exponential functions plot a straight line on semi-logarithmic graph paper.

ATTENUATION COEFFICIENTS

An attenuation coefficient is a measure of the quantity of radiation that is attenuated by a given thickness of an ab-

Figure 5–2 Attenuation of monochromatic radiation plotted on linear (A) and semi-logarithmic graph paper (B)

sorber. The name of the coefficient is determined by the units that are used to measure the thickness of the absorber. Four attenuation coefficients are described in classical texts on radiological physics, but only two are important in diagnostic radiology—the linear and mass attenuation coefficients.

Linear Attenuation Coefficient (μ)

The linear attenuation coefficient is the most important coefficient for diagnostic radiology. It is a quantitative measurement of attenuation per centimeter of absorber, so it tells us how much attenuation we can expect from a certain thickness of tissue. Since we measure our patients in centimeters, it is a practical and useful attenuation coefficient. In the next section, after we have discussed the mass attenuation coefficient, you will understand why the linear coefficient is more useful. It is symbolized by the Greek letter μ.

The unit of the linear attenuation coefficient is per centimeter, and thus the name **linear** attenuation coefficient, because a centimeter is a linear measurement. The expression per cm is the same as 1/cm and it is usually written cm^{-1}.

It is important that you realize that **the linear attenuation coefficient (μ) is for monochromatic radiation,** and that it is specific both for the energy of the x-ray beam and for the type of absorber. Water, fat, bone, and air all have different linear attenuation coefficients, and the size of the coefficient changes as the energy of the x-ray beam changes. When the energy of the radiation is increased, the number of x rays that are attenuated decreases, and so does the linear attenuation coefficient.

The mathematics involved in the derivation of the exponential equation for x-ray attenuation is beyond the scope of this book. The formula is:

$$N = N_0 e^{-\mu x}$$

N = Number of transmitted photons
N_0 = Number of incident photons
e = Base of natural logarithm
μ = Linear attenuation coefficient
x = Absorber thickness (cm)

This is a classical equation, and it has the same format as the equation for the decay of radionuclides. In fact, most people find it easier to think in terms of radionuclide decay, so we will digress for a moment. Radionuclides decay at an exponential rate. This rate is usually measured and defined in terms of half life, which is the time that it takes a material to decay to one-half its original activity. For example, ^{131}I has a half life ($T_{1/2}$) of 8.04 days. If we started with 100 units of activity, at the end of 8.04 days we would have 50 units, and at the end of another 8.04 days we would only have 25 units. The equation for this exponential decay is as follows:

$$N = N_0 e^{-\lambda t}$$

N = Activity of remaining radionuclide
N_0 = Activity of original radionuclide
e = Base of natural logarithm (2.718)
λ = Decay constant (sec^{-1})
t = Time (sec)

The decay constant (λ) can be easily related to half life ($T_{1/2}$), which is a more familiar concept. After the elapsed time of one half life ($T_{1/2}$), the quantity of remaining activity is $N_0/2$. The exponential decay equation can be rewritten as follows:

$$\frac{N_0}{2} = N_0 e^{-\lambda T_{1/2}}$$

Dividing both sides by N_0, the equation becomes:

$$\tfrac{1}{2} = e^{-\lambda T_{1/2}}$$

We would then go to a table of exponential values and find the value of the exponent $\lambda T_{1/2}$, which makes $e^{-\lambda T_{1/2}}$ equal to 1/2; or more simply, we could just look up the logarithm of 1/2 in a table of natural logarithms. We would find this value to be -0.693. We can now rewrite the exponential decay equation as follows:

$$\lambda \cdot T_{1/2} = 0.693 \text{ or } \lambda = \frac{0.693}{T_{1/2}}$$

The decay constant (λ) for any radionuclide can be calculated if we know its half life. For example, the decay constant for ^{131}I ($T_{1/2}$ = 8.04 days) is as follows:

$$\lambda = \frac{0.693}{8.04 \text{ days}} = .086/\text{day}$$

The attenuation of monochromatic radiation is exactly the same. All we need do is substitute thickness (cm of absorber) for time (sec). The names are changed, but the concept remains the same. The decay constant (λ) becomes the linear attenuation coefficient (μ) and half life ($T_{1/2}$) becomes the half value layer (HVL). The product of the linear attenuation coefficient and half value layer is equal to 0.693:

$$\mu \times \text{HVL} = 0.693 \text{ or HVL} = \frac{0.693}{\mu}$$

The half value layer is the absorber thickness required to reduce the intensity of the original beam by one-half. It is a common method for expressing the quality of an x-ray beam. A beam with a high half value layer is a more penetrating beam than one with a low half value layer.

If the values from the attenuation of the x-ray beam in Figure 5–1 are used in the exponential attenuation equation, the linear attenuation coefficient can be calculated as follows:

$$N = N_0 e^{-\mu x}$$
N = 800 photons transmitted
N_0 = 1000 initial photons
x = 1 cm of water

$$800 = 1000 \, e^{-\mu(1)} = \frac{1000}{e^\mu}$$

$$e^\mu = \frac{1000}{800} = 1.25$$

$$\mu = 0.22/\text{cm}$$

The last step in the calculation requires a table of exponential values, or natural logarithms. After we have determined the linear attenuation coefficient, the half value layer of the beam can be calculated as follows:

$$\text{HVL} = \frac{0.693}{\mu} = \frac{0.693}{0.22} = 3.15 \text{ cm}$$

You can see from Figure 5–1 that the beam is reduced to one-half its original intensity in the fourth 1 cm block of water, which confirms our calculations.

Calculating a linear attenuation coefficient is not of much practical value to a diagnostic radiologist, but the equation can be used for other purposes. There are tables available[1] that list the linear attenuation coefficients for substances such as water, bone, sodium iodide, and most of the elements. With the linear attenuation coefficient from these tables, we can calculate the percentage of transmitted photons for a whole variety of photon energies and for whatever thickness of tissue we may choose.

Mass Attenuation Coefficient (μ/ρ)

Another useful attenuation coefficient that is deeply rooted in the physics literature is the mass attenuation coefficient. It was instituted to quantitate the attenuation of materials independent of their physical state. For example, water, ice and water vapor, the three physical states of H_2O, all have the same mass attenuation coefficient. It is obtained by dividing the linear attenuation coefficient by the density (ρ) and it is symbolized by μ/ρ. The unit for the x-ray absorber is grams per square centimeter (gm/cm^2), which is a mass unit, and thus the name **mass** attenuation coefficient. Figure 5–3 illustrates the meaning of a gram per square centimeter by comparing aluminum and water. The density of water is 1 gm/cm^3, so a square centimeter of water must be 1 centimeter thick to weigh 1 gram. The density of aluminum is 2.7 gm/cm^3, so a square centimeter of aluminum only has to be 0.37 cm thick to weigh 1 gram. The arithmetic is simple. The thickness is merely the reciprocal of the density, or 1 divided by the density. A square centimeter of water 1 cm thick and a square centimeter of aluminum 0.37 cm thick both contain 1 gm/cm^2.

The unit of the mass attenuation coefficient is per gm/cm^2. It can be expressed

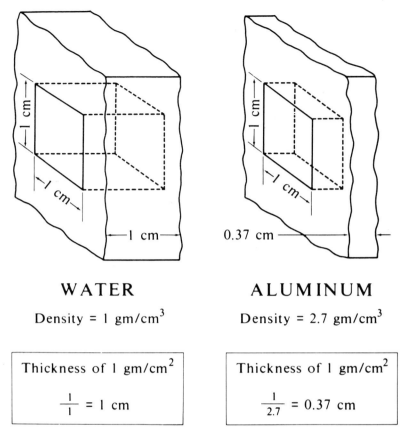

WATER

Density = 1 gm/cm^3

Thickness of 1 gm/cm^2
$\frac{1}{1}$ = 1 cm

ALUMINUM

Density = 2.7 gm/cm^3

Thickness of 1 gm/cm^2
$\frac{1}{2.7}$ = 0.37 cm

Figure 5–3   Thickness of 1 gm/cm² of water and of aluminum

in several ways: per gm/cm² or 1/gm/cm² or cm²/gm; usually it is written cm²/gm.

A brief review should help to avoid confusion about units. When we talk about either the linear or mass attenuation coefficient, there are two separate units for each; i.e., one for the absorber and the other for the coefficient. The units for the absorber are cm for the linear attenuation coefficient and gm/cm² for the mass attenuation coefficient. The units for the coefficients themselves are cm^{-1} for the linear and cm²/gm for the mass attenuation coefficient. The unit of the coefficient is the reciprocal of the unit of the absorber.

A simple way to understand the relationship between the linear and mass attenuation coefficients is to compare the

coefficients for water, ice, and water vapor as shown in Figure 5–4. The values in the illustration are for a 50-keV monochromatic beam. The linear attenuation coefficient for water is 0.214 cm^{-1}, and a 1-cm thickness of water absorbs 20% of the incident beam. The same thickness of ice absorbs 18.5%, since ice is a little less dense than water. Water vapor has very little density and a 1-cm thickness absorbs almost nothing. Density has a profound effect on x-ray attenuation at all energy levels.

The mass attenuation coefficient for water in Figure 5–4 is 0.214 cm²/gm, which is the same as the linear attenuation coefficient. They must be the same, since the density of water is 1, and the mass

50 keV		Density (gm/cm^3)	Thickness of 1 gm/cm^2
Linear Attenuation Coefficient (cm^{-1})	Mass Attenuation Coefficient (cm^2/gm)		
0.214	0.214	1	WATER 1 cm
0.196	0.214	0.917	ICE 1.09 cm
0.000128	0.214	0.000598	WATER VAPOR 1670 cm

Figure 5–4   Comparison of linear and mass attenuation coefficients for water, ice, and water vapor

attenuation coefficient is obtained by dividing the linear attenuation coefficient by the density (μ/ρ). The mass attenuation coefficient is the same for water, ice, and water vapor, which is logical since 1 gram of all three has exactly the same amount of mass. However, the thickness of 1 gm/cm^2 of water is 1 cm, ice 1.09 cm, and water vapor 1670 cm. These thicknesses will all attenuate the same amount of x ray (i.e., 20%) since they all contain the same amount of mass. As you can see in Figure 5–4, the mass attenuation coefficient is independent of the density of the absorber. The coefficients for water, ice, and water vapor are all the same, but their densities vary considerably.

To say that a gram of water and a gram of water vapor both absorb the same amount of radiation is true, but the statement has no meaning to a diagnostic radiologist. In fact, it is misleading. We just do not deal with gm/cm^2 of patient. We measure a patient's thickness in centimeters, and 1 cm of water absorbs a great deal more x ray than 1 cm of water vapor. When the effect of density is removed from the value of an attenuation coefficient, it is misleading in diagnostic radiology.

FACTORS AFFECTING ATTENUATION

Four factors determine the degree of attenuation of an x-ray beam as it passes through matter. One involves the nature of the radiation, and three involve the make-up of the matter.

RADIATION	MATTER
Energy	Density
	Atomic number
	Electrons per gram

Increasing the radiation energy increases the number of transmitted photons (and decreases attenuation); while increasing the density, atomic number, or electrons per gram of the absorber decreases the number of transmitted photons (and increases attenuation).

Relationships between Density, Atomic Number and Electrons per Gram

We will examine each of the four factors that affect attenuation separately, but first we must digress to review the relationships between density (ρ), atomic number (Z), and electrons per gram (e/gm).

Density and Atomic Number

The relationship between density and atomic number is complex, and no simple rule will cover all situations. In general, elements with high atomic numbers are denser than elements with low atomic numbers, but there are exceptions. Gold and lead provide a good example:

	ATOMIC NUMBER	DENSITY (gm/cm³)
Gold	79	19.3
Lead	82	11.0

There is no relationship between atomic number and density when different physical states of matter are considered. Water has an effective atomic number of 7.4 regardless of its state (ice, liquid, or vapor), but its density is different in each of these three forms.

Density and Electrons per Gram

Whenever a factor is expressed in the units per gram, the concept of volume is eliminated. Since density depends upon volume (weight per unit volume), there is no relationship between density and electrons per gram. A gram of water has the same number of electrons, regardless of whether they are compressed together in a 1-cm cube as a liquid, or spread out over 1670 cm³ as a vapor.

Atomic Number and Electrons per Gram

The number of electrons per gram is really a function of the number of neutrons in the atom. If the elements did not have neutrons, all materials would have 6.0 × 10²³ e/gm. Table 5–1 shows the relationships between atomic number and electrons per gram for various substances important in diagnostic radiology. Hydrogen, which has no neutrons, has 6.0 × 10²³ e/gm, which is twice as many as any other element. The elements found in soft tissue—carbon, nitrogen, and oxygen—all have 3.0 × 10²³ e/gm, and the higher atomic elements have even fewer e/gm. In

Table 5–1. Electrons Per Gram for Several Elements Important in Diagnostic Radiology

ELEMENTS	ATOMIC NUMBER	NUMBER OF ELECTRONS PER GRAM
Hydrogen	1	6.00×10^{23}
Oxygen	8	3.01×10^{23}
Calcium	20	3.00×10^{23}
Copper	29	2.75×10^{23}
Iodine	53	2.51×10^{23}
Barium	56	2.45×10^{23}
Lead	82	2.38×10^{23}

general, elements with low atomic numbers have more electrons per gram than those with high atomic numbers.

The Effects of Energy and Atomic Number on Attenuation

Energy and atomic number, in combination, determine the percentage of each type of basic interaction; so in this sense, their effects on attenuation are inseparable. Table 5–2 shows the percentage of photoelectric reactions for various radiation energies in water, bone, and sodium iodide. You can easily calculate the percentage of Compton reactions by subtracting the percentage of photoelectric reactions from 100 (ignoring the small contribution from coherent scattering). As the radiation energy increases, the percentage of photoelectric reactions decreases for water and bone; as the atomic number increases, the percentage of photoelectric reactions increases. With very low energy radiation (20 keV), photoelectric attenuation predominates, regardless of the atomic number of the absorber. As the radiation energy is increased, Compton scattering becomes more important until eventually it replaces the photoelectric effect as the predominant interaction. With high atomic number absorbers, like sodium iodide, the photoelectric effect is the predominant interaction throughout the diagnostic energy range.

The linear attenuation coefficient is the sum of the contributions from coherent scattering, photoelectric reactions and Compton scattering.

$$\mu = \mu_{coherent} + \mu_{P.E.} + \mu_{Compton}$$

For example, at 40 keV, the linear attenuation coefficient for water is .24 cm^{-1}. Of this total, .018 is from coherent scattering, .18 is from Compton scattering and the remaining .042 is from photoelectric attenuation. For water, the mass and linear attenuation coefficients are the same because the density of water is 1. However, for other materials, the mass and linear attenuation coefficients are different, but the principle is exactly the same.

If we know the relative percentage of each type of interaction, we can predict the total amount of attenuation (or transmission). Attenuation is always greater when the photoelectric effect predominates. Perhaps the difference between photoelectric and Compton attenuation will be easier to understand with an analogy. Suppose we take a flat stone and slide it along the ground at a high speed. If we slide the stone over a rough surface, such as a concrete sidewalk, friction will stop it in a short distance. If we slide the stone over a frozen pond, friction is reduced, and the stone will travel a much greater distance. In this analogy, the x-ray beam is the moving stone and attenuation is the friction that stops the stone. Photoelectric attenuation is like the concrete sidewalk and Compton attenuation is like the frozen pond. The photoelectric effect attenuates a beam much more rapidly than Compton scattering.

Energy

Besides its influence on the type of basic interaction, energy has its own effect on attenuation. Even when all of the basic

Table 5–2. Percentage of Photoelectric Reactions

RADIATION ENERGY	WATER $\overline{Z} = 7.4$	COMPACT BONE $\overline{Z} = 13.8$	SODIUM IODIDE $\overline{Z} = 49.8$
20 keV	65%	89%	94%
60 keV	7%	31%	95%
100 keV	2%	9%	88%

interactions are of one type, attenuation decreases as the radiation energy increases. Table 5–3 shows the percentage of photons transmitted through a 10-cm thick water phantom with various radiation energies. As you can see, the percentage of transmitted photons increases as the energy of the beam increases. With low-energy radiation (20 keV), most of the interactions are photoelectric, and few photons are transmitted. As the energy of the radiation increases, photoelectric attenuation becomes less important and completely ceases at 100 keV. However, even when all attenuation is from Compton scattering, the percentage of transmitted photons continues to increase as the radiation energy increases. A larger percentage of photons is transmitted with a 150-keV than with a 100-keV beam.

As the energy of the radiation increases, photoelectric attenuation decreases sharply, while Compton attenuation decreases only slightly. In the low-energy range, a massive quantity of photoelectric attenuation is superimposed on a background of Compton attenuation. As the energy of the radiation increases, photoelectric attenuation diminishes until the background of Compton attenuation is all that is left. Once this happens, increasing the beam energy will cause only a slight decrease in attenuation (and slight increase in transmission).

As a general rule, the higher the energy of the radiation, the larger the percentage of transmitted photons, regardless of the type of basic interaction. The only exception to this rule occurs with high atomic number absorbers, which we will discuss next.

Atomic Number

Usually, as the radiation energy increases, x-ray transmission increases (and attenuation decreases), but with high atomic number absorbers, transmission may actually decrease with increasing beam energy. This apparent paradox occurs because there is an abrupt change in the likelihood of a photoelectric reaction as the radiation energy reaches the binding energy of an inner-shell electron. A photon cannot eject an electron unless it has more energy than the electron's bind-

Table 5–3. Percent Transmission of Monochromatic Radiation Through 10 cm of Water

ENERGY (keV)	PERCENT TRANSMISSION (10-cm WATER PHANTOM)
20	0.04
30	2.5
40	7.0
50	10.0
60	13.0
80	16.0
100	18.0
150	22.0

Table 5–4. Percent Transmission of Monochromatic Radiation Through 1 mm of Lead

ENERGY (keV)	PERCENT TRANSMISSION
50	0.016
60	0.40
80	6.8
88	12.0
—K-EDGE FOR LEAD—	
88	0.026
100	0.14
150	0.96

ing energy. Thus, a lower-energy photon is more likely to be transmitted than a higher-energy photon, provided one has slightly less and the other slightly more energy than the binding energy of the electron.

Table 5–4 shows the percentage of transmission of monochromatic radiation through 1 mm of lead. A sudden change in transmission occurs at 88 keV, which is the binding energy of the K-shell electron. This is called the **K-edge.** With a radiation energy just below the K-edge, a fairly large percentage of the photons is transmitted (12%), while just above the K-edge, transmission drops to nearly zero. Of course, the same thing is true for the low atomic number elements at the K-edge, but the energies involved are usually less than 1 keV, far below the useful diagnostic energy range.

Figure 5–5 shows a plot of the mass attenuation coefficients of tin and lead

Figure 5–5   Comparison of the mass attenuation coefficients for tin and lead

over the range of energies used in diagnostic radiology. Remember, the higher the attenuation coefficient, the lower the number of transmitted photons. **Gram for gram, tin is a better absorber of x rays than lead between 29 and 88 keV.** This has a practical application. We are not usually concerned about attenuation per gram, but when we are carrying the gram on our back as a protective apron, our perspective changes. Because tin attenuates more radiation per unit weight than lead, it has recently come into use for this purpose. A lighter tin apron gives the same protection as a standard lead apron, or if you have a strong back, you can use the same weight of tin for the apron and have more protection.

The commonly used contrast agents barium and iodine were selected because of their low toxicity. However, a better choice could not have been made if they were selected for their physical properties. Both have ideal K-shell binding energies (iodine, 32 keV; barium, 34 keV). These binding energies are approximately the same as the mean energy of most diagnostic x-ray beams, so many interactions occur at the K-shell level. Attenuation is more intense than it would be for a higher atomic number element such as lead. Most photons in a polychromatic beam are less energetic than the 88-keV K-shell binding energy of lead.

Table 5–5 shows the atomic numbers and K-edges of most of the elements that are important in diagnostic radiology. When maximum x-ray absorption is desired, the K-edge of an absorber should be closely matched to the energy of the x-ray beam. For example, xeroradiography employs a selenium plate with a K-edge of 12.7 keV as the x-ray absorber. This low K-edge makes selenium an excellent absorber for the low energy radiation (30 to 35 kVp) used for mammography. However, selenium would be a poor choice as an absorber for a high energy beam, such as the 350 kVp that is used for chest radiography with a Field Emission unit. For high energy radiation, tungsten, with a K-edge of 69.5 keV, is a much better absorber. As we shall see later, the success of the rare earth intensifying screens and cesium iodide image intensifier is in large part related to excellent matching of their K-edges to beam energies.

Table 5–5. Atomic Numbers and K-Edges of Elements Important in Diagnostic Radiology

ELEMENT	SYMBOL	ATOMIC NUMBER (Z)	K-EDGE (keV)
Hydrogen	H	1	.013
Beryllium	Be	4	.11
Carbon	C	6	.28
Nitrogen	N	7	.40
Oxygen	O	8	.53
Sodium	Na	11	1.1
Aluminum	Al	13	1.6
Silicon	Si	14	1.8
Sulfur	S	16	2.5
Chlorine	Cl	17	2.8
Potassium	K	19	3.6
Calcium	Ca	20	4.0
Iron	Fe	26	7.1
Copper	Cu	29	9.0
Zinc	Zn	30	9.7
Germanium	Ge	32	11.1
Selenium	Se	34	12.7
Bromine	Br	35	13.5
Yttrium	Y	39	17.0
Molybdenum	Mo	42	20.0
Silver	Ag	47	25.5
Cadmium	Cd	48	26.7
Tin	Sn	50	29.1
Iodine	I	53	33.2
Cesium	Cs	55	36.0
Barium	Ba	56	37.4
Lanthanum	La	57	39.0
Gadolinium	Gd	64	50.2
Tantalum	Ta	73	67.5
Tungsten	W	74	69.5
Gold	Au	79	80.7
Lead	Pb	82	88.0

The Effect of Density on Attenuation

Tissue density is one of the most important factors in x-ray attenuation, and a difference in tissue densities is one of the primary reasons why we see an x-ray image. Density determines the number of electrons that are present in a given thickness, so it determines the tissue's stopping power. The relationship between density and attenuation is linear. If the density of a material is doubled, attenuation doubles. This is easiest to understand in terms of a gas whose density can be changed by compression. If a quantity of gas in a closed container is doubled, the number of electrons doubles. The same thickness of material now has twice as much mass, and it will attenuate twice as many photons.

The Effect of Electrons per Gram on Attenuation

The number of Compton reactions depends upon the number of electrons in a given thickness. Absorbers with many electrons are more impervious to radiation than absorbers with few electrons. Unfortunately, the number of electrons is usually expressed in the unit e/gm (a mass unit) rather than e/cm³ (a volume unit). In order for the number of electrons per gram to have meaning, we must know the density of the material. Density determines the number of electrons that will be present in a given thickness, and this is what determines x-ray attenuation as we think of it in clinical radiology. By multiplying electrons per gram and density, we get electrons per cubic centimeter.

$$\frac{e}{gm} \times \frac{gm}{cm^3} = \frac{e}{cm^3}$$

Now we are talking about a unit we can understand. A cubic centimeter represents a thickness of 1 cm, and this is the unit we use to measure our patient's thickness.

Table 5–6 summarizes the relationships between density, e/gm, and e/cm³ for air, fat, water, and bone.

Table 5–6.   Comparison of Physical Characteristics of Air, Fat, Water, and Bone

	EFFECTIVE ATOMIC NUMBER	DENSITY (gm/cm³)	ELECTRONS PER GRAM	ELECTRONS PER cm³
AIR	7.64	0.00129	3.01×10^{23}	0.0039×10^{23}
FAT	5.92	0.91	3.48×10^{23}	3.27×10^{23}
WATER	7.42	1.00	3.34×10^{23}	3.34×10^{23}
BONE	13.8	1.85	3.0×10^{23}	5.55×10^{23}

When Compton reactions predominate, the number of e/cm³ becomes the most important factor in attenuation, so even though bone has fewer e/gm than water, bone still attenuates more radiation, because it has more e/cm³.

The number of electrons per gram can be calculated by the equation:

$$N_o = \frac{NZ}{A}$$

N_o = Number of e/gm
N = Avogadro's number (6.02×10^{23})
Z = Atomic number
A = Atomic weight

When comparing one element with another, we can disregard Avogadro's number, since it is a constant and affects all elements equally. Then, the relative number of electrons per gram becomes the simple ratio:

$$\frac{Z}{A} \text{ or } \frac{\text{Number of Electrons}}{\text{Weight of the Atom}}$$

The weight of the atom is the sum of the weights of the protons and neutrons. The number of electrons and protons is equal, so the only factor that varies independently is the number of neutrons, which add mass without affecting the number of electrons. As the atomic number increases, the number of neutrons increases faster than the number of electrons. Hydrogen has no neutrons, and it has twice as many electrons per gram as any other element. Oxygen has one neutron per electron, and half as many electrons per gram as hydrogen. Lead has

more neutrons than electrons, so it has even fewer electrons per gram than oxygen. In general, the high atomic number elements have about 20% fewer electrons per gram than the low atomic number elements. Table 5–1 shows the number of electrons per gram for various elements important in diagnostic radiology.

ATTENUATION OF POLYCHROMATIC RADIATION

The attenuation of polychromatic radiation is more complex than the attenuation of monochromatic radiation. Polychromatic beams contain a whole spectrum of photons of various energies (see Fig. 2–17, p. 26), the most energetic being determined by the peak kilovoltage (kVp) used to generate the beam. **In general, the mean energy of polychromatic radiation is between one-third and one-half of its peak energy.** A 100-kVp beam has a mean energy of approximately 40 kV. This will vary somewhat depending upon filtration.

As polychromatic radiation passes through an absorber, the transmitted photons undergo a change in both quantity and quality. The number of photons decreases because some are deflected and absorbed out of the beam, just as they are with monochromatic radiation. However, in contrast to monochromatic radiation, the quality of the beam also changes. Quality changes because the lower-energy photons are more readily attenuated than the higher-energy photons. As the low-energy photons are removed from the beam, the mean energy of the remaining photons increases.

Figure 5–6 Attenuation of polychromatic radiation

The attenuation of polychromatic radiation is shown schematically in Figure 5–6. The x-ray beam begins with 1000 photons having a mean energy of 40 kV. The first centimeter of absorber (water) reduces the number of photons by 35% and increases their mean energy to 47 kV. The second centimeter of water reduces the number of photons only 27%, since now the remaining photons are a little more energetic, and

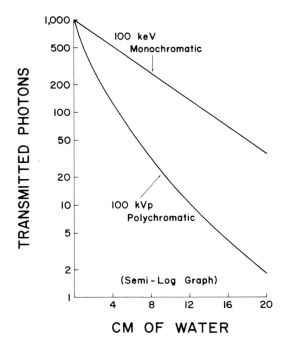

Figure 5–7 Comparison of the attenuation of polychromatic and monochromatic radiation

increases their mean energy to 52 kV. If the process is continued long enough, eventually the mean energy of the beam will approach its peak energy.

When the percentage of transmission of polychromatic radiation is plotted on semilogarithmic graph paper, it plots a curved line as shown in Figure 5–7. The initial slope of the curve is steep as many low-energy photons are attenuated by the first few centimeters of water. Eventually, the slope of the curve becomes similar to the slope for a monochromatic beam as the mean energy of the polychromatic radiation approaches its peak energy.

ATTENUATION IN DIAGNOSTIC RADIOLOGY

The photons in an x-ray beam enter a patient with a uniform distribution and emerge in a specific pattern of distribution. The transmitted photons carry the x-ray image, but their pattern also carries the memory of the attenuated photons. The transmitted and attenuated photons are equally important. If all photons were transmitted, the film would be uniformly black; if all photons were attenuated, the film would be uniformly white. In neither case would there be an x-ray image. Image formation depends upon a differential attenuation between tissues. Some tissues attenuate more x rays than other tissues, and the size of this differential determines the amount of contrast in the x-ray image.

To examine differential attenuation, we will begin with a radiograph of a hand, so we only have to consider two tissue types, bone and soft tissue. Figure 5–8 shows the linear attenuation coefficients of compact bone and water. Water is used to represent the soft tissues. Remember, the higher the linear attenuation coefficient, the greater the attenuation. As you can see, x-ray attenuation is greater in bone than in water, so the bones show up as holes in the transmitted photon pattern. We see these holes as white areas on a film. With a 20-keV x-ray beam, water has a linear

Figure 5–8   Linear attenuation coefficients for water and compact bone

attenuation coefficient of 0.77 cm⁻¹ and bone 4.8 cm⁻¹. Bone has a greater linear attenuation coefficient by a factor of 6. With such a large differential, the x-ray image will display a great deal of contrast. At an x-ray beam energy of 100 keV, differential attenuation is not nearly as large. Bone still attenuates more x rays than water, but now the difference is only by a factor of 0.6, so image contrast is considerably reduced.

Figure 5–8 illustrates another point. The total linear attenuation coefficient is actually made up of three separate coefficients, one for each of the basic interactions—coherent scattering, photoelectric effect, and Compton scattering. Each contributes its own component to the total linear attenuation coefficient. At low photon energies (20 keV) most of the difference in x-ray attenuation between bone and soft tissue results from a difference in the number of photoelectric reactions. More photoelectric reactions occur be-

cause bone contains calcium which has a relatively high atomic number. At high photon energies (100 keV) the difference in x-ray attenuation between bone and soft tissues is almost entirely the result of the difference in the number of Compton reactions. Few photoelectric reactions occur in either bone or soft tissue at 100 keV. **When Compton reactions predominate, differential attenuation is entirely dependent upon differences in density.** The reason is that denser materials have more electrons available to undergo reactions.

Figure 5–9 shows the Compton linear attenuation coefficient for water, bone, and sodium iodide. The number of Compton reactions decreases only slightly with increasing x-ray energies. As the energy of an x-ray beam is increased from 20 keV to 100 keV, the Compton linear attenuation coefficient for bone decreases about 20% (while the photoelectric linear attenuation coefficient decreases more than 99%).

Figure 5–9   Compton linear and mass attenuation coefficients for water, compact bone, and sodium iodide.

The shaded portion of Figure 5–9 shows the Compton mass attenuation coefficient. Remember, the mass attenuation coefficient indicates the amount of attenuation per gram, and it is not dependent upon density. As you can see, a gram of water attenuates more x rays than a gram of either bone or sodium iodide by Compton reactions. The reason is that water has more electrons per gram because it contains two atoms of hydrogen. Sodium iodide has even fewer electrons per gram than bone, because of the high atomic number of iodine, so a gram of sodium iodide attenuates fewer photons by Compton reactions than a gram of either water or bone. Nevertheless, even when Compton scattering is the only type of basic interaction, there is still a difference in x-ray attenuation between water, bone, and sodium iodide in favor of the higher atomic number absorber, but the difference is entirely dependent upon density.

Fat and water are always difficult to differentiate radiographically. The effec-tive atomic number of water (7.4) is slightly greater than fat (5.9), so they can be dif-ferentiated by photoelectric attenuation, with low energy techniques. With higher energy radiation, when Compton attenua-tion predominates, differentiation be-tween fat and water depends upon density and the number of electrons per gram. Water has a greater density, but fewer electrons per gram. The net results, the number of electrons per cubic centimeter, are nearly the same for both water and fat (Table 5–6). Water has approximately 2% more e/cm^3, which is too small a difference to demonstrate with only Compton reac-tions. A significant difference in attenua-tion between fat and water can only be demonstrated effectively with low energy techniques.

SCATTER RADIATION

Our discussion of attenuation has only dealt with primary radiation, which either passes through the patient unchanged or is completely removed from the useful beam.

The primary radiation carries the x-ray image. Now enters the villain—scatter radiation. It has nothing worthwhile to offer. Scatter radiation detracts from film quality and contributes no useful information.

How important is scatter radiation? How much of the density on an x-ray film is from scatter radiation? Several factors determine its importance. In most of our routine work, it is important, frequently making up from 50 to 90% of the total number of photons emerging from the patient. The reason for the large number of scattered photons will be more apparent if we consider the fate of a diagnostic x-ray beam. With thick parts, like the abdomen, only 1% of the photons in the initial beam reach the film. The rest are attenuated, the majority by Compton scattering. Fortunately, most of them do not reach the film. Nevertheless, those that reach the film make a major, and undesirable, contribution to total film blackening.

It would be more accurate to refer to all undesirable radiation as secondary radiation, which includes photons and electrons that might contribute to film fog. However, in actual practice, none of the electrons (photoelectric or recoil) has enough energy to reach the film, and the only characteristic radiation with sufficient energy to cause a problem occurs during contrast examinations with barium and iodine. The only secondary radiation of any significance comes from Compton scattering, and it has become common practice to refer to all undesirable radiation as scatter radiation, which is fairly accurate.

Factors Affecting Scatter Radiation

Three factors determine the quantity of scatter radiation. These are as follows:
1. Kilovoltage (kVp)
2. Part thickness
3. Field size

Scatter radiation is maximum with high-kVp techniques, large fields, and thick parts, and unfortunately, this is what we usually deal with in diagnostic radiology. We rarely have any control over part thickness and frequently must use large fields. The only variable we can control is kVp, but even here we have less control than we would like since patient doses go up sharply with low-kVp techniques.

Field size is the most important factor in the production of scatter radiation. A small x-ray field (usually called a narrow beam) irradiates only a small volume of tissue, so it generates only a small number of scattered photons. Most of them miss the film because they have a large angle of escape. Figure 5–10 shows the angle of escape for a scattered photon originating at point P. As you can see, the escape angle is much larger than the narrow angle encompassed by the primary beam. So the quantity of scatter radiation from a narrow beam is small to begin with, and most of it never reaches the plane of the film. For this

Figure 5–10 Angle of escape for scattered photons

reason, narrow-beam attenuation is the method that is used to measure the attenuation of primary radiation, and the terms **narrow-beam** and **primary** radiation are used synonymously.

As the x-ray field is enlarged, the quantity of scatter radiation increases rapidly at first, and then gradually tapers off until finally it reaches a plateau, or saturation point. A further increase in field size does not change the quantity of scatter radiation that reaches the film. The total number of scattered photons in the field increases, but the number that reach any particular point on the film remains constant. For example, consider the central point of a circular field 4 cm in diameter. Scattered photons originating from the periphery of the field can easily penetrate 2 cm of tissue to reach the field's center. However, if the field is increased to a 30-cm circle, most scatter photons do not have sufficient range to penetrate the 15 cm of tissue between the field's margin and center. So even though more scattered photons are generated in large fields, they do not increase the quantity reaching any particular area. The saturation point for scatter radiation occurs with a field approximately 30 × 30 cm, only a 12-inch square, which is not a large field for diagnostic radiology.

The quantity of scatter radiation reaches a saturation point with increasing **part thickness,** just as it does with increasing field size. The total number of scattered photons keeps increasing as the part becomes thicker, but photons originating in the upper layers of the patient do not have sufficient energy to reach the film. Unfortunately, we have little control over part thickness, and except for the occasional use of a compressed band, we must accept the patient as he is.

The effect of **kilovoltage** (kVp) on the production of scatter radiation is probably not as important as part thickness, and certainly it is not as important as field size. In the low-energy range (20 to 30 keV), where the photoelectric effect predomi-

nates, very little scatter radiation is produced. As the radiation energy increases, the percentage of Compton reactions increases, and so does the production of scatter radiation. After Compton scattering becomes the predominant interaction, scatter radiation production tends to plateau, just as it does with increasing field size and part thickness. The energy where the plateau occurs depends upon the atomic number of the tissue. But the plateau is not as well defined as it is with field size and part thickness. Even after Compton reactions predominate, the quantity of scatter radiation continues to increase with increasing beam energy, because more photons scatter in the forward direction and their greater energy allows them to penetrate greater thicknesses of tissue to reach the film.

Since we have so little control over the production of scatter radiation, we must find ways of keeping it from the x-ray film after it has been generated. The most important of these is the x-ray grid, which we will discuss in Chapter 8.

SUMMARY

Attenuation is the reduction in the intensity of an x-ray beam as it traverses matter by either the absorption or deflection of photons from the beam. The attenuation of monochromatic radiation is exponential; i. e., each layer of absorber attenuates the same percentage of the photons remaining in the beam. The attenuation of polychromatic radiation is not exponential. A large percentage of the low-energy photons are attenuated by the first few centimeters of absorber, so the quality (mean energy) of the remaining photons increases as the beam passes through an absorber.

The amount of attenuation depends upon the energy of the radiation and three characteristics of the tissue: atomic number, density, and electrons per gram. Increasing the radiation energy increases the number of transmitted photons, while increasing the atomic number, density, or electrons per gram decreases transmission. Energy and atomic number, together, determine the relative percentage of photoelectric and Compton reactions. With low-energy radiation, and high atomic number absorbers, a large amount of photoelectric attenuation is superimposed upon a small background of Compton attenuation. As the energy of the radiation is increased, photoelectric attenuation diminishes until the background of Compton attenuation is all that remains.

Density is one of the most important factors affecting attenuation, and radiographic image contrast is largely dependent upon differences in tissue density. The high contrast between air and soft tissues is entirely because of density differences. The number of electrons per gram plays a lesser role. Generally, as the atomic number increases, the number of electrons per gram decreases, but the decrease is more than compensated by an even greater increase in density. So high atomic number elements attenuate more radiation, even though they have fewer electrons per gram.

The amount of scatter radiation reaching an x-ray film increases with increasing field size, part thickness, and kilovoltage.

REFERENCE

1. Hubbell, J. H.: *Photon Cross Sections, Attenuation Coefficients, and Energy Absorption Coefficients from 10 keV to 100 GeV*. National Bureau of Standards, Handbook 29, August 1969.

CHAPTER 6

Filters

Filtration is the process of increasing the mean energy of polychromatic radiation by passing it through an absorber. Diagnostic x-ray beams are composed of photons that have a whole spectrum of energies; i.e., they are polychromatic. Their mean energy is from one-third to one-half of their peak energy, thus many of the photons fall in the lower-energy range. As polychromatic radiation passes through a patient, most of the lower-energy photons are absorbed in the first few centimeters of tissue, and only the higher-energy photons penetrate through the patient to form the radiographic image. Since the patient's radiation dose is dependent upon the number of absorbed photons, the first few centimeters of tissue receive much more radiation than the rest of the patient. This tissue can be protected by absorbing the lower-energy photons from the beam before they reach the patient by interposing a filter material between the patient and the x-ray tube. Filters are usually sheets of metal, and their only function in diagnostic radiology is to reduce the patient's radiation dose.

In a radiological examination the x-ray beam is filtered by absorbers at three different levels. Beginning at the x-ray source, these are as follows:
1. The x-ray tube and its housing **(inherent filtration)**
2. Sheets of metal placed in the path of the beam **(added filtration)**
3. The patient

INHERENT FILTRATION

Filtration resulting from the absorption of x rays as they pass through the x-ray tube and its housing is called **inherent filtration.** The materials responsible for inherent filtration are the glass envelope enclosing the anode and cathode, the in-

Table 6–1. Inherent Filtration for a Typical Diagnostic X-Ray Tube

ABSORBER	THICKNESS (mm)	ALUMINUM EQUIVALENT (mm)
Glass Envelope	1.40	0.78
Insulating Oil	2.36	0.07
Bakelite Window	1.02	0.05
Total		0.90

(From Trout, E. D.: The life history of an x-ray beam, Radiol. Tech. *35*, 161, 1963.)

sulating oil surrounding the tube, and the window in the tube housing. Inherent filtration is measured in **aluminum equivalents;** i.e., the thickness of aluminum that would produce the same degree of attenuation as the thickness of the material in question. Table 6–1 shows the inherent filtration of a typical diagnostic x-ray tube. It usually varies between 0.5- and 1.0-mm aluminum equivalent, and the glass envelope is responsible for most of it.

In a few special circumstances, unfiltered radiation is desirable. Since filtration increases the mean energy of an x-ray beam, it decreases tissue contrast. The decrease is insignificant in the higher-energy range, but with lower-energy radiation, under 30 kVp, this loss of contrast may be detrimental to image quality. Beryllium window tubes are designed to produce an essentially unfiltered beam. The exit portal of the glass envelope is replaced with beryllium (atomic number of 4), which is more transparent to low-energy radiation than glass. The radiation from these tubes has a minimum of inherent filtration, and it is excellent for soft-tissue radiography, particularly mammography.

ADDED FILTRATION

Added filtration results from absorbers that are placed in the path of the x-ray beam. Ideally, a filter material should absorb all low-energy photons and transmit all high-energy photons. Unfortunately, no such material exists. However, a material can be selected to absorb principally low-energy radiation, by utilizing the proclivity of photoelectric attenuation for low-energy photons. Attenuation is most intense when the photoelectric effect is the predominant interaction and diminishes when Compton reactions predominate. The energy of the radiation that is filtered from the beam can be regulated by selecting a material with an appropriate atomic number. Aluminum and copper are the materials usually selected for diagnostic radiology. Aluminum, with an atomic

number of 13, is an excellent filter material for low-energy radiation and a good general-purpose filter. Copper, with an atomic number of 29, is a better filter for high-energy radiation. However, it is inconvenient to change filters between examinations, and there is a risk of forgetting to make the change. For practicality, most radiologists prefer to use a single filter material, usually aluminum.

Copper is never used by itself as the only filter material. It is always used in combination with aluminum as a **compound filter.** A compound filter consists of two or more layers of different metals. The layers are arranged so that the higher atomic number element, copper, faces the x-ray tube and the lower atomic number element, aluminum, faces the patient. Most of the filtration occurs in the copper, and the purpose of the aluminum is to absorb the characteristic radiation from copper. Photoelectric attenuation in copper produces characteristic radiation with an energy of about 8 keV, which is energetic enough to reach the patient and significantly increase skin doses. The aluminum layer absorbs this characteristic radiation. Its own characteristic radiation has so little energy (1.5 keV) that it is absorbed in the air gap between the patient and filter.

Filter Thickness

After selecting a filter material, usually aluminum, the next step is to determine the appropriate thickness for the filter. The percentage of x-ray attenuation with 1, 2, 3, and 10 mm of aluminum for photons of various energies is shown in Table 6–2. Two millimeters of aluminum absorb virtually all photons with energies less than 20 keV, so that most of the advantages of filtration are achieved by this thickness. A filter of more than 3 mm of aluminum offers no advantage; in fact, excess filtration has definite disadvantages. In Table 6–2, the column on the right shows the percentage of photons at-

Table 6–2. Percent Attenuation of Monochromatic Radiation by Various Thicknesses of Aluminum Filtration

PHOTON ENERGY (keV)	PERCENTAGE OF PHOTONS ATTENUATED			
	1 mm ALUMINUM	2 mm ALUMINUM	3 mm ALUMINUM	10 mm ALUMINUM
10	100	100	100	100
20	58	82	92	100
30	24	42	56	93
40	12	23	32	73
50	8	16	22	57
60	6	12	18	48
80	5	10	14	39
100	4	8	12	35

tenuated by 10 mm of aluminum, clearly excessive filtration. The effect is an overall attenuation of the beam, primarily by the absorption of high-energy photons, all of the low-energy photons having already been absorbed by lesser thicknesses of aluminum. The quality of the beam is not significantly altered, but its intensity is greatly diminished. This lengthens the time required to make an exposure, which increases the likelihood of the patient's moving during the examination.

The National Council on Radiation Protection and Measurements[1] recommends the following total filtration for diagnostic radiology. The figures include both inherent and added filtration.

Operating kVp	Total Filtration
Below 50 kVp	0.5 mm aluminum
50 to 70 kVp	1.5 mm aluminum
Above 70 kVp	2.5 mm aluminum

The effect of aluminum filtration on a 90-kVp polychromatic x-ray beam is shown graphically in Figure 6–1. The unfiltered beam is composed of a spectrum of photons, many of which have energies in the 10 to 20 keV range. The highest point in the curve occurs at 25 keV. Filtration reduces the total number of photons in the x-ray beam (area under the curve), but more important, it selectively removes a large number of low-energy photons.

The intensity on the low-energy side of the curve (left) is reduced considerably more than the intensity on the high-energy side of the curve (right), and the highest point in the curve is shifted from 25 to 35 keV. The overall effect is an increase in the mean energy of the x-ray beam.

Copper filters are always at least 0.25 mm thick, and they are backed with a 1.0 mm layer of aluminum. Thinner copper filters are not practical, since minor variations in thickness are difficult to eliminate, and produce a serious lack of uniformity in the transmitted radiation.

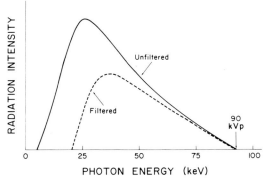

Figure 6–1 Energy and intensity of unfiltered and filtered polychromatic radiation

Table 6–3. Exposure Dose to the Skin for Comparable Density Radiographs of a Pelvic Phantom (18 cm Thick) With Various Thicknesses of Aluminum Filtration

ALUMINUM FILTRATION	60 kVp	
	EXPOSURE DOSE TO SKIN (MILLIROENTGENS)	PERCENT DECREASE IN EXPOSURE DOSE
None	2,380	—
0.5 mm	1,850	22
1.0 mm	1,270	47
3.0 mm	465	80

(From Trout, E. D., Kelley, J. P. and Cathey, G. A.: The use of filters to control radiation exposure to the patient in diagnostic roentgenology, Amer. J. Roentgen., *67, 942,* 1952).

Effect of Filters on Patient Exposure

Trout and his co-workers[2] demonstrated the degree of patient protection afforded by filters with a series of tests, one of which is summarized in Table 6–3. In this particular experiment, they made multiple radiographs of an 18-cm thick pelvic phantom using a 60-kVp x-ray beam. The initial radiograph was made without a filter and then repeated with increasing thicknesses of aluminum filtration. Exposure times were adjusted to produce films of equal density, and the radiation dose to the skin over the pelvis was measured for each exposure. As you can see in Table 6–3, the decrease in patient exposure was remarkable, up to 80% with 3 mm of aluminum filtration. These percentages are for a specific examination, but they should give you some insight into the degree of protection you can expect from adequate filtration.

Effect of Filters on Exposure Factors

The major disadvantage of filtration is a reduction in the intensity of the x-ray beam. Filters absorb some photons at all energy levels, and we must compensate for the loss of higher-energy photons by increasing exposure factors, usually by in-

Table 6–4. Exposure Times for Comparable Density Radiographs of a Pelvic Phantom (18 cm Thick) for Low and High Energy Radiation With Various Thicknesses of Aluminum Filtration

ALUMINUM FILTRATION	60 kVp · 100 mA		130 kVp · 100 mA	
	EXPOSURE TIME (SECONDS)	PERCENT INCREASE IN EXPOSURE TIME	EXPOSURE TIME (SECONDS)	PERCENT INCREASE IN EXPOSURE TIME
None	1.41	—	0.12	—
0.5 mm	1.61	14	0.12	0
1.0 mm	1.64	17	0.12	0
3.0 mm	2.14	52	0.12	0

(From Trout, E. D., Kelley, J. P. and Cathey, G. A.: The use of filters to control radiation exposure to the patient in diagnostic roentgenology, Amer. J. Roentgen., *67, 942,* 1952.)

creasing time. The percentage that the exposure time must be increased depends upon the initial energy of the x-ray beam, as shown in Table 6–4. The table is based on one of the experiments of Trout and his co-workers[2] in which they measured the percentage of increase in exposure time required to produce films of equal density with various thicknesses of aluminum filtration. With low-energy radiation, represented by 60 kVp in Table 6–4, exposure time had to be increased up to 50% with 3 mm of aluminum, but with high-energy radiation, represented by 130 kVp in the table, added filtration did not necessitate any increase in the exposure time. Even when it is necessary to increase exposure time because of filtration, the patient receives less radiation than he would from an unfiltered beam. The x-ray tube puts out more photons during longer exposures, but the filter absorbs many of them, and the total number reaching the patient actually decreases.

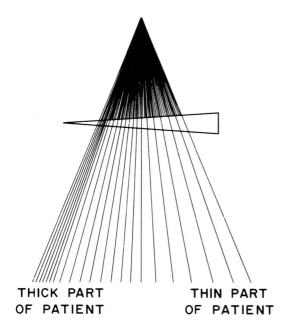

THICK PART
OF PATIENT

THIN PART
OF PATIENT

Figure 6–2 Wedge filter

Wedge Filters

Wedge filters are occasionally used in diagnostic radiology to obtain films of more uniform density when the part being examined diminishes greatly in thickness from one side of the field to the other. The filter is shaped like a wedge. The relationship between the filter and patient is shown in Figure 6–2. When one side of the patient is considerably thicker than the other, the wedge compensates for the difference. Less radiation is absorbed by the thinner part of the filter, so more is available to penetrate the thicker part of the patient. Wedge filters have been used extensively in x-ray therapy, but their value has never been exploited in diagnostic radiology. They are occasionally used for lateral views of the pregnant abdomen in an attempt to obtain films of uniform density.

SUMMARY

Filters are sheets of metal placed in the path of the x-ray beam near the x-ray tube housing for the purpose of absorbing low-energy radiation before it reaches the patient. Their only function is to protect the patient from useless radiation, and they perform their function remarkably well, frequently reducing skin exposures by as much as 80%. Aluminum is usually selected as the filter material for diagnostic radiology. Most high-energy photons are transmitted through aluminum, while low-energy photons are absorbed by photoelectric interactions. The photoelectric effect selectively absorbs low-energy photons because of its dependence upon energy and atomic number. The National Council on Radiation Protection and Measurement recommends an equivalent of 2.5 mm of aluminum permanent filtration for diagnostic x-ray beams of energies greater than 70 kVp. Some higher energy useful photons are absorbed by filtration, and exposure factors must be increased to compensate for this loss. When filters are used in examinations employing lower energy radiation, exposure time may have to be increased up to 50%; however, with higher energy radiation, no adjustment in exposure factors is usually required. Filters are simple and inexpensive. Nowhere else in all of radiology do we gain so much for so little money.

REFERENCES

1. *Medical X-Ray and Gamma-Ray Protection for Energies up to 10 MeV*. Washington, D. C.: National Council on Radiation Protection and Measurements. Report No. 33, 1968.
2. Trout, E. D., Kelley, J. P., and Cathey, G. A.: The use of filters to control radiation exposure to the patient in diagnostic roentgenology. Amer. J. Roentgen. *67*, 942, 1952.

CHAPTER 7

X-ray Beam Restrictors

An x-ray beam restrictor is a device that is attached to the opening in the x-ray tube housing for the purposes of regulating the size and shape of an x-ray beam. Beam restrictors can be classified into three categories:

1. Aperture diaphragms
2. Cones and cylinders
3. Collimators

APERTURE DIAPHRAGMS

The simplest type of x-ray beam restrictor is an aperture diaphragm. It consists of a sheet of lead with a hole in the center, and the size and shape of the hole determine the size and shape of the x-ray beam. Its principal advantage is its simplicity. Lead is soft, so the aperture can be easily altered to any desired size or shape. The principal disadvantage of an aperture diaphragm is that it produces a fairly large penumbra at the periphery of the x-ray beam as shown in Figure 7–1A. The center of the x-ray field is exposed by the entire focal spot, but the periphery of the field (P in the illustration) "sees" only a portion of

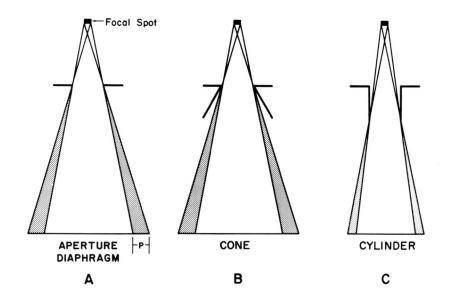

Figure 7–1 Aperture diaphragm (A), cone (B), and cylinder (C)

the focal spot; this partially exposed area is called the **penumbra.** The width of the penumbra can be reduced by positioning the aperture diaphragm as far away from the x-ray target as possible. This is usually accomplished by attaching the diaphragm to the end of a cone.

CONES AND CYLINDERS

The second type of x-ray beam restrictor comes in two basic shapes, conical and cylindrical. The flared shape of a cone would seem to be the ideal geometric configuration for an x-ray beam restrictor, but, the flare of the cone is usually greater than the flare of the x-ray beam, in which case the base-plate that attaches the device to the tube housing is the only part that restricts the x-ray beam (Figure 7–1B). When used in this way, it is little more than an aperture diaphragm. Beam restriction with a cylinder takes place at the far end of the barrel, so that there is less penumbra, as shown in Figure 7–1C. Cylinders may be equipped with extensions to increase their length in order to give even better beam restriction. A major disadvantage of aperture diaphragms, cones, and cylinders is the severe limitation they place upon the number of available field sizes. Even a large assortment cannot approach the infinite variety of field sizes needed in diagnostic radiology, and changing them is inconvenient.

COLLIMATORS

The collimator is the best all around x-ray beam restrictor. It has two advantages over the other types: (1) it provides an infinite variety of rectangular x-ray fields; (2) a light beam shows the center and exact configuration of the x-ray field. Two sets of shutters control the beam dimensions. They move together as a unit so that the second shutter aligns with the first to "clean up" its penumbra as shown in Figure 7–2. The shutters function as two adjustable aperture diaphragms. Each shutter consists of four, or more, lead

plates, as shown in Figure 7–3. These plates move in independent pairs. One pair can be adjusted without moving the other, which permits an infinite variety of square or rectangular fields. When the shutters are closed, they meet at the center of the x-ray field.

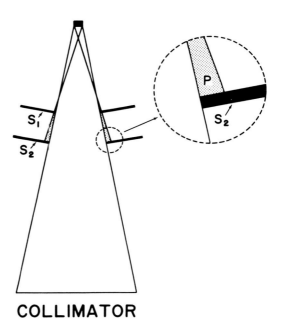

COLLIMATOR

Figure 7–2   Alignment of collimator shutters

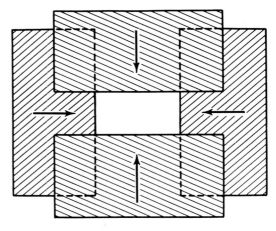

Figure 7–3   Collimator shutters (top view)

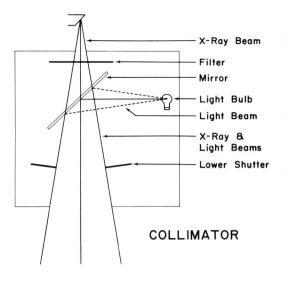

- X-Ray Beam
- Filter
- Mirror
- Light Bulb
- Light Beam
- X-Ray & Light Beams
- Lower Shutter

COLLIMATOR

Figure 7–4 Alignment of light and x-ray beams

The x-ray field is illuminated by a light beam from a light bulb in the collimator. The light beam is deflected by a mirror mounted in the path of the x-ray beam at an angle of 45°, as shown in Figure 7–4. The target of the x-ray tube and light bulb should be exactly the same distance from the center of the mirror. As the light beam passes through the second shutter opening, it is collimated to coincide with the x-ray beam. The distance from the mirror in the collimator to the target of the x-ray tube is critical. The collimator must be mounted so that the x-ray target and light bulb are exactly the same distance from the center of the mirror. If the collimator is mounted too far from the x-ray target, the x-ray source will be further from the second shutter than the light source, and the x-ray beam will be smaller than the light beam.

The last function of a collimator is to identify the center of the x-ray field. This is accomplished by painting a cross-line on a thin sheet of plexiglass mounted on the end of the collimator. The light beam that illuminates the radiographic field also shows its center.

Collimators have a back-up system for identifying field size should the light bulb burn out. The x-ray field size for various target-film distances is indicated by a calibrated scale on the front of the collimator.

A federal regulation requires automatic collimators on all new x-ray installations. Automatic collimators are the same as other collimators except that their shutters are motor-driven by electronic sensors in the film holder. These sensors measure the film cassette and relay its size back to the collimator motor. The motor then positions the shutters to exactly match the size of the x-ray field and cassette. Their sole purpose is to protect the patient from needless radiation.

Testing X-ray Beam and Light Beam Alignment

The alignment of the x-ray beam and light beam should be checked periodically, since the mirror tends to get out of adjustment from daily use. The only equipment needed to test alignment are four L-shaped wires (pieces of paper clips work nicely), a 14 × 17-inch x-ray film in a cassette, and a small lead letter "R." Place the film on the top of the x-ray table, open the collimator shutter to a convenient size

Figure 7–5 Test film of light and x-ray beam alignment

(10 × 10 inch), carefully position the L-shaped wires at the corner of the light field, and place the "R" in the lower right corner. Then make an x-ray exposure (40 inch, 3.3 mAs, 40 kVp) to mark the position of the x-ray field on the film. Without touching the film or wires, enlarge the field size to 12 × 12 inch and expose the film for the second time (same exposure factors).

Figure 7–5 shows a test film taken with a collimator whose mirror is out of adjustment. The dark center shows the position of the x-ray beam, and the wires indicate the position of the light beam. The second exposure (with an enlarged field) is made to assure visibility of all the wires. The wire in the left lower corner of the illustration would not have been visible on the film without the second exposure.

In order to adjust a misaligned mirror, return the processed x-ray film to its original position on the x-ray table. The "R" in the lower right corner assists in orienting the film properly. Position the light beam to the images of the wires, as you did earlier for the film exposure, and adjust the mirror in the collimator until the light beam coincides exactly with the x-ray field (dark area on the film). Then repeat the test to make sure that the mirror adjustment has correctly aligned the light and x-ray beams.

FUNCTIONS OF X-RAY BEAM RESTRICTORS

Collimators and other x-ray beam restrictors have two basic functions; to protect the patient and to decrease scatter radiation.

While patient protection is the principal reason for using collimators today, it is interesting to note that the old-time radiologists restricted x-ray beams before they knew anything about the harmful effects of low doses of radiation. They used small fields because they obtained better films with small fields. Since they had no grids, their only means of controlling scatter radiation was to limit field size. So they collimated their x-ray beams and obtained excellent films.

Patient Protection

The mechanism by which collimators protect the patient is obvious; that is, the smaller the x-ray field, the smaller the volume of the patient that is irradiated. If a 20 × 20-cm field is collimated to 10 × 10 cm, the area of the patient that is irradiated decreases from 400 to 100 cm², a fourfold decrease in area and a corresponding decrease in volume. A decrease in field size is especially significant, because area is a square function. Trimming only a few centimeters off the edge of the field significantly decreases the exposed volume of the patient.

The ideal shape for a radiographic field for maximal patient protection has never been established. Initially, all x-ray beam restrictors were round (cones) and now they are usually square or rectangular (collimators). It was argued that x-ray fields should not be round, while x-ray films are rectangular. Round fields expose portions of the patient that are not even included

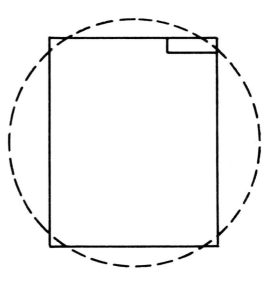

Figure 7–6 Overlap of a round field on a rectangular film

on the film, as shown in Figure 7–6; so x-ray beam restrictors were made square. But the ideal field shapes should be dictated by the shape of the part being examined, and not by the shape of either the film or collimator. Some parts are better examined with round fields; i.e., gallbladders and paranasal sinuses. Certainly a circular field that is completely encompassed by the film is the best-shaped field when a round part is being examined.

Problems frequently arise, especially on board examinations, regarding beam restrictor sizes. These problems can be solved by setting up proportions between the comparable sides of similar triangles as shown in Figure 7–7. For example, if an aperture diaphragm (A) is 25 cm from the x-ray target and the target film distance (B) is 100 cm, what size aperture (a) should be used to produce a 15 cm x-ray field (b) for a gallbladder examination? Using proportional triangles, the aperture hole should be:

$$\frac{a}{15} = \frac{25}{100} \text{ or } a = 15 \times \frac{25}{100} = 3.75 \text{ cm}$$

Decreased Scatter Radiation with Collimators

The quantity of scatter radiation reaching an x-ray film depends upon field size; i.e., the larger the field, the more scatter radiation. Figure 7–8 shows the general shape of the curves that are obtained when the number of transmitted primary and scattered photons is plotted against field size. The exact contribution from scatter depends upon the thickness of the part being examined and the energy (kVp) of the x-ray beam. The amount of primary radiation at the plane of the film is independent of field size. The number of

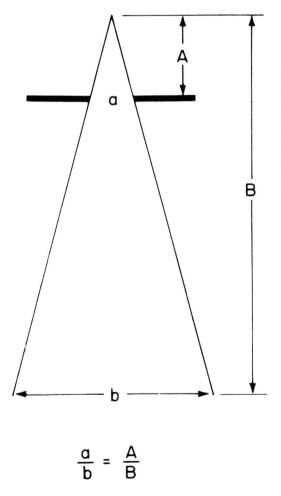

$$\frac{a}{b} = \frac{A}{B}$$

Figure 7–7 The sizes of the aperture and x-ray field are proportional to the target-aperture and target-film distances

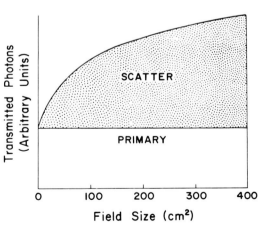

Figure 7–8 Transmitted radiation for various sizes of x-ray fields

transmitted primary photons, per unit area, is the same for a 1 × 1-cm field and a 30 × 30-cm field, so the number of primary photons in Figure 7–8 plots a straight line.

The number of scattered photons reaching the x-ray film depends upon field size. Small x-ray fields generate little scatter radiation. As the field size is enlarged, the amount of scatter radiation increases rapidly at first, and then tapers off with larger fields. After the x-ray field reaches a size of about 30 × 30 cm, the total quantity of scatter radiation is near its maximum. Since collimators are only successful in decreasing scatter radiation with small fields, we should restrict the size of our x-ray beams as much as possible.

A final fact to remember about collimators is that they affect exposure factors. Small fields produce little scatter radiation, so the total quantity of blackening on the x-ray film decreases as the field size decreases. In order to keep film density constant, as you decrease the size of the x-ray field, you must increase the exposure factors.

SUMMARY

There are three types of x-ray beam restrictors: aperture diaphragms, cones (cylinders), and collimators. Their basic function is to regulate the size and shape of the x-ray beam. Closely collimated beams have two advantages over larger beams. First, a smaller area of the patient is exposed, and since area is a square function, a decrease of one-half in x-ray beam diameter effects a fourfold decrease in patient exposure. Second, well-collimated beams generate less scatter radiation and thus improve film quality. By decreasing the amount of scatter radiation, collimators also affect exposure factors. As the x-ray field size is decreased, the exposure factors must be increased to maintain a constant film density.

Collimators are the best general-purpose beam restrictors. They offer two advantages over the other types: (1) the x-ray field is illuminated, which permits accurate localization on the patient; and (2) the x-ray field can be adjusted to an infinite variety of rectangular shapes and sizes.

CHAPTER **8**

Grids

The radiographic grid consists of a series of lead foil strips separated by x-ray transparent spacers. It was invented by Dr. Gustave Bucky in 1913, and it is still the most effective way of removing scatter radiation from large radiographic fields. Figure 8–1 shows how a grid functions. Primary radiation is oriented in the same axis as the lead strips and passes between them to reach the film unaffected by the

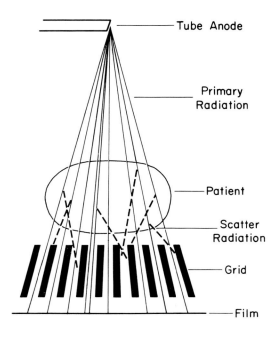

Figure 8–1 Grid function

grid. Scatter radiation arises from many points within the patient, and it is multidirectional, so that most of it is absorbed by the lead strips, and only a small amount passes between them.

The interspaces of grids are filled either with aluminum or some organic compound. The main purpose of the interspace material is to support the thin lead foil strips. Aluminum interspace grids can probably be manufactured more precisely, and they are structurally stronger than grids with organic interspacers. Patient exposures are higher with aluminum because it absorbs more primary radiation, but it also absorbs more secondary radiation, thus contrast improvement is probably better. At the present time both materials are used, and there is no clear-cut differentiation as to which is better.

TERMINOLOGY

Grid ratio is defined as the ratio between the height of the lead strips and the distance between them. Figure 8–2 is a cross-sectional scale drawing of a grid with a ratio of 8. The lead strips are approximately 0.05 mm thick, so that they may appropriately be considered lead foil. The interspaces are much thicker than the lead strips. Grid ratios are usually expressed as two numbers, such as 10:1, with the first number the actual ratio and the second number always 1. The grid ratio is a

$$r = \frac{h}{D} = \frac{2.0}{0.25} = 8$$

r — GRID RATIO

h — HEIGHT OF LEAD STRIPS

D — DISTANCE BETWEEN LEAD STRIPS

Figure 8–2　Cross section of a grid

Figure 8–3　Linear grid

parameter widely used to express a grid's ability to remove scatter radiation. Ratios usually range from 4 to 16. Generally the higher the ratio, the better the grid functions. Grid ratios are indicated on the top of grids by manufacturers.

Grid pattern refers to the orientation of the lead strips in their longitudinal axis. It is the pattern of the grid that we see from a top view. The two basic grid patterns are linear and crossed.

In a **linear grid** the lead strips are parallel to each other in their longitudinal axis, as shown in Figure 8–3. Most x-ray tables are equipped with linear grids. Their major advantage is that they allow us to angle the x-ray tube along the length of the grid without loss of primary radiation from grid "cutoff."

A crossed grid is made up of two superimposed linear grids which have the same focusing distance, as shown in Figure 8–4. The grid ratio of crossed grids is equal to the sum of the ratios of the two linear grids. A crossed grid made up of two 5:1 linear grids has a ratio of 10:1, and functions about the same as a linear grid with a 10:1 ratio. Crossed grids cannot be used with oblique techniques requiring angulation of the x-ray tube, and this is their biggest disadvantage.

A **focused grid** is a grid made up of lead strips that are angled slightly so that they focus in space, as shown in Figure 8–5.

Figure 8–4　Crossed grid

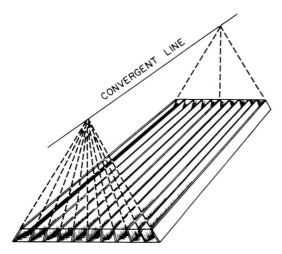

Figure 8–5 Focused linear grid

A focused grid can be either linear or crossed, since the focusing refers to the cross-sectional plane of the lead strips. Most grids are focused. Linear focused grids converge at a line in space called the **convergent line.** Crossed grids converge at a point in space called the **convergent point.** The **focal distance** is the perpendicular distance between the grid and the convergent line or point. In practice, grids have a focusing range which indicates the distance within which the grid can be used without a significant loss of primary radiation. The **focusing range** is fairly wide for a low ratio grid and narrow for a high ratio grid. A 5:1 grid focused at 40 inches has a focusing range of approximately 28 to 72 inches, while a 16:1 grid focused at 40 inches has a range of only 38 to 42 inches. Focal ranges are indicated on the top of grids by manufacturers.

A **parallel grid** is one in which the lead strips are parallel when viewed in cross-section. They are focused at infinity, so they do not have a convergent line. These grids can only be used effectively with either very small x-ray fields or long target-grid distances. They are frequently used in fluoroscopic spot film devices, but otherwise have little use in modern radiology.

Lines per inch is the number of lead strips per inch of grid. It can be calculated by adding the thickness of the lead strips and interspaces and dividing this sum into 1. Since the thickness of the lead strips and interspaces is usually expressed in millimeters, the answer must be multiplied by 25.4, which is the number of mm/in. The final equation is as follows:

$$\text{Lines/in.} = \frac{25.4}{D + d}$$

D = thickness of interspaces (mm)
d = thickness of lead strips (mm)

A grid (grid-front) cassette is a special x-ray cassette, usually used for portable radiography, with a grid built into the front of the cassette. Most grid cassettes are focused and have a fairly low grid ratio (4:1 to 8:1).

EVALUATION OF GRID PERFORMANCE

Grids are used to improve contrast by absorbing secondary radiation before it reaches the film. The "ideal grid" would absorb all secondary radiation and no primary radiation. It would give maximum film contrast without an unnecessary increase in patient exposure. However, the ideal grid does not exist, and the design of all grids is a compromise. The price of better film contrast is increased patient exposure. We must always compromise one for the other. Grids with high ratios give maximum contrast, but the improved contrast is not always worth the increased patient exposure. In every clinical situation, we must weigh these two factors. In order to help in grid selection and design, several tests have been devised to evaluate grid performance. These tests also help us understand the way a grid functions. We will discuss three methods of evaluating performance:

1. Primary transmission (Tp)
2. Bucky factor (B)
3. Contrast improvement factor (K)

Primary Transmission (Tp)

Primary transmission is a measurement of the percentage of primary radiation transmitted through a grid. Ideally, a grid should transmit 100% of the primary radiation, since it carries the radiographic image. The equipment for measuring primary transmission is shown in Figure 8–6. The x-ray beam is collimated to a narrow pencil of radiation, and the phantom is placed a great distance from the grid. With this arrangement, no scatter radiation reaches the grid. A small amount is pro-duced in the phantom, but it diffuses out of the beam in the large air-gap between the phantom and the grid.

Two measurements must be made to determine the percent of primary transmission. The first measurement is made with the grid in place to determine the intensity of the radiation transmitted through the grid, and the second measurement is made after removal of the grid to determine the intensity of the radiation directed at the grid. A simple ratio of the intensity with the grid to the intensity without the grid gives the fractional transmission, which is multiplied by 100 to give the percentage of transmission.

$$Tp = \frac{Ip}{I'p} \times 100$$

Tp = Primary transmission (%)
Ip = Intensity with grid
I'p = Intensity without grid

Table 8–1 shows the primary transmission for eight different grids. There is a significant loss of primary radiation with grids. For the eight grids tested, the primary transmission varied between 57 and 72.5% and was generally lower for crossed grids.

The primary transmission that is measured experimentally is less than would be anticipated. If the geometric relationship between the lead strips and the x-ray target is accurate, so that there is no grid cutoff, and if no primary radiation is absorbed in the interspaces, then the percentage of the grid's surface area that is made up of interspaces will be the percentage of anticipated primary transmission. This merely determines the percent of the grid surface area that is not lead, and is as close as we will ever come to an ideal grid. The equation for calculating the anticipated primary transmission is as follows:

$$Calc. \ Tp = \frac{D}{D + d} \times 100$$

Calc. Tp = Anticipated primary transmission (%)
d = Thickness of lead strips
D = Thickness of interspaces

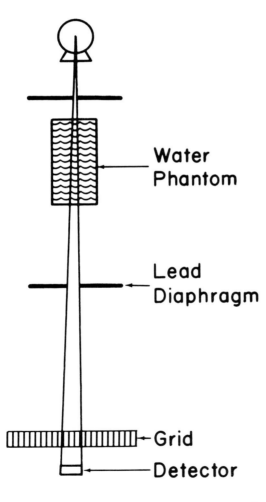

Figure 8–6 Apparatus for measuring primary transmissions (Tp)

Table 8–1. Primary Transmission (Tp)

GRID NO.	GRID RATIO	LEAD STRIP THICKNESS—d (μ)	INTERSPACE THICKNESS—D (μ)	PRIMARY TRANSMISSIONS (%)
1	3.4	50	320	67.5
2	2 × 3.1*	50	350	57
3	11	30	220	69
4	7	60	290	72.5
5	6	80	370	72.5
6	9	50	380	67
7	2 × 7*	50	370	72.5
8	**15**	**60**	**390**	**64**

*Crossed grids
Modified from Hondius Boldingh (ref. 1)

The measured primary transmission is always less than the calculated primary transmission. The example in Figure 8–7 will help to demonstrate the magnitude of this difference. The dimensions are for grid number 8 in Table 8–1, which is a 15:1 grid with an experimentally determined primary transmission of 64%. Its lead strips are 60μ thick and its interspaces are 390μ wide. The calculated primary transmission is 87%, which is 23% more than the measured primary transmission. The difference is largely the result of absorption by the interspace material. Also, there is probably some loss in primary radiation because of manufacturing imperfections in the focusing of the lead strips.

Bucky Factor (B)

The Bucky factor is the ratio of the incident radiation falling on the grid to the transmitted radiation passing through the grid. It is a practical determination, since it indicates how much we must increase exposure factors when we change from a non-grid to a grid technique. It also tells us how much the patient's exposure dose is increased by the use of a grid. The Bucky factor is similar to primary transmission (Tp), except for one difference. Primary transmission indicates only the amount of primary radiation absorbed by a grid, while the Bucky factor indicates the absorption of both primary and secondary radiation. It is determined with a large x-ray field and a thick phantom as shown

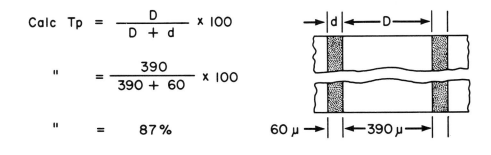

$$\text{Calc } Tp = \frac{D}{D + d} \times 100$$

$$" = \frac{390}{390 + 60} \times 100$$

$$" = 87\%$$

Figure 8–7 Anticipated primary transmission

Figure 8–8 Apparatus for measuring the Bucky factor (B)

Table 8–2. Bucky Factor (B)

GRID RATIO	70 kVp	120 kVp
No Grid	1	1
5:1	3	3
8:1	3.5	4
12:1	4	5
16:1	4.5	6

From Liebel Flarsheim (ref. 2)

in Figure 8–8. The transmitted radiation is measured with the grid in place, and the incident radiation after the grid has been removed. The equation for calculating the Bucky factor is as follows:

$$B = \frac{\text{Incident radiation}}{\text{Transmitted radiation}}$$

The Bucky factor is a measure of the total quantity of radiation absorbed from an x-ray beam by a grid, so in part, it is a measure of the grid's ability to absorb scatter radiation. Table 8–2 shows the Bucky factors for several different grids with two different energies of radiation. Generally, high-ratio grids absorb more scatter radiation and have larger Bucky factors than low-ratio grids. The size of the Bucky factor also depends upon the energy of the x-ray beam. High-energy beams generate more scatter radiation and place a greater demand on a grid's performance than low-energy radiation. The Bucky factor for the 16:1 grid in Table 8–2

increases from 4.5 to 6 as the radiation energy increases from 70 to 120 kVp. More scatter radiation is generated by the 120-kVp beam, and the 16:1 grid successfully absorbs it. However, the 5:1 grid in Table 8–2 is not as efficient. Its Bucky factor is the same for both 70 and 120 kVp radiation. Low-ratio grids do not absorb scatter radiation from high-energy beams as well as high-ratio grids.

While a high Bucky factor is desirable from the point of view of film quality, it is undesirable in two other respects. **The higher the Bucky factor, the greater the exposure factors and radiation dosage to the patient.** If the Bucky factor for a particular grid-energy combination is 5, then exposure factors and patient exposure both increase 5 times over what they would be for the same examination without a grid.

Contrast Improvement Factor (K)

The contrast improvement factor is the ratio of the contrast with a grid to the contrast without a grid.

$$K = \frac{\text{Contrast with a grid}}{\text{Contrast without a grid}}$$

This is the ultimate test of grid performance, since it is a measure of a grid's ability to improve contrast, which is its primary function.

Unfortunately, the contrast improvement factor is dependent upon kVp, field size, and phantom thickness. This is understandable, since these three factors de-

Table 8–3. Contrast Improvement Factor (K)

GRID NO.	GRID RATIO	LEAD CONTENT (mg/cm²)	CONTRAST IMPROVEMENT FACTOR (K)
1	3.4	170	1.95
2	2 × 3.1*	310	1.95
3	11	340	2.1
4	7	390	2.1
5	9	460	2.35
6	15	460	2.6
7	2 × 7*	680	2.95
8	15	900	2.95

*Crossed grids
Modified from Hondius Boldingh[1]

termine the amount of scatter radiation. The larger the quantity of scatter radiation, the poorer the contrast, and the lower the contrast improvement factor. To permit comparison of different grids, the contrast improvement factor is usually determined at 100 kVp with a large field and a phantom 20 cm thick as recommended by the International Commission on Radiologic Units and Measurements.[3] Table 8–3 shows the contrast improvement factor for eight different grids. It is more closely related to the lead content of the grid than any other factor. Generally, the higher the grid ratio, the higher the contrast improvement factor, but grid ratio is not as reliable an indicator as lead content.

While the contrast improvement factor of a particular grid is dependent on kVp, field size, and part thickness, the relative quality of two grids appears to be independent of these factors. A grid that has a high contrast improvement factor at 100 kVp will have a high factor at 50 or 130 kVp. In comparing two grids, the one that performs better with low-energy radiation will also perform better with high-energy radiation.

Figure 8–9 Relationship between grid ratio, lines per inch, and lead content of a grid

LEAD CONTENT OF GRIDS

The lead content of a grid is expressed in gm/cm². An easy way to understand what this means is to imagine cutting a grid up into 1-cm squares and then weighing one square. Its weight in grams is the lead content of the grid (ignoring the interspace material). The amount of lead in a grid is a good indicator of its ability to improve contrast provided the grid is well designed. Poor design would be a solid sheet of lead.

There is a definite relationship between the grid ratio, lead content, and number of lines per inch, as shown in Figure 8–9. If the grid ratio remains constant and the number of lines per inch is increased, the lead content must decrease. The only ways to increase the number of lines per inch is by decreasing the thickness of either the lead strips or interspaces. If the lead strips are made thinner, as they are in Figure 8–9B, the number of lines per inch increases without affecting grid ratio, because the thickness of lead strips is not considered in determining grid ratio. However, when the lead strips are made thinner, there is only a small increase in the number of lines per inch at a cost of a large decrease in lead content. If the number of lines per inch is increased by decreasing the width of the interspaces, as in Figure 8–9C, then the lead strips must be made shorter to keep the grid ratio constant, and again, the lead content of the grid decreases. This puts a limitation on the number of lines per inch a grid may have and still be effective. If a 10:1 grid could be constructed with 1000 lines per inch, it would be only 0.2 mm thick, and it would have too little lead to be of any real value.

In practice, when grids are constructed with many lines per inch, both the thickness and height of the lead strips are decreased. These grids are thinner, and improve contrast less than grids of comparable ratios with fewer lines per inch. A 133-line 10:1 grid improves contrast about the same as an 80-line 8:1 grid.

Figure 8–10   Grid cutoff

GRID CUTOFF

The primary disadvantage of grids is that they increase the amount of radiation that the patient receives. Another disadvantage is that they require careful centering of the x-ray tube because of the danger of grid cutoff. Grid cutoff is the loss of primary radiation that occurs when the images of the lead strips are projected wider than they would be with ordinary magnification, as shown in Figure 8–10. It is the result of a poor geometric relationship between the primary beam and the lead foil strips of the grid. Cutoff is complete and no primary radiation reaches the film when the projected images of the lead strips are thicker than the width of the interspaces. The resultant radiograph will be light in the area where the cutoff occurs. With linear grids there may be uniform lightening of the whole film, one edge of the film, or both edges of the film, depending on how the cutoff is produced. The amount of cutoff is always greatest with high-ratio grids and short grid-focusing distances. There are four situations that produce grid cutoff:

1. Focused grids used upside down.
2. Lateral decentering (grid angulation).
3. Focus-grid distance decentering.
4. Combined lateral and focus-grid distance decentering.

Upside-down Focused Grid

All focused grids have a tube-side, which is the side of focus of the lead strips. When a focused grid is used upside down, there is severe peripheral cutoff with a dark band of exposure in the center of the film and no exposure at the film's periphery.

Figure 8–11A illustrates how cutoff occurs, and Figure 8–11B shows the resultant radiograph. The higher the grid ratio, the narrower the exposed area. When a crossed grid is used upside down, only a small square in the center of the film is exposed.

Lateral Decentering

Lateral decentering results from the x-ray tube being positioned lateral to the convergent line but at the correct focal distance, as shown in Figure 8–12A. All of

Figure 8–11A   Cutoff from an upside-down focused grid

Figure 8–11B   Radiograph resulting from an upside-down focused grid

Figure 8–12A   Cutoff from lateral decentering

Figure 8–12B   Series of radiographs resulting from increasing amounts of lateral decentering

Table 8–4. Loss of Primary Radiation from Lateral Decentering for Grids Focused at 40 Inches

GRID RATIO	PERCENT LOSS OF PRIMARY RADIATION					
	INCHES OF LATERAL DECENTERING					
	1	2	3	4	5	6
5	13	25	38	50	63	75
6	15	30	45	60	75	90
8	20	40	60	80	100	—
10	25	50	75	100	—	—
12	30	60	90	100	—	—
16	40	80	100	—	—	—

the lead strips cut off the same amount of primary radiation, so there is **a uniform loss of radiation over the entire surface of the grid, producing a uniformly light radiograph.** This is probably the most common kind of grid cutoff, but it cannot be recognized by inspection of the film. All we see is a light film which is usually attributed to incorrect exposure factors. Figure 8–12B shows a series of film strips that were all taken with the same exposure factors, but with increasing amounts of lateral decentering. The x-ray tube was centered at the convergent line for the film strip on the left, and then laterally decentered 1, 2, and 3 inches for the next three strips. The films become progressively lighter as the amount of lateral decenter-ing increases, but the exposure is still uniform. The center and both edges of the film are equally exposed, and it's impossible to recognize the cutoff from inspection of the film.

Three factors affect the magnitude of cutoff from lateral decentering. They are grid ratio, focal distance, and the amount of decentering. The equation for calculating the loss of primary radiation with lateral decentering is as follows:

$$L = \frac{rb}{f_0} \times 100$$

L = Loss of primary radiation (%)
r = Grid ratio
b = Lateral decentering distance (inches)
f_0 = Focal distance of grid (inches)

Table 8–5. Loss of Primary Radiation from Lateral Decentering for Grids Focused at 72 Inches

GRID RATIO	PERCENT LOSS OF PRIMARY RADIATION					
	INCHES OF LATERAL DECENTERING					
	1	2	3	4	5	6
5	7	14	21	28	35	42
6	8	17	25	33	42	50
8	11	22	33	45	56	67
10	14	28	42	56	70	83
12	17	33	50	67	83	100
16	22	45	67	90	100	—

The amount of cutoff increases as the grid ratio and decentering distance increase; and cutoff decreases as the focal distance increases, as shown in Tables 8–4 and 8–5. The loss of primary radiation for any given amount of lateral decentering can be minimized with low-ratio grids and a long focal distance. With a 5:1 grid focused at 72 inches, there is a 14% loss of primary radiation with 2 inches of lateral decentering. If the grid ratio is increased to 16:1, the loss of primary radiation increases to 45%; and if the focal distance is then decreased to 40 inches, the loss of primary radiation goes up to 80%. When exact centering is not possible, as in portable radiography, low-ratio grids and long focal distances should be used whenever possible. It takes 8 inches of lateral decentering for 100% cutoff of primary radiation with a 5:1 grid focused at 72 inches, while it takes only 2.5 inches of lateral decentering for complete cutoff with a 16:1 grid focused at 40 inches.

Off-level Grids

When a linear grid is tilted, as it frequently is in portable radiography, there is a uniform loss of primary radiation across the entire surface of the grid, as illustrated in Figure 8–13. The effect on the film is the same as the effect of lateral decentering.

Focus-grid Distance Decentering

In focus-grid distance decentering, the target of the x-ray tube is correctly centered to the grid, but it is positioned above or below the convergent line. If the target is above the convergent line, it is called **far** focus-grid distance decentering; if the target is below the convergent line, it is called **near** focus-grid distance decentering. The results are the same, but they differ in magnitude. The cutoff is greater with near than with far focus-grid distance decentering. Figures 8–14 and 8–15 show the cutoff getting progressively greater with increasing distance from the film center. The central portion of the film is not affected, but the periphery is light. Since the fractional loss of radiation is not uniform, it must be calculated for a point, which actually represents two parallel lines running the length of the grid on either side of the center line. The loss of primary radiation is directly proportional to the grid ratio and distance from the center line.

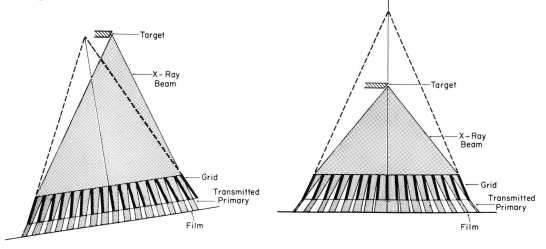

Figure 8–13   Cutoff from an off-level grid

Figure 8–14   Cutoff from near focus-grid distance decentering

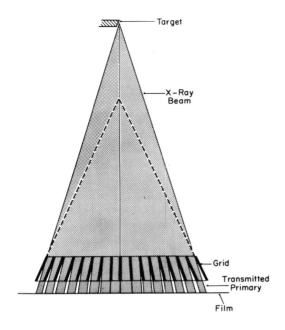

Figure 8–15   Cutoff from far focus-grid distance decentering

The equations for calculating the loss of primary radiation from near and far focus-grid distance decentering are as follows:

Near Focus-Grid Distance Decentering	Far Focus-Grid Distance Decentering
$L = rc\left(\dfrac{1}{f_1} - \dfrac{1}{f_0}\right) \times 100$	$L = rc\left(\dfrac{1}{f_0} - \dfrac{1}{f_2}\right) \times 100$

L = Loss of primary radiation at point c (%)
r = Grid ratio
f_0 = Grid focusing distance
f_1 = Target-grid distance (below convergent line—inches)
f_2 = Target-grid distance (above convergent line—inches)
c = Distance from center of grid (inches)

Table 8–6 shows the extent of cutoff at various distances from the center of grids focusing at 40 inches with a 10-inch focus-grid distance decentering error. The left half of the table indicates near (30 inches) and the right half far (50 inches) focus-grid distance decentering. The loss of primary radiation increases as the grid

ratio increases, and as the distance from the center of the grid increases; the loss is greater with near than with far focus-grid distance decentering. At the margin of a 14-inch wide film (7 inches from grid center), the loss of primary radiation is 35% for a 6:1 grid and 94% for a 16:1 grid with near focus-grid distance decentering. With far focus-grid distance decentering, the loss at the film margin decreases to 21% for a 6:1 grid and 64% for a 16:1 grid.

Parallel grids are focused at infinity so, of course, they are always used with near focus-grid distance decentering, as shown in Figure 8–16. They usually have a low grid ratio to minimize cutoff. The only time there is not significant cutoff is with long target-grid distances or small fields. A film taken with a parallel grid has a dark center and light edges because of near focus-grid distance decentering.

Combined Lateral and Focus-grid Distance Decentering

The most commonly recognized kind of grid cutoff is from combined lateral and focus-grid distance decentering. It is prob-

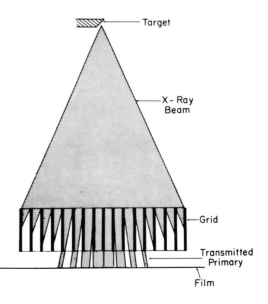

Figure 8–16   Cutoff from a parallel grid

Table 8-6. Loss of Primary Radiation from Near and Far Focus-Grid Distance Decentering for a Grid Focused at 40 Inches

	PERCENT LOSS OF PRIMARY RADIATION							
GRID RATIO	TARGET AT 30 INCHES				TARGET AT 50 INCHES			
	INCHES FROM GRID CENTER				INCHES FROM GRID CENTER			
	1	3	5	7	1	3	5	7
6	5	15	25	35	3	9	15	21
8	7	20	33	47	4	12	20	28
10	8	25	42	58	5	15	25	35
12	10	30	50	70	6	18	30	42
16	13	40	66	94	8	32	48	64

ably not as common as lateral decentering alone, but lateral decentering cannot be recognized as such on the resultant radiograph. Combined decentering is easy to recognize. It causes an uneven exposure resulting in a film that is light on one side and dark on the other side. There are two kinds of combined decentering depending upon whether the tube target is above or below the convergent line. The amount of cutoff is directly proportional to the grid ratio and decentering distance, and inversely proportional to the focal distance of the grid. With high-ratio grids and large decentering errors, there is a large loss of primary radiation. With long focus-grid distances, there is less loss of primary radiation.

Combined lateral and focus-grid distance decentering above the convergent line is illustrated in Figure 8–17. The projected images of the lead strips directly

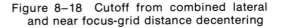

Figure 8–17 Cutoff from combined lateral and far focus-grid distance decentering

Figure 8–18 Cutoff from combined lateral and near focus-grid distance decentering below the tube target are broader than those on the opposite side, and the film is light on the near side. Cutoff is greatest on the side directly under the x-ray tube. Combined lateral and focus-grid distance decentering below the convergent line is illustrated in Figure 8–18. The projected images of the lead strips are broader on the side opposite the tube target than on the same side, and the film is light on the far side. Cutoff is least on the side under the x-ray tube. With equal decentering errors the amount of cutoff is greater with combined decentering below the convergent line than with combined decentering above the convergent line.

MOVING GRIDS

The moving grid was invented by Dr. Hollis E. Potter in 1920, and for many years a moving grid was called a Potter-Bucky grid. In recent years the name has been shortened to Bucky grid, which is unfortunate, since the name of the inventor is omitted. Grids are moved to blur out the shadows cast by the lead strips. Most moving grids are reciprocating, which means they continuously move 1 to 3 cm back and forth throughout the exposure. They start moving when the x-ray tube anode begins to rotate. Older grids move only in one direction and must be cocked for each exposure. They also have timers which are set for a little longer than the exposure time in order to avoid grid lines. These single-stroke grids are inconvenient and seldom used in modern equipment.

Moving grids are advantageous because they eliminate grid lines from the film. Many years ago this was important, since the lead strips were thick and unevenly spaced. However, with better manufacturing methods grids have improved so that grid lines are not nearly as distracting, and many radiologists now prefer stationary grids.

If you are using a moving grid and want to avoid grid lines, you must take two precautions. First, the grid must move fast enough to blur its lead strips. If it moves too slowly, you will see either the grid lines themselves or random density variations in the film that are just as distracting as the lines. Second, the transverse motion of the grid should not be synchronous with the pulses of the x-ray generator. When this happens, the shadow of each lead strip is superimposed on the shadow of its neighbor. Each pulse produces a faint image of the lead strip on the film. Between pulses, the grid moves one interspace distance so that the next lead strip is over the position of the preceding strip, and with a new pulse, the two images are superimposed. Thus, even though the grid moves, the grid lines will be distinct.

Moving grids have several disadvantages. They are costly, subject to failure, may vibrate the x-ray table, and put a limit on the minimum exposure time since they move slowly. An even more serious disadvantage is that they increase the patient's radiation dose. There are two reasons for this. The first is lateral decentering. Since the grid moves 1 to 3 cm during the exposure, the tube is not centered directly over the center of the grid during most of the exposure. This lateral decentering may result in a loss of as much as 20% of the primary radiation with a high-ratio grid and a short focusing distance. The second cause of increased patient exposure is more difficult to understand. The photons are spread out uniformly on the film by a moving grid. With the identical number of photons per unit area, a film is 15% darker

Figure 8–19 Analogy between water level and film density for moving and stationary grids

with a stationary grid, because the photons are concentrated between the lead strips. Figure 8–19 attempts to illustrate how this happens. The total quantity of density (blackness) on the film is represented by the water level in Figure 8–19A. This is the amount of density that is spread out uniformly over the film by a moving grid. In Figure 8–19B, a grid is immersed into the water to represent the grid lines on a film. Now all of the water is concentrated between the grid lines, and the water level rises just as the amount of blackness on the film rises. The total quantity of density on the film is the same with both moving and stationary grids, but with stationary grids the film is made up of many narrow voids (grid lines) containing no density, interspersed with black lines carrying all of the density.

Rotating Grids

Grid lines can be eliminated by rotating a round linear grid, a technique used in serial angiography. A reciprocating grid stops to change directions and the exposure may occur at this time. A rotating grid moves continuously throughout the exposure sequence so it is better suited for serial filming. An angular velocity of 600 revolutions per minute eliminates grid lines even with short exposures.[4] The grid is brought up to this velocity by blowing a jet of air into small cups around the grid's periphery.

The cut-off characteristics of rotating grids are different than those of stationary or reciprocating grids. Figure 8–20 shows an aerial view of a rotating grid stopped in three positions. At each position the lead strips converge to a line in space, but as the grid rotates, the line continuously changes its orientation and effectively becomes a point—the convergent point. In the illustration, the x-ray tube is centered at point A and its position and the position of the convergent point remain constant as the grid rotates. With the grid stopped in position 1, the x-ray tube falls on the

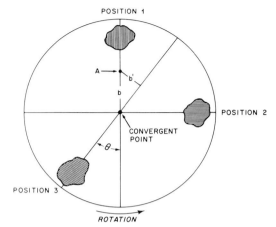

Figure 8–20   Rotating grid stopped in 3 positions

convergent line, so there is no lateral decentering. At position 2, lateral decentering (b) is maximum, and at position 3 it is intermediate (b') between the other two positions. Every 90°, the decentering error changes from zero to a maximum as the cosine of the angle θ. The average positive value of the cosine is $2/\pi$, or 0.64.[5] For any given decentering error, and for all types of decentering (lateral, distance and combined), the loss of primary radiation (cutoff) is 36% less for a rotating grid than a comparable stationary grid. Rotating grids are not suitable for oblique radiographic techniques since they converge to a point rather than a line.

GRID SELECTION

There is no simple rule to guide the clinician in choosing a grid for any particular situation. A compromise is always involved. The price of increased "cleanup" with high-ratio grids is a considerable increase in patient exposure and an increase in the criticalness of x-ray tube centering. You must weigh the value of a better-quality radiograph against your moral obligation to keep the patient's exposure at a minimum. There is little to be gained using

Figure 8–21   Fractional transmission of scatter radiation through grids (Courtesy of Sven Ledin and The Elema Shoenander Co.)

high-ratio grids in the low-kVp range. Usually, **8:1 grids will give adequate results below 90 kVp. Above 90 kVp, 12:1 grids are preferred.** Crossed grids are only used when there is a great deal of scatter radiation, such as in biplane cerebral angiography.

The efficiency of scatter radiation absorption by various grids is shown in Figure 8–21, which is a graph plotting the fractional transmission of scatter radiation against grid ratio. There is little decrease in transmitted scatter beyond an 8:1 ratio grid, and almost no change between 12:1 and 16:1. For this reason 12:1 grids are preferable to 16:1 grids for routine radiography. The improvement in film quality in going from a 12:1 to a 16:1 grid is not worth the greater patient exposure.

AIR GAP TECHNIQUES

The x-ray grid is the most important means of reducing scatter radiation with large radiographic fields, but under certain circumstances an alternate method, an air gap, produces comparable results with less patient exposure. The basic principle of the air gap technique is quite simple. Scatter radiation arising in the patient from Compton reactions disperses in all directions, so the patient acts like a large light bulb as shown in Figure 8–22A. In the illustration, scattered photons are shown radiating out from a point source, but the point actually represents a tiny block of tissue. Each ray represents a separate scattering event, and numerous scatterings within the small block produces the array shown. The closer the patient is to the film, the greater the concentration of scatter per unit area. With an air gap (AG), the concentration decreases because more scattered photons miss the film. The name "air filtration" has been applied to air gap techniques, but this is a misnomer. **Scatter radiation decreases because scattered photons miss the film, and not from filtration.** Negligible quantities of radiation are absorbed in the gap, and the beam is not appreciably hardened, so the name air filtration should be discarded.

There is no strong bias for forward scattering in the diagnostic energy range, so the distribution of Compton scattering is nearly random. A photon is almost as likely to scatter at 90° as at 45°, or 180°. With increasing energy, more photons scatter in the forward direction, but the increase is negligible in the diagnostic range. When the energy of the incident photon is increased from 10 keV to 140 keV, a much greater change than is likely in clinical radiology, the most probable angle of scatter only changes from 53° to 45°.[6] With a strong forward bias, as in megavoltage therapy, air gaps are ineffective as a means of controlling scatter radiation.

Figure 8–22 B and C compares the distribution of scattered radiation arising from superficial tissue blocks on opposite sides of the patient. More radiation reaches the film from scattering near the exit surface (B), because the film intercepts

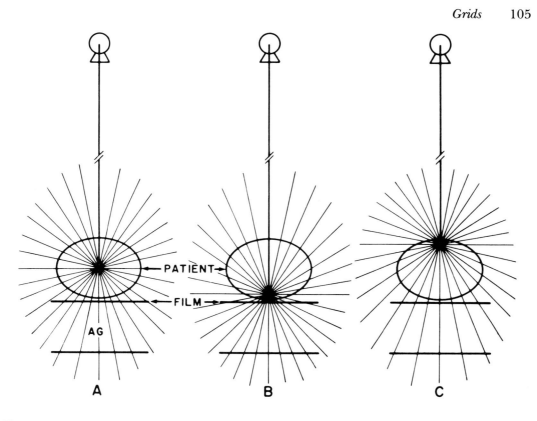

Figure 8–22   Air gap (AG) techniques

a larger angle of the scattered "beam." The angle of interception is smaller for scattering occurring on the input side of the patient (C), since a natural "gap" separates the film from the scattering site. The difference in the contribution from the two sides is even greater than the illustration implies. Many scattered photons from the input surface (C) are absorbed during their long journey through the patient; whereas those originating near the exit surface (B) have only a short escape distance. As a result of these two factors, a greater angle of capture and less tissue attenuation, most of the scattered photons reaching the film arise in the immediately adjacent superficial tissue layers, an ideal arrangement for an air gap technique. You can see from the illustration that the air gap is most effective in removing scatter radiation when the scatter originates close to the film (B).

Optimum Gap Width

Air gap techniques are used in two clinical situations, magnification radiography and chest radiography. With magnification techniques the object-film distance is optimized for the screen-focal spot combination and the air gap reduces the scatter radiation to acceptable levels as an incidental bonus. In chest radiography the air gap is used in lieu of a grid and techniques are designed around the air gap. For example, image sharpness deteriorates as the gap widens, so the focal-film distance is usually lengthened from 6 to 10 feet to restore sharpness. Air gaps and grids have the same function—to remove as much scatter radiation and as little primary radiation as possible. As a measure of performance, gap width is analogous to grid ratio. A larger air gap, like a higher ratio grid, removes a larger percentage of scatter radiation.

Figure 8–23 shows the ratio of scatter to primary radiation with air gap widths from ⅝ to 15 inches for three different absorber thicknesses. A ratio of 5 means that 5 scattered photons reach the film for each primary photon. At the ideal ratio of zero, all of the transmitted photons are primary. As the gap increases, the ratio of secondary to primary radiation decreases, but the change is gradual without an abrupt transition point. The optimum gap width is a matter of judgement. The following four guidelines should be used to select a gap width:

1. The thicker the part, the more advantageous a larger gap. Figure 8–23 shows that a change from a 1 inch to a 15 inch width produces a more marked de-

Table 8–7. Comparative Contrast Improvement Factors for Grid and Air Gap Techniques (100 kVp, 30 × 30 cm Field)

ABSORBER THICKNESS (CM OF WATER)	CONTRAST IMPROVEMENT FACTOR			
	AIR GAP		GRID	
	5 IN	10 IN	7:1	15:1
10	1.39	1.81	1.50	1.85
20	1.37	2.21	2.10	2.85

Data from Gould and Hale[6]

crease in scatter radiation for a 22-cm phantom than a 10-cm phantom.

2. The first inch of air gap improves contrast more than any subsequent inch. The increase from a 1- to a 2-inch gap improves contrast more than an increase from a 14- to a 15-inch gap.

3. Image sharpness deteriorates with increasing gap width unless the focal-film distance is increased to compensate for the greater magnification. An increase in focal-film distance from 6 to 10 feet is customary in chest radiography to compensate for this loss of sharpness. A further increase in focal-film distance is usually not physically possible because of space limitations, or technically feasible at an acceptable exposure time because of the heat tolerance of the x-ray tube. Remember, a 50% increase in distance doubles the exposure factors.

4. If the gap is widened by moving the patient away from the film with a fixed focal-film distance, the patient is closer to the x-ray tube and his exposure increases. The increase can be corrected by a comparable increase in the focal-film distance, but this may not be a possible alternative for the reasons stated above.

Table 8–7 shows that a 5-inch air gap approaches the performance of a light (7:1) grid for thin patients. A 10-inch gap is the same as a heavy (15:1) grid for thin patients, but not as good for thicker patients. The final decision on air gap width is

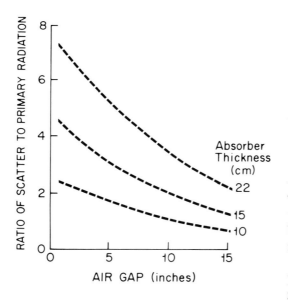

Figure 8–23   Ratio of scatter to primary radiation for various air gaps and absorber thicknesses

usually made empirically. Changing widths from patient to patient is inconvenient. Experience has shown that a 10-inch gap and a 10-foot focal-film distance with an energy from 110 to 150 kVp produces satisfactory results.

Exposure Factors with Air Gaps

Figure 8–24 compares a 6-foot focal-film distance with a grid to a 10-foot focal-film distance with a 10-inch air gap. The exposure factor, patient exposure and transmitted primary radiation are all assigned a value of one for the grid technique which is used as the standard for comparison. In this example, the primary transmission of the grid is 65%, and the experimental design was chosen to produce films of equal density (same total number of photons) and contrast (same ratio of primary to secondary photons). The x-ray tube exposure must be increased for the air gap technique because of the larger focal-film distances (FFD). Applying the

inverse square law (constant kVp), exposures would have to be increased 2.8 times ($120^2 \div 72^2 = 2.8$), but the actual increase is somewhat less since only 65% of the primary photons are transmitted through the grid. The increase is 1.8 times ($2.8 \times .65 = 1.8$), a substantial difference that taxes the heat capacity of the x-ray tube.

Patient exposures are usually less with air gaps than grids, because grids absorb primary photons. With the grid technique shown in Figure 8–24, 1.54 primary photons must pass through the patient for each one reaching the film ($1.0 \div .65 = 1.54$); the difference (35%) is absorbed in the grid. Only 1.19 primary photons need pass through the patient with the air gap technique to produce a comparable concentration per unit area of film; the difference ($1.19 - 1.0 = .19$ or 19%) is lost by inverse square. The air gap loses less primary radiation, so the patient's exposure is less. If the patient exposure is unity with the grid, it will be 0.77 with the air gap ($1.19 \div 1.54 = .77$), a significant but not dramatic savings.

Magnification with Air Gaps

Two factors determine the amount of magnification, the object-film distance and the focal-film distance. Magnification is greatest with a short focal-film distance and a long object-film distance. As a general rule, image sharpness deteriorates with magnification. The objective with an air gap technique is to preserve image sharpness by lengthening the focal-film distance until magnification returns to pre-air gap levels. However, some deterioration is inevitable for parts close to the film. Figure 8–25 shows that the objective is not accomplished with a 120-inch focal-film distance, at least not for a 10-inch air gap and a reasonable size (10-inch thick) patient. Magnification is less with the 72-inch focal-film distance for all object-film distances up to 15 inches. The longer focal-film distance produces a more uniform magnification from the front to the

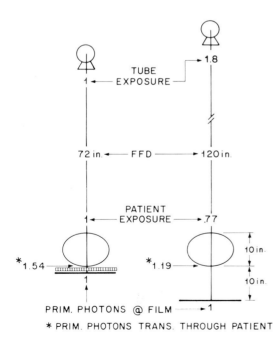

Figure 8–24 Comparison of grid and air gap techniques for chest radiography

Figure 8–25 Magnification with 72 inch (no air gap) and 120 inch (air gap) focal-film distances (FFD)

back of the patient, a desirable characteristic. This uniformity is preserved with lesser air gaps. With a 5-inch gap, the curve would maintain its slope, but slide down the magnification scale to cross the 72-inch curve at a shorter object-film distance. Experienced chest radiographers do not feel that image sharpness deteriorates noticeably with air gap techniques.

SUMMARY

Radiographic grids consist of lead foil strips separated by x-ray transparent spacers. They are used to absorb scatter radiation and improve radiographic image contrast. The grid ratio is defined as the ratio of the height of the lead strips to the distance between them, and it is the simplest way of characterizing a grid. Grids come in two patterns, linear and crossed. Crossed grids consist of two superimposed

linear grids; their great disadvantage is that they cannot be used with oblique techniques. Most grids are focused to a line in space called a convergent line, but they can be used over a variable range of distances called the focal range.

Three tests have been devised to evaluate grid performance. (1) Primary transmission is a measurement of the percentage of primary radiation transmitted through a grid (usually between 60 and 70%). (2) The Bucky factor is a measurement of the total radiation (primary and scatter) absorbed by a grid. It indicates how much exposure factors must be increased because of grids, and also how much more radiation the patient receives. Bucky factors range from 3 to 7 depending upon the grid ratio. (3) The contrast improvement factor is a measurement of a grid's ability to improve contrast, and it is the best test of grid performance. Generally, high-ratio grids with a high lead content have the highest contrast improvement factors.

The grid ratio, lead content, and number of lines per inch are all interrelated. A grid with many lines per inch (over 100) is generally thinner and has a lower lead content than a grid of comparable ratio with fewer lines per inch.

Grid cutoff is the loss of primary radiation that occurs when the images of the lead strips are projected wider than they would be with ordinary magnification. The amount of cutoff with a particular decentering error is greatest with high-ratio grids that have a short focusing distance. Lateral decentering is the most common error, and it causes a uniform loss of primary radiation, so it is impossible to recognize on the film. With focus-grid distance decentering, the film is light on both sides; while with combined lateral and focus-grid distance decentering, the film is light only on one side.

Moving grids eliminate the image of the lead strips from the film, and this is their chief advantage. Generally, exposure factors are a little greater with moving grids than with stationary grids, because of a lateral decentering error during a portion of the exposure, and because the exposure is spread out over the entire surface of the film. With properly positioned stationary grids, there is no decentering error, and the exposure is concentrated between the lead strips. Rotating a linear grid eliminates grid lines, effectively changes the convergent line to a point, decreases cutoff by 36% for a given decentering error, and makes the grid unsatisfactory for oblique techniques.

Grid selection involves a compromise between film quality and patient exposure. High-ratio grids produce films with better contrast at a cost of increased patient exposure. Generally, low-ratio grids are adequate for low-energy radiation; 8:1 grids should be used with energies less than 90 kVp, and 12:1 grids for higher-energy radiation.

Air gaps are an alternative method of eliminating scatter radiation with large radiographic fields. The intensity of scatter radiation is maximum at the patient's surface and diminishes rapidly at increasing distance from the surface. If the film is placed at a distance, the scatter simply misses the film. Focal-film distances are increased with air gap techniques in an attempt to maintain image sharpness, and as a consequence, x-ray exposure factors are greater with the air gaps than grids. However, patient exposures are generally less with air gaps, because the grid absorbs some primary radiation.

REFERENCES

1. Hondius Boldingh, W.: Grids to reduce scattered x-ray in medical radiography. Philips Research Reports Supplement #1. Eindhoven, Netherlands: Philips Research Laboratories, 1964.
2. *Characteristics and Applications of X-ray Grids.* rev. ed. Liebel Flarsheim Co., 1968.
3. *Methods of Evaluating Radiological Equipment and Materials.* National Bureau of Standards, Handbook 89, August 1963.
4. Amplatz, K.: Simple Bucky diaphragm for high speed angiography. Invest. Radiol. *2*, 387, 1967.
5. Bull, K. W., Curry, T. S. III, Dowdey, J. E., and Christensen, E. E.: The cutoff characteristics of rotating grids. Radiol. *114*, 453, 1975.
6. Gould, R. G. and Hale, J.: Control of scattered radiation by air gap techniques: applications to chest radiography. Amer. J. Roentgen. *122*, 109, 1974.

CHAPTER 9

Intensifying and Fluoroscopic Screens

The x-ray photons making up the radiographic image cannot be seen by the human eye. This information is converted into a visual image by one of two methods. A photographic emulsion can be exposed to the x rays directly. More commonly, the energy of the x rays is converted into radiation in the visible-light spectrum, and this light may be used to expose x-ray film (radiography or photofluorography), or the light may be viewed directly (fluoroscopy). The sensitivity of film to direct x-ray exposure is low. Direct exposure of film would require prohibitively large patient x-ray doses for most examinations. Therefore, almost all radiographic film examinations require that the radiographic image be converted into light at some stage by a luminescent screen.

FLUORESCENCE

Luminescence refers to the emission of light by a substance. It can be caused by varying kinds of stimuli (e.g., light, chemical reactions, or ionizing radiation). The term **fluorescence** is applied to that form of luminescence produced when light is emitted instantaneously (within 10^{-8} seconds of the stimulation). If the emission of light is delayed beyond 10^{-8} seconds, the term **phosphorescence** is used.

Fluorescence, as used in radiology, is **the ability of crystals of certain inorganic salts** (called phosphors) **to emit light when excited by x rays.** For many years the crystals, or phosphors, of importance in radiology were **calcium tungstate** (the phosphor in intensifying screens) and zinc cadmium sulfide (the phosphor in fluorescent and photofluorographic screens). Recent advances in technology have resulted in introduction of a number of new phosphors which include cesium iodide in image intensifier tubes, and several new intensifying screen phosphors including barium fluorochloride, barium strontium sulfate, yttrium, and the rare earths gadolinium and lanthanum.

Theories concerning the mechanism of luminescence are discussed in several textbooks of x-ray physics and will not be repeated here. The process is basically one in which a relatively small number of high-energy photons (x rays) is changed into a larger number of photons with much lower energy (light). At energies used in diagnostic radiology, almost all x-ray absorption in the screen is due to the photoelectric effect in the high atomic number elements of the phosphor.

INTENSIFYING SCREENS

Intensifying screens are used because they **decrease the x-ray dose** (less mAs) to the patient, yet still afford a properly exposed x-ray film. Also, the reduction in exposure allows use of short exposure times, which becomes important when it is necessary to minimize patient motion.

The x-ray film used with intensifying

screens has photosensitive emulsion on both sides. The film is sandwiched between two intensifying screens in a cassette, so that the emulsion on each side is exposed to the light from its contiguous screen (light from one screen will be almost completely absorbed by the emulsion nearest it). Remember, the screen functions to absorb the energy (and information) in the x-ray beam that has penetrated the patient, and to convert this energy into a light pattern which has (as nearly as possible) the same information as the original x-ray beam. The light, then, forms a latent image on x-ray film. The transfer of information from x-ray beam to screen light to film results in some loss of information. In this and following chapters we will discuss some of the factors involved in the degradation of information and the things that can be done to keep this to a minimum.

Construction

An intensifying screen has four layers:
1. A base, or support, made of plastic or cardboard.
2. A reflecting layer (TiO_2).
3. A phosphor layer ($CaWO_4$).
4. A plastic protective coat.

The total thickness of a typical intensifying screen is about 15 or 16 mils (1 mil = 1/1000 inch = .0254 mm).

Base

The screen support, or base, may be made of high-grade cardboard or a polyester plastic. The base of Du Pont intensifying screens is a polyester plastic (Mylar*) which is 10 mils thick (10 mils = 254 microns). Kodak X-OMATIC and LANEX screens have a similar (Estar**) base 7 mils thick.

Reflecting Coat

The light produced by the interaction of x-ray photons and phosphor crystals is

*Mylar is a trademark fo E. I. du Pont de Nemours and Co.
**Estar is a trademark of Eastman Kodak Company.

emitted in all directions. Much of the light is emitted from the screen in the direction of the film. However, many light photons are also directed toward the back of the screen (i.e., toward the base layer) and would be lost as far as photographic activity is concerned. The reflecting layer acts to reflect light back toward the front of the screen. The reflecting coat is made of a white substance, such as titanium dioxide (TiO_2), and is spread over the base in a thin layer, about 1 mil thick. Some screens do not have a reflecting layer (e.g., Kodak X-OMATIC fine and regular).

Phosphor Layer

The phosphor layer, containing phosphor crystals is applied over the reflecting coat or base. The crystals are suspended in a plastic (polymer) containing a substance to keep the plastic flexible. We will discuss the phosphor in more detail later. The thickness of the phosphor layer is about 4 mils for par-speed screens. The thickness of the phosphor layer is increased 1 or 2 mils in high-speed screens, and is decreased slightly in detail screens.

Protective Layer

The protective layer applied over the phosphor is made of a plastic, largely composed of a cellulose compound that is mixed with other polymers. It forms a layer about 0.7 to 0.8 mil thick. This layer serves three functions: (1) it helps prevent static electricity, (2) gives physical protection to the delicate phosphor layer, and (3) provides a surface which can be cleaned without damaging the phosphor layer.

Figure 9–1 Par-speed x-ray intensifying screen (cross-section)

Figure 9–1 shows a cross section of a typical par-speed intensifying screen with a plastic base. Unlike the highly mechanized operation of x-ray film production, screens are largely a product of hand labor.

Phosphor

The original phosphor used in x-ray intensifying screens was **crystalline calcium tungstate** ($CaWO_4$). New (since about 1973) screen phosphor technology is being developed to increase screen speed over that available with calcium tungstate, and has resulted in the introduction of a bewildering variety of screens and corresponding films. Let us first consider calcium tungstate, then review some of the new phosphors.

Natural calcium tungstate (scheelite) is no longer used because synthetic calcium tungstate of better quality is produced by fusing sodium tungstate and calcium chloride under carefully controlled conditions. The first commercial calcium tungstate screens were made in England and Germany in 1896; they were first made in the United States in 1912. The calcium tungstate crystal must be absolutely free of any contaminant if it is to fluoresce properly. **It produces light primarily in the blue region of the visible spectrum,** with a wavelength range of 3500 to 5800 Å (1 angstrom = .0001 microns = .00000001 cm), with a peak wavelength of about 4300 angstroms (430 millimicrons) which is seen by the eye as a violet color. Although the eye is not sensitive to light of this wavelength, x-ray film emulsion exhibits maximum sensitivity to light from calcium tungstate screens. Figure 9–2 diagrams the spectrum of calcium tungstate fluorescence, the response of the eye to light of different wavelengths, and the sensitivity of x-ray film. Film sensitivity is seen to be high throughout most of the range of light emitted by the screen, a fact which insures maximum photographic effect. Note that the film does not exhibit photosensitivity to red light, so red light

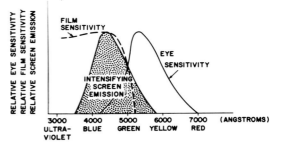

Figure 9–2 The spectral emission of a calcium tungstate x-ray intensifying screen compared to the spectral sensitivity of x-ray film and the eye

can be used in the darkroom without producing any photographic effect on the film.

Intensifying Action of Screens

An intensifying screen is used because it is able to convert a few absorbed x-ray photons into a lot of light photons. The **efficiency with which the phosphor converts x rays to light is termed the intrinsic efficiency of the phosphor**, and is more properly defined as the ratio of the light energy generated by the crystal to the x-ray energy absorbed. The intrinsic efficiency of calcium tungstate is about 5%. If one knows the energy of the absorbed x-ray photon, the wavelength of the emitted light, and the intrinsic efficiency of the phosphor, the number of light photons generated is easily calculated. For example, assume a 50 keV x-ray photon (50,000 electron volts) is absorbed in a calcium tungstate screen which emits most of its light at a wavelength of 4,300 Å. The energy in electron volts (eV) of this light photon is calculated by:

$$\lambda \text{ (wavelength)} = \frac{12.4}{keV}$$

$$4{,}300 = \frac{12.4}{keV}$$

$$keV = \frac{12.4}{4{,}300} \cong .003$$

$$eV = 3$$

The energy of a 4,300 Å blue light photon is about 3 eV. At 100% intrinsic efficiency, a 50,000 eV x-ray photon would produce about 17,000 light photons of 3 eV energy:

$$\frac{50,000}{3} \cong 17,000$$

Since the intrinsic efficiency of calcium tungstate is only 5%, the actual number of light photons emitted by this phosphor is about 850 (17,000 × .05 = 850). One reason some new intensifying screen phosphors are faster than calcium tungstate is that the new phosphor has a higher intrinsic efficiency (up to 20%).

The ability of light emitted by the phosphor to escape from the screen and expose the film is termed the screen efficiency. For typical screens about half the generated light gets to the film, the rest is absorbed in the screen and is wasted. In the previous example, only half the 850 light photons generated would be able to escape from the screen and expose the film.

To examine the manner in which the screen amplifies the photographic effect of x rays, let us consider the case of a film-screen combination, compared to a film alone, each irradiated by one thousand 50 keV x-ray photons. Of the 1000 photons, a high speed calcium tungstate screen will absorb 40% (we will discuss this aspect in more detail later), or 400. Each of the 400 x-ray photons will produce 850 light photons, for a total of 340,000 light photons. Half of these light photons (170,000) will escape the screen and expose the film. Let us assume that 100 light photons are needed to form one latent-image center. The screen-film system in our example has caused the formation of 1700 latent-image centers. We will consider the concept of the latent image in the next chapter. At this point, let us simply define a latent-image center as the end product of the photographic effect of light or x rays on the film emulsion. It is possible to measure the magnitude of the photographic effect of an exposure by counting the number of latent-image centers formed as a result of that exposure. In the case of x rays exposing film directly, only about 5% of the x-ray photons are absorbed by the film, so our example will cause 50 x-ray photons to react with the film emulsion. It is usually considered that one latent-image center is formed for each x-ray photon absorbed by a film emulsion. The result of the same 1000 x-ray photons acting directly on film is to produce only 50 latent-image centers, versus 1700 latent-image centers resulting from the use of intensifying screens. In our example, the ratio of the photographic effect of screen versus non-screen, or direct, exposure is 34 to 1. If kVp remains constant, direct film exposure will require 34 times as many mAs as a film-screen exposure. A review of the example of the intensifying effect of screens is presented in Table 9–1. Stated another way, patient exposure is

Table 9–1. Comparison of the Photographic Effect of 1000 X-Ray Photons Used With and Without Intensifying Screens

	X-RAY PHOTONS ABSORBED BY SCREEN	X-RAY PHOTONS ABSORBED BY FILM	LIGHT PHOTONS GENERATED	LIGHT PHOTONS REACHING FILM	LATENT-IMAGE CENTERS FORMED
INTENSIFYING SCREEN	400	—	340,000	170,000	1700
DIRECT EXPOSURE	—	50	—	—	50

decreased greatly when intensifying screens are used. A measure of this decrease in exposure is termed the intensification factor of the screen. **The intensification factor of a screen is the ratio of the x-ray exposure needed to produce the same density on a film with and without the screen** (intensification factor is commonly determined at a film density of 1.0).

$$\text{INTENSIFICATION FACTOR} = \frac{\text{Exposure required when screens are not used}}{\text{Exposure required with screens}}$$

The intensification factor of $CaWO_4$ screens will increase with increasing energy (kVp) of the x-ray beam (Figure 9–3). The K-absorption edges of silver and bromine in the film are 26 keV and 13 keV respectively, while the K-absorption edge of tungsten is 69.5 keV. Photoelectric absorption of low-kVp x rays will be relatively greater in film because of the low-keV K-absorption edge of silver and bromine. High-kVp x rays will be more abundantly absorbed by the photoelectric process in calcium tungstate screens. For this same reason, a heavily filtered x-ray beam will increase the screen intensification factor

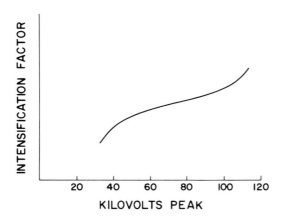

Figure 9–3 Variation of the intensification factor with kVp

by removing the low-energy components of the beam. Thus,. $CaWO_4$ intensifying screens are relatively faster in radiography of a thick body part, such as the lumbar spine, than when an extremity is examined. That is, only higher-energy x rays can penetrate the thick part and reach the screen.

There will actually be a small number (3 or 4%) of x-ray photons directly absorbed by the film when a screen-film combination is exposed. This direct action of x rays would create so few latent-image centers compared to those caused by the fluorescence of the screen that it may be ignored as having no detectable influence on total film response to the exposure.

Speed of Calcium Tungstate Intensifying Screens

Several factors determine how "fast" or "slow" a calcium tungstate screen will be; these include **thickness of the phosphor layer, size of the phosphor crystals,** presence or absence of **light-absorbing dye** in the phosphor layer, and the **efficiency of fluorescence** of the crystal. Of course, the faster screen will allow a lower x-ray exposure to the patient, but a price for this speed must be paid. **The speed of a calcium tungstate screen and its ability to record detail are in reciprocal relationship;** high speed means less detail. These screens are classified as fast, medium (par-speed), and slow (detail), with intensification factors in the range of 100, 50, and 35 respectively.

The size of the calcium tungstate crystal is of some importance in determining speed. The fluorescent emission of calcium tungstate crystals increases with size. High-speed screens have larger crystals than those of slow-speed (often called detail) screens. However, difference in crystal size is not the only factor involved in determining screen speed. A fast screen may be twelve times as fast as a slow (detail) screen, but the crystals in the fast screen are only about twice as large as the crystals in the slow screen. Recently, the speed of calcium tungstate screens has been increased by increasing the efficiency of the crystal in converting the energy of the absorbed x-ray photon into light. Even the smallest crystals in the slowest screens are very large compared to the size of the silver halide grains in the film emulsion. Phosphor particle size ranges from 4 microns (slow screen) to 8 microns (fast screen). The size of the silver halide crystal in an x-ray film emulsion is about 1 micron. Consequently, any screen lacks the ability to record fine detail when compared to x-ray film.

A thicker phosphor layer will result in a faster screen because the thick layer will absorb more x-ray photons than a thin layer. Thick screens will be faster, but will cause a decrease in the clarity of the image recorded on the film. This decrease in image clarity is due primarily to **diffusion of light** in the phosphor layer. If a thick phosphor layer is employed, an x-ray photon may be absorbed in the phosphor at some distance from the film. **The light photons generated by this absorbed x-ray photon are emitted in all directions.** Not all of the light will reach the film, but that which does will expose an area of the film which is much larger than the size of the

Figure 9–5 Unsharp image borders produced by light diffusion in intensifying screens

calcium tungstate crystal that emitted the light (Figure 9–4). In addition, some light scattering takes place in the screen, and further increases the area of illumination. The resultant light diffusion obviously causes images to have less sharp borders. Consider Figure 9–5. If an x-ray beam is directed onto a film-screen combination which has a thick lead block covering half the film, one would expect one-half of the film to be exposed and one-half to be entirely unexposed, with the line between the two areas being very sharp. If the x-ray beam were to expose film alone (without screens), the line between exposed and unexposed areas would be very sharp. However, if the film is sandwiched between intensifying screens, the border is less sharp because some light will diffuse into the area under the edge of the lead block and cause exposure of film in an area which actually receives no x-ray exposure. This light which diffused under the edge of the lead block is not available to expose that portion of the film which is not covered by the block. The final result is the production of a more gradual change in density, which is unlike the ideal abrupt transition from black to unexposed (clear) film. Attempts to measure the magnitude

Figure 9–4 Screen unsharpness is caused by light diffusion in the intensifying screen

of this problem of light diffusion and scattering will lead us to consideration of the concepts of line spread function and modulation transfer function in Chapter 13.

A thin screen causes less light diffusion than a thick one because light photons are produced closer to the film. Another way to decrease light diffusion is to incorporate a substance which absorbs light in the screen. The substance is commonly a yellow dye, but the question of which color is most effective has not been resolved (the 3M Alpha 4 screen has a pink dye). The light photons which emerge from the crystal immediately adjacent to the film will obviously travel the shortest distance before leaving the phosphor layer. Scattered photons must travel longer distances in the phosphor layer, and thus they have a better chance of being absorbed by the dye. The dye will decrease the speed of the screen because it decreases the amount of light emitted. Light-absorbing dyes are included in screens designed to produce greater detail.

Resolving Power

The maximum number of line pairs per millimeter which can be resolved by the screen-film system is called the **resolving power**. A **line pair** means a line and a space. For example, two lines (or two line pairs) per mm means that there are two lines and two spaces per mm. Each line is ¼ mm wide, and each space is ¼ mm wide, thus making each line pair ½ mm wide. A more detailed discussion of resolving power will be presented in Chapter 13. X-ray film is able to record up to 100 line pairs per mm, but the slowest screens can record only a little over 10.

Temperature Effect

X-ray screens fluoresce more brilliantly at low temperature. At extremes of temperature this may have clinical significance. At 95°F, an increase in exposure of about 25% may be necessary to produce the same film density as a similar radiograph done at 70°F.

Screen-Film Contact

The cassette in which the intensifying screens are mounted provides a light-tight container for the film. It also serves to hold the film in tight contact with the screens over its entire surface. With good film-screen contact a dot of light produced in the screen will be recorded as a comparable dot on the film. If contact is poor, this dot of light will diffuse before it reaches the film, so that its radiographic image is unsharp.

There is a simple method for testing film-screen contact. A piece of wire screen is placed on the cassette, and a radiograph of the wire screen is made. The sharpness of the image of the wire in all regions of the film is compared, and any areas of poor film-screen contact become obvious, for the image of the wire appears fuzzy. The wire screen should be made of iron, brass, or copper (aluminum and plastic screens fail to absorb enough x rays) and should have a heavier wire than that used in ordinary window screen. It is best to mount the test wire screen between two pieces of plastic, composition board, or cardboard. Poor film-screen contact is produced rapidly by rough handling of the cassette, but eventually any cassette will wear out with routine use.

Cleaning

Intensifying screens must be kept clean. Any foreign material, such as paper or blood, on the screen will block light photons and produce an area of underexposure on the film corresponding to the size and shape of the soiled area. Cleaning will eliminate the "high spots" on a screen; these high points are the major source of excessive wear. The cause of screen failure is mechanical attrition. Under normal conditions of use, x-ray photons will not damage screens. Screens are best cleaned with a solution containing an antistatic compound and a detergent; the solution should be applied gently (never rub vigorously) with a soft lint-free cloth. The cassette should never be closed after cleaning until it is absolutely dry.

NEW PHOSPHOR TECHNOLOGY

It is usually agreed that the maximum useful speed of calcium tungstate screens has been achieved. New screen phosphors have permitted greater speed, but this changing technology is complex and perplexing.

Increasing Screen Speed

We must first consider how intensifying screen speed can be increased. There are three possible ways. The phosphor layer can be made thicker to absorb more of the x-ray beam. The phosphor may have a higher conversion efficiency of x rays to light. The phosphor may be able to absorb the x-ray beam more effectively. To review, there are three possible ways to increase screen speed:

1. Thicker phosphor layer
2. Higher conversion efficiency phosphor
3. Higher absorption phosphor

Before entering this long discussion of new phosphor technology, please review Table 9–2 which catalogs many of the non-calcium tungstate screens available by manufacturer, phosphor composition, and color of light emitted by the phosphor.

Thicker Phosphor Layer

Thick phosphor layers absorb more of the x-ray beam than thin layers. This is the major way in which the speed of calcium tungstate screens is increased. A pair of Du Pont par speed $CaWO_4$ screens absorbs about 20% of the x-ray beam. A pair of Du Pont Hi Plus screens absorbs about 40% of the x-ray beam (and is twice as fast as par speed). However, the Hi Plus screens are not 2 times as thick as par, they are about 2.3 times as thick as the par screens. Why is this? If 100 x-ray photons struck a pair of par screens, 80 photons would be transmitted through the screens (20 are absorbed). A second set of par screens placed in the path of the 80 transmitted photons would absorb 20%, or 16 photons, allowing 64 to

Table 9–2. Some of the Non-Calcium Tungstate Intensifying Screen Phosphors

MANUFACTURER	NAME	PHOSPHOR	SPECTRAL EMISSION
Du Pont	Quanta II	Barium fluorochloride	Blue
	Quanta III	Lanthanum oxybromide	Blue
Kodak	X-Omatic Regular	Barium strontium sulfate	Blue
	Lanex	Gadolinium and Lanthanum oxysulfide	Green
3 M	Alpha 4	Gadolinium and Lanthanum oxysulfide	Green
	Alpha 8	Same	Green
U.S. Radium	Rarex B	Yttrium oxysulfide	Blue
	Rarex B G	Yttrium and Gadolinium oxysulfide	Blue
General Electric	Blue Max 1	Lanthanum oxybromide	Blue
	Blue Max 2	Lanthanum oxybromide	Blue

Table 9–3. Relative Speed of Various CaWO₄ Screens

CALCIUM TUNGSTATE SCREEN (DU PONT CRONEX)	RELATIVE SPEED
Detail	1
Fast Detail	2
Par	4
Hi-Plus	8
Lightning Plus	12

pass through. Thus, a double thickness of par speed screens does not absorb 40% of the x-ray beam. It is possible to continue to increase the speed of CaWO₄ screens by increasing screen thickness, but unsharpness caused by light diffusion in the thick phosphor layer becomes unacceptable. Thus, **calcium tungstate screens may be considered a compromise between speed** (needing thick screens) **and sharpness** (needing thin screens). Because of the emphasis being given new screen phosphors, it is not difficult to overlook the fact that currently available CaWO₄ screens offer a wide range of speeds. For example, Table 9–3 lists the Du Pont family of CRONEX* CaWO₄ intensifying screens which cover a range of 12 in speed.

Conversion Efficiency

In 1972, reports describing rare earth oxysulfide phosphors for use in intensifying screens were published.[9] This work was supported by a contract from the Atomic Energy Commission to the Lockheed Corporation, and this class of phosphors is sometimes referred to as the Lockheed rare earth phosphors. Rare earth intensifying screens have been commercially available since about 1973.

Chemists divide the periodic table of the elements into four basic groups: alkaline earths, rare earths, transition elements and

non-metals. The term rare earth developed because these elements are difficult and expensive to separate from the earth and each other, not because the elements are scarce. The rare earth group consists of elements of atomic number 57 (lanthanum) through 71 (lutetium), and includes gadolinium (atomic number 64) and europium (atomic number 63). Because lanthanum is the first element, the rare earth group is also known as the lanthanide series. Lanthanum (La) and gadolinium (Gd) are used in the rare earth phosphors. A related phosphor, yttrium (Y), with atomic number 39, is not a rare earth but has some properties similar to the rare earths.

The rare earth phosphors are produced as crystalline powders of **terbium-activated gadolinium oxysulfide** (Gd_2O_2S:Tb) and **terbium-activated lanthanum oxysulfide** (La_2O_2S:Tb). Unlike CaWO₄, the rare earth phosphors do not fluoresce properly in the pure state. Maximum rare-earth light production occurs when approximately 0.3 atom-per cent terbium (another rare earth) replaces lanthanum or gadolinium.

The x ray to light conversion efficiency of rare earth phosphors is significantly greater than that of CaWO₄. It is generally correct to state that the x ray to light conversion efficiency of CaWO₄ is about 5%, while that of the rare earth phosphors is about 20%. Stated another way, one absorbed x-ray photon in a CaWO₄ intensifying screen will produce about 1000 light photons, the same photon absorbed in a rare earth screen will produce about 4000 light photons. The conversion efficiency of yttrium oxysulfide screens is about the same as gadolinium. In the literature, actual conversion efficiency figures quoted are $CaWO_4$ 3–5%, La_2O_2S:Tb 13%, Gd_2O_2S:Tb 18%, Y_2O_2S:Tb 18%. The Du Pont Quanta II screen has a phosphor of barium fluorochloride, europium activated (BaFCl:Eu) which also owes a part of its increased speed to a more efficient conversion of x-ray energy to light.

*CRONEX is a trademark of E. I. du Pont de Nemours and Co.

Higher Absorption Phosphor

The fraction of the x-ray beam absorbed by a pair of par speed $CaWO_4$ screens is about 20%, high speed $CaWO_4$ screens about 40%, and rare earth screens about 60%. The increased absorption in the faster $CaWO_4$ screens occurs because a thicker screen is used; the increased absorption in rare earth screens is a result of improvement in the absorption characteristics of the phosphor.

At diagnostic x-ray energies, absorption is almost entirely due to the **photoelectric effect** in the high atomic number elements of the phosphor. As discussed in Chapter 4, a photoelectric reaction is most likely to occur: (1) in elements with high atomic numbers, and (2) when the x-ray photon energy and the binding energy of the ejected K-shell electron are almost the same.

A phosphor with a higher atomic number would have higher absorption. However, since the atomic numbers of tungsten (74) and lead (82) are almost at the end of the periodic table, the potential for this type of improvement is limited. It is interesting to note that the improvement in the input phosphor of image intensifier tubes involved a change from zinc sulfide (atomic numbers 30 and 16) to cesium iodide (atomic humbers 55 and 53). Actually, the phosphors used in the new fast intensifying screens have an atomic number lower than tungsten. Table 9–4 lists some of the elements found in in-

Figure 9–6 Approximate x-ray absorption as a function of x-ray photon energy, in keV, in a calcium tungstate intensifying screen

tensifying screens, together with their atomic number (Z) and K-shell binding energy. Figure 9–6 diagrams the approximate x-ray absorption curve of a calcium tungstate screen. Notice that the screen is less absorbing as radiation energy increases until the 70 keV K-edge of tungsten is reached. In Figure 9–7 the approximate absorption curve of $Gd_2O_2S:Tb$ is added to the $CaWO_4$ curve. Up to 50 keV both phosphors absorb about the same. But at the 50.2 keV K-edge of Gd the rare earth screen develops an advantage of 4–5× over $CaWO_4$ which per-

Table 9–4. Atomic Number and K-Shell Binding Energy of Some Screen Phosphors

ELEMENT	ATOMIC NUMBER (Z)	K-SHELL BINDING ENERGY [keV]
Yttrium (Y)	39	17.05
Barium (Ba)	56	37.4
Lanthanum (La)	57	38.9
Gadolinium (Gd)	64	50.2
Tungsten (W) (Wolfram)	74	69.5

sists until the 70 keV K-edge of W is reached. It is apparent that Gd, which has a lower atomic number than W, enjoys an absorption advantage over W in the x-ray energy range of 50–70 keV because of the differences in photoelectric absorption related to the K-shell electron binding energies of these two elements. However, in diagnostic radiology a large percentage of x rays in the beam will have an energy less than 50 keV, making the advantage of gadolinium much less. This is the reason lanthanum is added to the phosphor of some rare earth screens (such as Kodak LANEX and 3M Alpha). Lanthanum, with its K-edge at 39 keV, effectively "closes the window" between 39 and 50 keV. In Figure 9–8 the approximate x-ray absorption curves of La_2O_2S, Gd_2O_2S, and $CaWO_4$ are compared. By combining the two rare earth phosphors, the rare earth screen has a significant absorption advantage over $CaWO_4$ in the 39 to 70 keV range. Figure 9–9 shows the approximate absorption of yttrium oxysulfide (U.S. Radium Rarex B

Figure 9–8 Comparison of the approximate x-ray absorption curves of $CaWO_4$, La_2O_2S and GdO_2S

Figure 9–7 Comparison of the approximate x-ray absorption as a function of x-ray photon energy, in keV, in $CaWO_4$ and GdO_2S

screens) compared to $CaWO_4$. Notice that $CaWO_4$ and Y_2O_2S match from 17 to 70 keV. While these two phosphors absorb x-ray energy about the same, the Y_2O_2S screen produces more light photons because of its higher x ray to light conversion efficiency (18% vs. 3 to 5%). The absorption of $BaFCl$ is almost the same as La_2O_2S, showing an absorption advantage over $CaWO_4$ from 38 keV (K-edge of Ba) to 70 keV (K-edge of W).

Let us summarize this section. The K-edges of Ba, La and Gd correspond closely to the maximum intensity of x rays in the primary beam. This causes much of the energy in the primary beam to fall in the region of increased absorption for these phosphors. This is the principal reason these phosphors have higher absorption of x rays used in diagnostic radiology as compared with $CaWO_4$, even though the atomic number (Z) of tungsten (74) is higher than that of barium (56), lanthanum (57) or gadolinium (64). The absorption for yttrium (39) is the same as tungsten from 17 to 70 keV, but yttrium is

Figure 9–9 Comparison of the approximate x-ray absorption curves of CaWO$_4$ and YOS

sity on a film used to record the exposure. The relative speeds shown are in comparison to par speed calcium tungstate screens being assigned a relative speed of 4 because they are 4 times as fast as a detail CaWO$_4$ screen. Thus, a relative speed of 16 means the screen is 4 times as fast as a par speed screen (i.e., requires ¼ as much mAs) or 16 times as fast as a detail screen. This concept will be discussed again in Chapter 11. The numbers in Table 9–5 are only approximations used for a general comparison, the values applicable to an individual installation may vary significantly from these values. In Chapter 11 we will discuss the films used with these screens, and in Chapter 13 we will examine potential problems associated with very fast screens.

Emission Spectrum

This section will deal with the wavelength (color) of light emitted by the various phosphors. This is an important consideration because **one must match the light output of the screen and the maximum sensitivity of the film used.**

The spectrum of light emitted by some of the new screen phosphors is quite differ-

"faster" because of a higher conversion efficiency.

Table 9–5 is an attempt to roughly compare the relative speed of some of the new screens. Relative speed may be defined as the reciprocal of the exposure (such as mAs) required to produce a specified den-

Table 9–5. Comparison of the Relative Speed of a Variety of Screens

MANUFACTURER	SCREEN	RELATIVE SPEED
Du Pont	Detail	1
	Par	4
	Lightning Plus	12
	Quanta II	16
	Quanta III	32
Kodak	Regular	7
	Lanex	32
U.S. Radium	Rarex B	16
	Rarex BG	32
General Electric	Blue Max 2	16
3 M	Alpha 4	16
	Alpha 8	32

Table 9–6. Spectral Emission of Several Screen Phosphors

PHOSPHOR	SPECTRAL EMISSION PEAK WAVELENGTH	EXAMPLE
Tungsten	430 nm	Du Pont Cronex family U.S. Radium T-2, TF-2
Barium Lead Sulfate	360 nm	Kodak X-Omatic Fine Du Pont Hi-Speed
Barium Strontium Sulfate	380 nm	Kodak X-Omatic Regular
Barium Fluorochloride	390 nm	Du Pont Quanta II

ent from that of $CaWO_4$, which produces a continuous spectrum of light in the blue region with a peak wavelength of about 4300 Angstroms (or 430 nm, with one nanometer = .000000001 meter), shown in Figure 9–2. Some of the non-calcium tungstate phosphors also produce light in the blue-violet range. Table 9–6 lists some of these phosphors. Natural silver halide films are maximally sensitive to light of this wavelength. Figure 9–10 shows in graphic

form the approximate spectral emission of the screen phosphors listed in Table 9–6, compared to the sensitivity of natural silver halide film (such as Du Pont Cronex films and Kodak X-omat films). Keep in mind that the speed of these screens covers a wide range.

We must now consider the light emission of the two rare earth phosphors $Gd_2O_2S:Tb$ and $La_2O_2S:Tb$. The spectral emission of the rare earth phosphors is

Figure 9–10 Approximate spectral emission of several different intensifying screen phosphors compared to the natural sensitivity of silver halide

produced by the terbium ion. The terbium emission is not a continuous spectrum (as is $CaWO_4$), but is concentrated in narrow lines with a very strong peak at 544 nm which is in the green light part of the spectrum. There are less intense emission peaks in the blue, blue-green, yellow and red areas. Since standard x-ray silver halide film will not absorb (i.e., is not sensitive to) light in the green area, a special film must be used with these screens. Such films are Kodak Ortho G and 3M Trimax film Type XD and XM. This subject will be explored in more detail in Chapter 11. Figure 9–11 is a graph of the spectral emission of the Kodak LANEX regular screen (which contains both Gd_2O_2S:Tb and La_2O_2S:Tb in its phosphor) and the sensitivity of Kodak Ortho G film. Since the sensitivity of natural silver halide film stops at about 500 nm, use of this film with rare earth screens would result in loss of much of the speed of these screens because the film would be insensitive to much of the light produced.

The spectral emission of yttrium oxysulfide screens is similar to the rare earth screens in that it shows line emission, but a large fraction of the emission from a Y_2O_2S:Tb screen falls within the sensitivity range of natural silver halide films. However, the principal emission of the terbium at 544 nm is still present. Yttrium oxysulfide screens may be used with natural silver halide films, but will exhibit even more speed when used with green sensitive films.

Response to Kilovoltage

For practical purposes, the speed of a calcium tungstate intensifying screen is the same throughout the entire range of kVp used in diagnostic radiology. For many years technologists have been accustomed to making adjustments in technique kVp, knowing that screen response would always be predictable no matter what kVp was used. In comparison to this linear $CaWO_4$ response to kVp, **the kilovoltage response of rare earth and barium screens is not linear.** These screens show maximum speed at about 80 kVp, with slightly less speed at low (50 to 60 kVp) and high (over 100 kVp) kilovoltages. The need for exposure technique adjustment because of screen speed variation with kVp is not great, and is usually of little practical importance unless kVp lower than 75 is used. It is advisable to establish constant kVp (with variable mAs) exposure technique charts when using non-calcium tungstate screens.

Phototimers

Most phototimers being used today will not work well with rare earth screens. Most of these phototimers have a response time of about 30 milliseconds (i.e., it takes 30 milliseconds for the phototimer to measure the radiation and terminate the exposure). With fast screens, a response time of 3 milliseconds is recommended.[3] In addition, the phototimer must be able to recognize differences in screen speed caused by variation in kVp. If a photomultiplier type

Figure 9–11 Approximate spectral emission of the Kodak LANEX Regular screen (rare earth) compared to the sensitivity of Kodak Ortho G film (this is similar to charts supplied through the courtesy of the Eastman Kodak Company)

phototimer is used, the fluorescent screen (photocathode) used in the photomultiplier tube will probably have to be the same phosphor as used in the intensifying screen. It is also probable that ionization chamber type phototimers can be made to work satisfactorily. Use of phototimers with very fast screens will usually require special consideration, and one should plan for appropriate changes in advance.

Screen Asymmetry

Some intensifying screens, such as the Kodak LANEX Regular rare earth screens, have a thinner phosphor layer on the front screen than on the back screen. With this very fast screen a significant fraction of the incident x-ray beam is absorbed by the front screen. Thus, a thicker back screen is required if it is to absorb the same number of photons as the front screen (i.e., fewer x rays arrive at the back screen, so it must absorb a larger percentage of its part of the beam). Asymmetry also helps produce equality in sharpness of the image produced by the front and back screens. Because of the differential absorption of x rays in the thickness of the screen phosphor, more x rays are absorbed (and light produced) in that portion of the screen closest to the source of the x rays. This means that x rays absorbed by the front screen are more likely to cause light production near the base (and reflecting coat) of the screen, and this light produced deep in the phosphor will undergo significant diffusion before reaching the film. X-ray absorption in the back screen, for the same reason, will be greater nearer the film (or screen protective coat) and produce light near the outer surface of the screen which will not undergo much diffusion before reaching the film. For very fast screens, sharpness of the rear screen would be better than that of the front screen for screens of equal thickness.

To review, some companies make front and back screens asymmetrical to cause: (1) equal amounts of light production by each screen and (2) equal sharpness of the image produced by each screen.

Quantum Mottle

Quantum mottle, commonly called "noise," results from statistical fluctuation in the number of x-ray photons absorbed by the intensifying screens to form the light image which is recorded on film. With the fast screens and films now available it is possible to use a film-screen system so fast (i.e., the screen does not have to absorb many x rays) that noise makes the resulting image unsatisfactory. This subject will be reviewed in painful detail in Chapter 13. At this time, we only wish to emphasize that any discussion of fast screens demands careful evaluation of system noise. One pays a price for speed.

FLUOROSCOPIC SCREENS

The major difference between fluoroscopic and intensifying screens is related to the wavelength of the fluorescent light. The light from the fluoroscopic screen must have a wavelength corresponding to the maximum sensitivity of the eye, which is from 5000 to 6000Å. From 1914 to 1933 cadmium tungstate was the phosphor used. In 1933 the Patterson Type B fluoroscopic screen was introduced in the United States. This screen was made of zinc cadmium sulfide, silver activated. Unlike calcium tungstate, which fluoresces in the pure state, crystals of zinc cadmium sulfide will luminesce effectively only if they contain a small amount of a metallic impurity called an activator. The activator used is silver, and a change in its concentration of as little as 1 part per million may change the color of light produced. Zinc sulfide has a natural blue fluorescence, but the addition of activators and cadmium can vary this color through the entire visible-color range to red. Both zinc sulfide and zinc cadmium sulfide are efficient in converting the energy of x rays into light, with a fluorescence efficiency of about 10 to 15%. The phosphor now used in fluoroscopic screens is silver-activated zinc cadmium sulfide which is synthesized to fluoresce in the yellow-green range, with a peak at about 5300 Å. The screen is similar in physical construction to intensifying screens, but the phosphor layer is thicker, averaging 7 to 8 mils. Phosphor particle size may vary from 25 to 40 microns. The resolving power of fluoroscopic screens is no more than 3 line pairs per mm.

When a fluoroscopic screen is viewed directly, the examiner must be protected from any x rays transmitted through the screen. This protection is afforded by lead glass, which is glass containing a large proportion of lead (about 60% by weight). This glass is transparent to visible light but effectively absorbs x rays. The protection afforded by this glass is expressed as its lead equivalent. By lead equivalent is meant the thickness of lead which will produce the same degree of attenuation of the x-ray beam as the lead glass in question. The recommended lead equivalent for a fluoroscopic screen (National Council on Radiation Protection and Measurements, Report No. 33) is as follows:

"The lead equivalent of the barrier of conventional fluoroscopes shall be at least 1.5 millimeters for equipment operating up to 100 kVp, at least 1.8 millimeters for equipment whose maximum operating potential is greater than 100 kVp and less that 125 kVp, and at least 2.0 millimeters for equipment whose maximum operating potential is 125 kVp or greater."

The edges of fluoroscopic screens are sealed watertight, so these screens require little care, compared to intensifying screens.

The input screens used in some x-ray image intensifiers contain zinc cadmium sulfide as the phosphor, and are similar to fluoroscopic screens. The input screen phosphor in the new generation of image intensifiers is composed of cesium iodide. The output screen of all image intensifiers is zinc cadmium sulfide.

PHOTOFLUOROGRAPHY

Photofluorography is frequently called mass miniature radiography. This is the method usually employed in projects such as mass chest x rays for tuberculosis control. In this technique the image of a fluorescent screen is recorded on film by means of a camera. The film used is of small size. Some units use cut film 4 inches by 4 inches in size. More commonly, roll film is used; the film is usually 70-mm wide, but may be 90 or 100 mm.

Two types of fluorescent screens are used. The phosphor may be silver-activated zinc sulfide, which emits a blue light (4400 Å), or zinc cadmium sulfide (the same as a fluoroscopic screen). Particle size and phosphor thickness are about the same as those employed in fluoroscopic screens, and resolving power ranges between 2 and 5 line pairs per mm. The film emulsion used with zinc sulfide screens must be blue sensitive and that for zinc cadmium sulfide yellow-green sensitive.

SUMMARY

Intensifying screens are used in diagnostic radiology because they reduce x-ray dose to the patient. Also, the lower exposures required (less mAs) allow the shorter exposure times needed to reduce motion unsharpness. Until about 1971, calcium tungstate was the phosphor used in most screens. New technology has resulted in very fast rare earth and other phosphors. There are three ways in which screens can be made "faster":

1. Thicker phosphor layer
2. Higher conversion efficiency phosphor
3. Higher absorption phosphor

$CaWO_4$ screen speed is determined largely by thickness of the phosphor layer. The newer fast phosphors exhibit a higher conversion efficiency. Higher absorption of x rays in the diagnostic range is a function of the matching of the K-absorption edge of the screen phosphor to the energy spectrum in the x-ray beam. The spectral emission of some phosphors requires that an appropriately sensitized film be used, or much of the light will be wasted. Intensifying screens are usually used in pairs, with a double emulsion x-ray film sandwiched between the two screens in a light-tight cassette. System noise becomes important when the fastest film-screen systems are used.

A fluoroscopic screen converts the x-ray image into light to be viewed by the eye and must fluoresce with a yellow-green light to which the eye is most sensitive. The phosphor used is silver-activated zinc cadmium sulfide. The input screen for the new generation of x-ray image intensifiers is cesium iodide.

REFERENCES

1. Alves, R. V. and Buchanan, R. A.: Properties of Y_2O_2S:Tb x-ray intensifying screens. Paper presented at the IEEE meeting in Miami, Dec. 1972. Lockheed Palo Alto Research Laboratory, Palo Alto, California 94304.
2. Balter, S., and Laughlin, J. S.: A photographic method for the evaluation of the conversion efficiency of fluoroscopic screens. Radiol. *86*, 145, 1966.
3. Bates, L. M.: Properties of radiographic films and intensifying screens which influence the efficacy of a film-screen combination. Contained in the syllabus of the joint BRH-ACR Conference "First Image Receptor Conference: Film/Screen Combinations," at Arlington, Virginia, Nov. 13–15, 1975. HEW Publication (FDA) 77–8003, p. 123.
4. Buchanan, R. A., Finkelstein, S. I., and Wickersheim, K. A.: X-ray exposure reduction using rare-earth oxysulfide intensifying screens. Radiol. *105*, 185, 1972.
5. Castle, J. W.: Sensitivity of radiographic screens to scattered radiation and its relationship to image contrast. Radiol. *122*, 805, 1977.
6. Coltman, J. W., Ebbighausen, E. G., and Alter, W.: Physical properties of calcium tungstate x-ray screens. J. Appl. Physics *18*, 530, 1947.
7. Holland, R. S.: Image Analysis. Contained in the syllabus of the AAPM 1975 Summer School, "The Expanding Role of the Diagnostic Radiologic Physicist", Rice University, Houston, Texas. July 27–Aug. 1, 1975, p. 103.
8. Lawrence, D. J.: Kodak X-OMATIC and LANEX screens and Kodak films for medical radiography. Radiography Markets Division, Eastman Kodak Company File No. 5.03, June 1976.
9. Ludwig, G. W. and Prener, J. S.: Evaluation of Gd_2O_2S:Tb as a phosphor for the input screen of x-ray image intensifier. IEEE Tran. N S 19, 3, 1972.
10. Meredith, W. J., and Massey, J. B.: *Fundamental Physics of Radiology*. Baltimore: Williams & Wilkins, 1968.
11. Morgan, R. H.: Characteristics of x-ray films and screens. Radiol. *49*, 90, 1947.
12. Patterson, C. V. S.: Roentgenography: fluoroscopic and intensifying screens (In) *Medical Physics*, Vol. 2. (O. Glasser, ed.) Chicago: Year Book Medical Publishers, 1950.
13. Patterson, C. V. S.: Roentgenography: fluoroscopic and intensifying screens (In) *Medical Physics*, Vol. 3. (O. Glasser, ed.) Chicago: Year Book Medical Publishers, 1960.
14. Patterson X-ray Screens: Sales Manual for Du Pont Patterson X-ray Screen Dealers. Wilmington, Del.: Photo Products Department, E. I. du Pont de Nemours and Co., Inc., 1952.
15. Properzio, W. S., and Trout, E. D.: The deterioration of x-ray fluoroscopic screens. Radiol. *91*, 439, 1968.
16. Roth, B.: X-ray Intensifying Screens. Contained in the syllabus of the AAPM 1975 Summer School, "The Expanding Role of the Diagnostic Radiologic Physicist", Rice University, Houston, Texas. July 27–Aug. 1, 1975, p. 120.
17. Stevels, A. L. N.: New phosphors for x-ray screens. Medicamundi *20*, 12, 1975.
18. Ter-Pogossian, M.: The efficiency of radiographic intensifying screens (In) *Technological Needs for Reduction of Patient Dosage from Diagnostic Radiology*. (M. L. Janower, ed.) Springfield: Charles C Thomas, 1963.
19. Thompson, T. T., Radford, E. L. and Kirby, C. C.: A look at rare-earth and high-speed intensifying screens. Applied Radiol. *6*, 71, 1977.

CHAPTER 10

Physical Characteristics of
X-ray Film and Film Processing

When an x-ray beam reaches the patient, it contains no useful medical information. After the beam passes through and interacts with the tissues in the part examined, it contains all the information which that particular radiographic examination can possess. This information is represented by variation in the number of x-ray photons in different areas of the emergent beam. We are unable to make direct use of the information in this form and must transfer it to a medium suitable for viewing by the eye. The method of transfer might involve a magnetic tape or disc, a fluoroscopic screen, or xerography. However, by far the most important material used to "decode" the information carried by the attenuated x-ray beam is photographic film. The film may be exposed by the direct action of x rays. More commonly, however, the energy of the x-ray beam is converted into light by intensifying screens, and this light is used to expose the film.

It is unfortunate that the transfer of information from the x-ray beam to the screen-film combination always results in a loss of information. In reviewing x-ray film, we must examine both the film and the various factors which influence the amount of information lost in the transfer process.

Figure 10–1 Cross-section of a double emulsion x-ray film

FILM

X-ray film is photographic film consisting of a photographically active, or radiation-sensitive, emulsion which is usually coated on both sides of a transparent sheet of plastic called the base. Firm attachment between the emulsion layer and the film base is achieved by a thin layer of adhesive. The delicate emulsion is protected from mechanical damage by layers known as the supercoating (Figure 10–1).

Film Base

The only function of the film base is to provide a support for the fragile photographic emulsion. Three characteristics of the base must be considered. First, it must not produce a visible pattern or absorb too much light when the radiograph is viewed. Second, the flexibility, thickness, and

Figure 10–2 Wrinkled emulsion resulting from shrinking of the film base

strength of the base must allow for ease of processing (developing) and produce a radiograph that "feels right" when handled (a film too "floppy" to "snap" under the hangers of a viewbox gets a cool reception). Third, the base must have **dimensional stability;** that is, the shape and size of the base must not change during the developing process or during the stored life of the film. Figure 10–2 illustrates a radiograph in which the base has slowly diminished in size over a period of 22 years. Notice how shrinking of the base has thrown the unshrinking emulsion into folds, producing a wrinkled appearance.

Original x-ray "plates" consisted of a glass plate with the emulsion coated on one side. It is no longer possible to make a "flat plate of the abdomen," because x-ray plates are not available. The onset of World War I cut off the supply of photographic glass from Belgium and additionally created a demand for a less fragile x-ray film for use by the

Army. Cellulose nitrate, previously used as a base for photographic film, was adapted to x-ray film in 1914. However, cellulose nitrate is quite flammable, and several fires were caused by improper handling and storage of the film. Because of this fire hazard a new "safety-base" film was urgently sought, and in 1924 a "safety" film with a cellulose triacetate base was developed. This **acetate**-base safety film (cellulose acetate will burn if held directly in a flame) is still widely used. In 1960, the first medical radiographic film using a polyester base was introduced. **Polyester** as a film base offers the advantage of improved dimensional stability, even when stored under conditions of varying humidity, and it is much stronger than acetate.

What is polyester? It is similar to Dacron* polyester fiber used in clothing. The raw materials, dimethyl terephthalate (DMT) and ethylene glycol, are brought together under conditions of low pressure and high temperature to form a molten polymer which is then literally stretched into sheets of appropriate size and thickness to form film base. Cronex* film, manufactured by E. I. du Pont de Nemours and Co. is an example of a polyester-base film, and the characteristics of polyester may be appreciated by examining a piece of "cleared" Cronex film.

Triacetate and polyester bases are clear and colorless. In 1933 the first commercialized blue tint was added to x-ray film in an effort to produce a film that was "easier" to look at, causing less eyestrain. Present x-ray film is tinted blue. The blue dye may be added to the film base or to the emulsion.

Triacetate base is about $8/1000$ inch (8 mils) thick, and polyester base is 7 mils thick. The slightly thinner polyester base has handling properties approximately equal to the thicker acetate.

Photographic emulsion would not adhere to the finished base if applied

*Dacron and Cronex are trademarks of E. I. du Pont de Nemours and Co., Inc.

directly. Therefore, a thin layer of adhesive substance is applied to the base to insure perfect union between base and emulsion.

Emulsion

The two most important ingredients of a photographic emulsion are **gelatin** and **silver halide.** The exact composition of the various emulsions is a closely guarded industrial secret. Most x-ray film is made for use with intensifying screens, and has emulsion coated on both sides of the base. Emulsion thickness will vary with film type but is usually no thicker than 0.5 mil. A thicker emulsion would not be useful because of the inability of light to penetrate to the deeper layers.

Gelatin

Photographic gelatin for x-ray film is made from bone, mostly cattle bone from India and Argentina. (Useless information: India and Argentina do not have better cows, but they have a lot of them. They also have inexpensive labor to process the bones.) Gelatin satisfies several exacting requirements better than any other suspension medium. It keeps the silver halide grains well dispersed and prevents the clumping of grains. Processing (developing and fixing) solutions can penetrate gelatin rapidly without destroying its strength or permanence, and gelatin is available in reasonably large quantity and uniform quality.

Silver Halide

Silver halide is the light-sensitive material in the emulsion. The halide in medical x-ray film is about 90 to 99% silver bromide and about 1 to 10% silver iodide (the presence of AgI produces an emulsion of much higher sensitivity than a pure AgBr emulsion). The silver iodo-bromide crystals are precipitated and emulsified in the gelatin under exacting conditions of concentration and temperature, as well as the sequence and the rate at which these chemicals are added. The method of precipitation determines crystal size, structural perfection, and the concentration of iodine. In general, the precipitation reaction involves the addition of silver nitrate to a soluble halide to form the slightly soluble silver halide:

$$AgNO_3 + KBr \longrightarrow AgBr + KNO_3$$

The silver halide in a photographic emulsion is in the form of small **crystals** suspended in the gelatin. The crystal is formed from ions of silver (Ag^+), ions of bromine (Br^-) and ions of iodine (I^-) arranged in a cubic lattice (Figure 10–3). These grains, or crystals, in a medical x-ray film emulsion are small, but still relatively large compared to fine-grain photographic emulsions. Crystal size might average 1.0

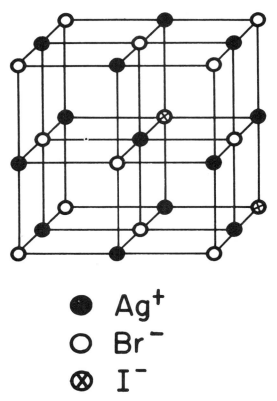

● Ag^+

○ Br^-

⊗ I^-

Figure 10–3 The silver iodo-bromide crystal lattice

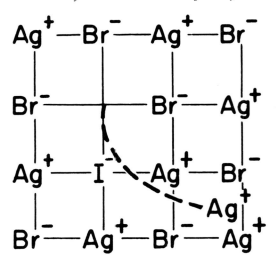

Figure 10–4   A point defect

to begin formation of the latent-image centers.

Latent Image

Metallic silver is black. It is silver which produces the dark areas seen on a developed radiograph. We must explain how exposure of the sensitized silver iodobromide grains in the film emulsion to light (from x-ray intensifying screens), or to the direct action of x rays, initiates the formation of atomic silver to form a pattern. The energy absorbed from a light photon gives an electron in the bromine ion enough energy to escape. The electron can move in the crystal for relatively large distances, so long as it does not encounter a region of impurity or fault in the crystal.

$$Br^- + \text{light photon} \longrightarrow Br + \text{electron}$$

A site of crystal imperfection, such as a dislocation defect, or an AgS sensitivity speck, may act as an electron trap where the electron is captured and temporarily fixed. The electron gives the sensitivity speck a negative charge, and this attracts the mobile interstitial Ag+ ions in the crystal. At the speck, the silver ion is neutralized by the electron to form a single silver atom.

$$Ag^+ + \text{electron} \longrightarrow Ag$$

This single atom of silver then acts as an electron trap for a second electron. The negative charge causes a second silver ion to migrate to the trap to form a two-atom silver nucleus. Growth of silver atoms at the site of the original sensitivity speck continues by repeated trapping of electrons and then neutralizing them with interstitial silver ions. The negative bromine ions that have lost electrons are converted into neutral bromine atoms which leave the crystal and are taken up by the gelatin of the emulsion. Figure 10–5 shows a schematic diagram of the development of a two-atom latent image according to the Gurney-Mott hypothesis.[6]

to 1.5 microns (1 micron = .001 millimeter) in diameter with about 6.3×10^9 grains per cubic centimeter of emulsion, and each grain contains an average of 1,000,000 to 10,000,000 silver ions.

The silver iodo-bromide grain is not a perfect crystal because a perfect crystal has almost no photographic sensitivity. There are several types of crystal defects. A point defect consists of a silver ion which has moved out of its normal position in the crystal lattice; these interstitial silver ions may move in the crystal (Figure 10–4). A dislocation is a line imperfection in the crystal, and may be thought of as a brick wall which contains one row in which the bricks are not the same size as all the other bricks, thus causing a strain in the wall structure. This may be the way in which the iodine ion strains the crystal.

Chemical sensitization of a crystal has several forms. Commonly, this is produced by adding a sulfur-containing compound, such as allylthiourea, to the emulsion which reacts with silver halide to form silver sulfide. The silver sulfide is usually located on the surface of the crystal and is referred to as the **sensitivity speck.** It is the sensitivity speck which traps electrons

Figure 10–5   Formation of the latent image

A single silver halide crystal may have one or many of these centers in which atomic silver atoms are concentrated. The presence of atomic silver is a direct result of the response of the grain to light exposure, but no visible change has occurred in the grain. However, these small clumps of silver can be seen with electron microscopy. These clumps of silver atoms are termed **latent-image centers** and are the sites at which the developing process will cause visible amounts of metallic silver to be deposited. The difference between an emulsion grain that will react with the developing solution and thus become a visible silver deposit and a grain that will not be "developed" is the presence of one or more latent-image centers in the exposed grain. At least two atoms of silver must be present at a latent-image center to make a grain developable; i.e., to become a visible deposit of silver. In practical terms, however, the minimum number to produce developability is probably between three and six. The more silver atoms which exist at a latent-image center, the greater is the probability that the grain will be developed. Some centers will contain several hundred silver atoms. Under the usual conditions, the absorption of one quantum of light by a silver halide grain will produce one atom of silver and one of bromine.

Direct X-ray Exposure

The photographic effect of direct absorption of x rays by the emulsion is not due to electromagnetic radiation itself, but it is caused by electrons emitted when the x-ray photon interacts with the silver halide in the emulsion. These electrons are derived from photoelectric absorption or Compton scattering and have rather long ranges in the emulsion. In fact, an electron produced in this way may react with many grains in an emulsion. The manner in which the energy of the electrons is imparted to the photographic emulsion is complex and will not be considered in detail. However, the final result is to free electrons from the bromide ion, producing bromine atoms and an electron which can move to a trapping site and begin the process of latent-image formation. The energy of one absorbed x-ray photon can produce thousands of silver atoms at latent-image sites in one or several grains. Even this large number of silver atoms is low considering the energy of the absorbed photon. Most of the energy of the absorbed photon is lost in processes which do not produce any photographic effect (such as losses to gelatin). Only 3 to 10% of the photon energy is used to produce photolytic silver. The photographic effect of direct x-ray exposure on an emulsion can be increased by a factor of almost 100 by proper chemical sensitization of the emulsion.

The sensitivity of film to direct x-ray exposure varies markedly (by a factor of 20 to 50) with the energy (kVp) of the x-ray beam. This x-ray spectral sensitivity is most important when considering use of film to measure x-ray exposure dose; i.e., film badge monitoring. Above 50 kVp, the efficiency with which absorbed x-ray photons are utilized to produce a photographic effect decreases significantly with increasing photon energy. At about 50 kVp, the average keV of the x rays produced will be close to the K-shell binding energy of silver (25.5 keV) and bromine (13.5 keV). This

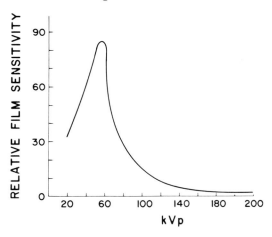

Figure 10–6   Film sensitivity varies with radiation quality

will cause the film to exhibit maximum photoelectric absorption of 50-kVp x rays. Figure 10–6 shows, in a rough graphic form, the way in which the x-ray sensitivity of film varies with kVp.

The sensitivity also varies greatly with the way in which the film is developed. The amount of blackening (density) on the developed film may be used as an indication of how much x-ray exposure (i.e., how many milliroentgens) the film has received. However, because the sensitivity of the film varies greatly with the energy (kVp) of the x rays, blackening of a simple piece of film does not give an accurate estimation of the exposure to which the film has been subjected. For example, a film subjected to an exposure of 50 mR at an x-ray energy of 50 kVp will, after development, exhibit a much higher density (amount of blackening) than will an identical film subjected to an exposure of 50 mR by 200-kVp x rays. The problem of variation of film sensitivity with radiation energy is partially solved by placing various metal filters in front of the film in an attempt to control the energy (kVp) of the x rays which reach different areas of the film. The accuracy of film badge monitoring of x-ray exposure is about ±20%. Film badge monitoring of personnel exposure offers several advantages over other methods, such as ionization chambers. The film badge provides a permanent record, it is small in size and weight, rugged and inexpensive.

Supercoating

Covering the emulsion is a thin layer, commonly gelatin, which serves to protect the emulsion from mechanical damage. In special types of film this supercoat, or antiabrasive coating, may contain substances which make the film surface smooth and slick. This is a desirable quality in film which must be transported through a cut-film rapid film changer.

FILM PROCESSING

Development

Development is a chemical process which amplifies the latent image by a factor of millions (about 100,000,000) to form a visible pattern of silver. The basic reaction is reduction (addition of an electron) of the silver ion which changes it into black metallic silver:

$$Ag^+ + e \longrightarrow Ag$$

The developer is the reducing agent. Development is generally an all or none phenomenon, an entire grain is developed (reduced) once the process begins. The process is usually initiated at the site of a latent-image speck (commonly on the surface of the grain). It is believed that the action of the silver atoms in the latent image is to accelerate (catalyze) the reduction of the silver ions in the grain by the developing chemicals. The silver in a grain which does not contain a latent image can be reduced by the developer, but at a much slower rate. Thus, **time is a fundamental factor in the developing process.** Development should be discontinued when the differential between exposed, developed grains and unexposed, undeveloped grains is at a maximum.

The developing solution contains two developing agents, either hydroquinone and metol (Elon* is the same agent as metol) or hydroquinone and phenidone. Two agents are used because of the phenomenon of **synergism,** or superadditivity. The mixture results in a development rate greater than the sum of the developing rate of each developing agent. Recently the hydroquinone-phenidone combination has become more important because the speed of this combination is of value in rapid (90 sec) processing of film. The reasons for development synergism are complex and not fully understood, so we will not explore the details.

The chemistry of developing is not our chief interest, but the formulas for the basic reactions help in gaining a good understanding of the process. The developing agent reduces silver ions to metallic silver, causing oxidation and inactivation of the developing agent and the liberation of hydrogen ions. For example:

* Elon is a trademark of Eastman Kodak Co.

| Developer (Hydroquinone) | + | Silver Ions | ⟶ | Oxidized Developer (Quinone) | + | Silver Atoms | + | Hydrogen Ions |

Developer + Silver ⟶ Oxidized + Silver + Hydrogen
(Phenidone) + Ions ⟶ Developer + Atoms + Ions

Notice that the reaction must proceed in an alkaline solution. When hydroquinone is oxidized to quinone, two electrons are liberated to combine with the two silver ions to form metallic silver. The reaction of phenidone is similar (see diagram).

The silver which is formed is deposited at the latent-image site, gradually enlarging this initially microscopic black spot into a single visible black speck of silver in the emulsion.

In addition to **developing agents,** the developing solution contains (1) an **alkali** to adjust the pH, (2) a **preservative** (sodium sulfite), and (3) **restrainers,** or antifoggants.

The **alkali** adjusts the hydrogen ion concentration, which greatly affects the developing power of the developing agents, especially hydroquinone. In addition, the alkali serves as a buffer to control the hydrogen ions liberated during the development reaction. Most radiographic developers function at a pH range of 10 to 11.5. Typical alkalies include sodium hydroxide, sodium carbonate, and borates (sodium metaborate and sodium tetraborate).

Sodium sulfite is added for two reasons. The oxidation products of the developing agents decompose in alkaline solution and form colored materials which can stain the emulsion. These products react rapidly with sodium sulfite to form a colorless, soluble substance. In addition, sodium sulfite acts as a preservative. In alkaline solution, the developing agent will react with oxygen from the air. The sulfite acts as a preservative by decreasing the rate of oxidation, especially of hydroquinone.

Fog is defined as the **development of unexposed silver halide grains** which do not contain a latent image. In a complex manner, dilute concentrations of soluble bromide (potassium bromide) decrease the rate of fog formation. To a lesser degree the bromide also decreases the rate of development of the latent image. Phenidone is not as sensitive to bromide concentration as metol. With phenidone developers an organic restrainer must also be added to prevent the developing of unexposed grains by this active developing agent.

The bromide ions released by the reduction of silver ions to silver atoms pass into the developing solution. In large part, it is this increase in bromide concentration that limits the life of developing solutions.

Replenishment

We have seen that, during use, developing solutions consume developing agents and preservatives, but acquire hydrogen ions and bromide ions. Replenishing solutions which are used to maintain the activity of the developer must be free of bromide, contain alkaline agents and buffers, and to a lesser extent, restore depleted preservative and developing agents.

Fixing

Only part of the silver halide in the emulsion is reduced to silver during developing. The remaining silver halide impairs both the immediate usefulness and permanence of the developed radiograph. Therefore, it must be removed, but the fixing solution must remove silver halide without damaging the image formed by metallic silver.

The solubility of silver halide (we will use silver bromide as an example) in a water solution is controlled by the concentration of silver and halide ions. Silver bromide is only slightly soluble in water. The product of the silver and bromide ions in solution is always constant for any given temperature and may be expressed by the equation:

Silver ion × Bromide ion = Constant

If the concentration of silver ions could be reduced, the concentration of bromide ions would have to increase, which means that more silver bromide would have to dissolve from the emulsion. Thus, the solubility of silver halide would increase. The function of the fixing agent is to form water-soluble complexes in which silver ions are tightly bound. The soluble complex so formed effectively removes silver ion from solution.

Two agents form satisfactory stable complexes with silver ions: cyanides and thiosulfates. Cyanides are poisonous and not generally used. **Thiosulfate** in the form of the sodium or ammonium salt is the common fixing agent or "hypo." Why is it called hypo? In earlier chemical nomenclature, the compound we call sodium thiosulfate ($Na_2S_2O_3$) was given the name hyposulfite of soda, and "hypo" it remains to photographers. At least three silver thiosulfate complexes are formed in the fixing solution; their identities need not concern us. A typical reaction might be:

Silver Bromide + Sodium Thiosulfate $\longrightarrow$ Silver Thiosulfate Complex + Sodium Bromide

The ammonium thiosulfate salt is the more active and is used in fixer supplied as a liquid concentrate.

In addition to thiosulfate, the fixing solution contains a substance to harden the gelatin. Hardening results in a decrease in the swelling of gelatin, making it tougher and more resistant to abrasion. The hardener is usually a chromium or aluminum compound. The fixing bath also contains an acid, stabilizers, and a buffer to maintain the acid pH level.

An incompletely fixed film is easily recognized because it has a "milky" or cloudy appearance. This is a result of the dispersion of transmitted light by the very small silver iodo-bromide crystals which have not been dissolved from the emulsion.

Washing

After developing and fixing, the film must be well washed with water. Washing serves primarily to remove the fixing-bath chemicals. Everyone has seen an x-ray film which has turned brown with age. This is the result of incomplete washing. Retained hypo will react with the silver image to form brown silver sulfide, just as silverware acquires a brown tarnish when exposed to the hydrogen sulfide produced by cooking gas. The general reaction is:

Hypo + Silver $\longrightarrow$ Silver Sulfide (Brown) + Sodium Sulfite

SUMMARY

X-ray film is a photographic film coated with emulsion on both sides of the film base. The light-sensitive material in the emulsion is a silver iodo-bromide crystal. X-ray film is only slightly sensitive to direct x-ray exposure. It is designed to be most sensitive to light in the blue-violet spectrum, which is the light emitted by calcium tungstate intensifying screens. Impurities in the silver halide crystal structure increase the light sensitivity of the film emulsion. Light, or x-ray, exposure causes the grains in the emulsion to develop an invisible latent image. The developing process magnifies the latent image to produce a visible pattern of black metallic silver.

The sensitivity of x-ray film to direct x-ray exposure varies with the kVp of the x-ray beam.

REFERENCES

1. Baines, H., and Bomback, E.S.: *The Science of Photography.* 2nd ed. London: Fountain Press, 1967.

2. Fuchs, A.W.: Evolution of roentgen film. Amer. J. Roentgen. *75,* 30, 1956.

3. James, T.H., and Higgins, G.C.: *Fundamentals of Photographic Theory.* 2nd ed. New York: Morgan and Morgan, Inc., 1968.

4. Martin, F.C., and Fuchs, A.W.: The historical evolution of roentgen-ray plates and films. Amer. J. Roentgen. *26,* 540, 1931.

5. Mees, C.E.K., and James, T.H.: *The Theory of the Photographic Process.* 3rd ed. New York: The Macmillan Co., 1969.

6. Neblette, C.B.: *Photography, Its Materials and Processes.* 6th ed. New York: Van Nostrand, 1962.

CHAPTER 11

Photographic Characteristics of X-ray Film

INTRODUCTION

The diagnostic accuracy of a radiographic film examination depends, in part, on the visibility of diagnostically important information on the film. Understanding the relationship between the exposure a film receives and the way the film responds to the exposure is essential to intelligent selection of proper exposure factors and type of film to provide maximum information content of the radiograph.

What is meant by the term "exposure" of an x-ray film or film-screen combination? Exposure is proportional to the product of the milliamperes of x-ray tube current and the exposure time. Thus, an exposure of 100 milliamperes for 1 second is expressed as 100 milliampere-seconds, usually written 100 mAs. An exposure of 100 mAs could also be produced by using 50-mA tube current for 2 seconds, 200 mA for ½ second, 500 mA for ⅕ second, etc. In this chapter, film exposure is assumed to mean exposure of the x-ray film by light from x-ray intensifying screens unless otherwise stated.

Exposure (mAs) of the x-ray film produces film blackening, or density. The quality of the x-ray beam (kVp) has more effect on image contrast. Two general, but not completely accurate, statements should be kept in mind:

mAs controls film density.
kVp controls image contrast.

This chapter will amplify the topic of the response of the x-ray film to exposure.

PHOTOGRAPHIC DENSITY

When the x-ray beam passes through body tissues, variable fractions of the beam will be absorbed, depending on the composition and thickness of the tissues and the quality (kVp) of the beam. The magnitude of this variation in beam intensity is the mechanism by which the x-ray beam acquires the information which it transmits to the film. This pattern of varying x-ray intensity has been called the x-ray image. Webster's Collegiate Dictionary defines an image as "a mental representation of anything not actually present to the senses." This definition is particularly applicable to the idea of the x-ray image. The x-ray image actually exists in space, but it cannot be seen or otherwise detected by the natural senses. The x-ray image is the pattern of information that the x-ray beam acquires as it passes through and interacts with the patient; i.e., the beam is attenuated by the patient. The x-ray image is present in the space between the patient and the x-ray film (or x-ray intensifying screen). The information content of the x-ray image must be transformed into a visible image on the x-ray film with as little loss of information as possible. We have seen how the energy of the x-ray beam may be used to produce a visible pattern of black metallic silver on the x-ray film, the degree

137

$$\text{DENSITY} = \text{LOG}_{10}\frac{I_o}{I_t}$$

Figure 11–1   Photographic density

of film blackening being directly related to the intensity of radiation reaching the film or intensifying screen. The measurement of film blackness is called photographic density; usually, only the word **density** is used. Density is expressed as a number. This number is actually a **logarithm,** using the common base 10. Photographic density is defined by an equation:

$$D = \text{Log}\frac{I_0}{I_t}$$

Where D is density, I_0 is light incident on a film and I_t is light transmitted by the film. Refer to Figure 11-1. If 10 arrows (photons) of light strike the back of the film, and only 1 photon passes through the film, then, $I_0 = 10$ and $I_t = 1$:

$$\text{Density} = \text{Log}\frac{10}{1} = \text{Log } 10 = 1$$

Note that $\dfrac{I_0}{I_t}$ measures the **opacity** of the film (the ability of film to stop light). The reciprocal of density, $\dfrac{I_t}{I_0}$, measures the fraction of light transmitted by the film and is called **transmittance.** Useful densities in diagnostic radiology range from about 0.3

(50% of light transmitted) to about 2 (1% of light transmitted). A density of 2 means that $\log\dfrac{I_0}{I_t} = 2$. Since the log of 100 = 2, $\dfrac{I_0}{I_t} = 100$. Thus, for every 100 light photons incident on the film, only 1 photon, or 1%, will be transmitted.

Table 11-1 lists some common values for opacity $\left(\dfrac{I_0}{I_t}\right)$, density $\left(\text{Log}\dfrac{I_0}{I_t}\right)$, and the percent of light transmission. Note that an increase in film density of 0.3 decreases transmitted light to one-half its previous value. For example, an increase in density from 0.6 to 0.9 decreases the percent of transmitted light from 25 to 12.5%. This emphasizes the fact that the number used to signify a certain density has no units, but is a logarithm. The number 0.3 is the logarithm of 2. Thus, an increase in density of 0.3 $\left(\text{Log}\dfrac{I_0}{I_t}\right)$ means an increase in opacity $\left(\dfrac{I_0}{I_t}\right)$ of 2; opacity is doubled by a density increase of 0.3.

Higher density means a blacker film (less light transmission). In routine x-ray work, a density of 2 (1% of light transmitted) is black when viewed on a standard viewbox,

Table 11–1. Percentage of Light Transmitted by X-Ray Films of Various Densities

OPACITY $\frac{I_0}{I_t}$	DENSITY $\text{Log}\frac{I_0}{I_t}$	PERCENT OF LIGHT TRANSMITTED
1	0	100
2	0.3	50
4	0.6	25
8	0.9	12.5
10	1.0	10
30	1.5	3.2
100	2	1
1,000	3	0.1
10,000	4	0.01

and a density of 0.25 to 0.3 (50% of light transmitted) is very light.

If an unexposed x-ray film is processed, it will demonstrate a density of about 0.12. This density consists of base density and fog. The plastic material used to make the film base absorbs a small amount of light. Also, the blue dye used to color some film base adds slightly to base density. Total base density will average about 0.07. A few of the silver halide grains in an x-ray film emulsion develop without exposure. These unexposed, but developed, grains comprise the density known as fog. Fog density of a fresh x-ray film averages about 0.05. We will refer to the subject of base and fog density several times in this chapter and in Chapter 13.

Why is density expressed as a logarithm? There are three primary reasons. First, logarithms conveniently express large differences in numbers on a small scale. For example, the difference in the light transmission represented by going from density = 1 (10% of light transmitted) to density = 2 (1% of light transmitted), is a factor of 10.

Second, the physiological response of the eye to differences in light intensities is logarithmic (Figure 11–2). Assume that a film having regions of density which equal 0.3, 0.6, and 0.9 is transilluminated by a

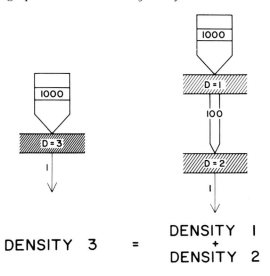

$$\text{DENSITY } 3 = \begin{matrix} \text{DENSITY } 1 \\ + \\ \text{DENSITY } 2 \end{matrix}$$

Figure 11–3 The density of superimposed films is the sum of the density of the individual films

light source of 1000 photons. The number of light photons transmitted will be 500, 250, and 125 respectively. The difference in transmitted light photons between density 0.3 and density 0.6 is 250 (500 to 250), but between density 0.6 and density 0.9 is only 125 photons (250 to 125). However, the eye will interpret density 0.3 as being exactly as much brighter than density 0.6, as density 0.6 is brighter than density 0.9. The eye has "seen" the equal differences in density rather than the unequal differences in the number of light photons transmitted.

The third reason for expressing density as a logarithm deals with the addition or superimposition of densities. If films are superimposed, the resulting density is equal to the sum of the density of each film. Assume two films, one of density 2 and one of density 1, which are superimposed and put in the path of a light source with an intensity of 1000 units (Figure 11–3). The film of density 1 absorbs 90% of the light (100 units are transmitted) and the film of density 2 absorbs 99% of these 100 units to finally allow 1 unit of light to be transmitted. We started with 1000 units

INCIDENT LIGHT (I_o)

X-RAY FILM

TRANSMITTED LIGHT (I_t)

	A	B	C
	D=0.3	D=0.6	D=0.9

$$\frac{I_o}{I_t} \qquad \frac{1000}{500} = 2 \quad \frac{1000}{250} = 4 \quad \frac{1000}{125} = 8$$

$$\log \frac{I_o}{I_t} = \text{DENSITY} \quad \log 2 = 0.3 \quad \log 4 = 0.6 \quad \log 8 = 0.9$$

Figure 11–2 The reduction in intensity caused by three films having densities of 0.3, 0.6, and 0.9

(I_0 = 1000) and ended with 1 unit of light (I_t = 1), so we may calculate density:

$$D = Log \frac{I_0}{I_t} = Log \frac{1000}{1} = 3$$

The effect of superimposing films with a density of 2 and 1 is the same as using a single film of density 3. Almost all the film used in radiology has two emulsions, one on each side of the base. The total density exhibited by the radiograph is the sum of the density of each emulsion.

CHARACTERISTIC CURVE

It is necessary to understand the relationship between the exposure a film receives and the density produced by the exposure. The relationship between exposure and density is plotted as a curve, known as the characteristic curve or H and D curve (named after F. Hurter and V. C. Driffield, who first published such a curve in England in 1890). The concept of the characteristic curve of an x-ray film exposed by light from x-ray intensifying screens is illustrated in Figure 11-4. Film density is plotted on the vertical axis, and the film exposure on the horizontal axis. The shape and location of this curve on the graph are important and will, we hope, take on some meaning as this chapter progresses.

Characteristic curves are derived by giving a film a series of exposures, developing the film, and plotting the resulting density against the known exposure. The actual exposure the film received may be measured in the laboratory, but such measurements are not of importance in the use and understanding of the characteristic curve (using medium-speed intensifying screens and 80-kVp x rays, a density of 1.0 on the x-ray film requires that about 3×10^4 x-ray photons hit each square mm of the screen). By **film exposure** we refer to the product of the intensity of the exposure (milliamperes of x-ray tube current) and time of exposure expressed in seconds. Exposure is expressed in terms of

Figure 11–4   Typical characteristic curve of a screen-type x-ray film, exposed with x-ray intensifying screens

milliampere-seconds, usually abbreviated mAs. One way to produce a characteristic curve is to expose different areas of a film with constant kilovoltage and milliamperage, while varying the time of exposure (e.g., with constant kVp and mA, doubling the time of exposure will double the mAs). The exposure is recorded as the relative exposure. The term **relative exposure** tends to create confusion. Actually, the radiologist and his technologist think in terms of relative exposure when evaluating radiographs. For example, if a radiograph of the abdomen exposed with factors of 70 kVp and 75 mAs is judged to be underexposed, the correction might involve increasing the mAs to 150. In other words, the correction involves doubling the exposure. The actual exposure (such as the number of milliroentgens or the number of x-ray photons per square mm) is not known, and need not be known. The relationship between the two exposures is

Figure 11–5 The relationship between relative exposure and the corresponding log relative exposure

important. One function of the characteristic curve is to allow one to predict how much change is necessary to correct an exposure error. For example, if a film with the characteristic curve shown in Figure 11-5 is underexposed, so that its average density is 0.35, the corresponding relative exposure is 4. If the exposure (mAs) is doubled (relative exposure is increased to 8), it can be predicted that average density will increase to about 0.8. The exposure is also recorded as the logarithm of the relative exposure. This is mainly for two reasons. First, use of a logarithmic scale allows a very wide range of exposures to be expressed in a compact graph. Second, use of log relative exposure makes analysis of the curve easier. Two exposures whose ratio is constant (e.g., one is twice the other) will always be separated by the same distance on the exposure scale, regardless of their absolute value. Refer to Figure 11-5, in which both the relative exposure and the log relative exposure are indi-

cated, and note that **an increase in the log relative exposure of 0.3 always represents a doubling of the relative exposure.**

Analysis of the characteristic curve of a particular x-ray film will give us information about the contrast, speed (sensitivity), and latitude of the film. First, note the following in Figure 11–6. Even at 0 exposure, the film density is not 0, but will usually be 0.2, or less. This density is made up by fog (development of unexposed grains of silver halide in the emulsion) and base density (opacity of the film base) which have been previously discussed. Therefore, total density on an exposed and developed film will include base and fog density. The minimum density caused by base and fog in a "fresh" film is about 0.12. To evaluate density produced by the exposure alone, one must subtract base and fog density from the total density. Second, note that at low density (toe) and at high density (shoulder), the film shows little change in density despite a relatively large change in log relative exposure

Figure 11–6 The regions of the characteristic curve

(Figure 11–6). The important part of the characteristic curve is between the toe and shoulder, and in this region the curve is almost a straight line. In this "straight line" portion, the density is approximately proportional to the log relative exposure. For example, if log relative exposure 1.1 produces a density of 1.0, and log relative exposure 1.3 produces a density of 2.0, we can predict that a density of about 1.5 will be produced by a log relative exposure of 1.2 (these figures correspond roughly to the characteristic curve of Figure 11–6).

Film Contrast

The information content of the invisible x-ray image is "decoded" by the x-ray film into a pattern of variations in optical density, or radiographic contrast. Radiographic contrast is the density difference between image areas in the radiograph. There are many definitions of contrast, but we will use the simple definition that contrast is the difference in density existing between various regions on the film. Radiographic contrast depends on subject contrast and film contrast. Subject contrast depends on the differential attenuation of the x-ray beam as it passes through the patient. The discussion of attenuation in Chapter 6 has already introduced the important aspects of subject contrast. Subject contrast was seen to be affected by the thickness, density, and atomic differences of the subject; the radiation energy (kVp); contrast material; and scatter radiation. The major theme of the remainder of this chapter will be the discussion of film contrast.

The information content of the x-ray image is the pattern of varying intensity of the x-ray beam caused by differential attenuation of x rays by the subject. Through areas of bone or opaque contrast material, few x rays reach the film, while many photons are transmitted through soft tissue, and the air around the patient stops almost no x-ray photons. The kVp must be selected with care so that the numbers of photons attenuated by bone and soft tissue are in the proper proportion to produce an x-ray image of high information content for the film intensifying screen to "decode." The correct kVp is tremendously important in producing proper subject contrast. This relationship (kVp and contrast) will be examined in detail in Chapter 13. Using the correct mAs causes the total number of x rays in each part of the attenuated x-ray beam to be sufficient to produce the correct film exposure, thus producing correct overall density in the processed film. Since exposure (mAs) determines the total number of x rays in the beam, mAs may be considered analogous to light in producing an ordinary photograph. Too little, or too much, mAs results in an underexposed or overexposed radiograph.

Subject contrast may be thought of as one factor which controls the log relative exposure which reaches the film. That is, film directly under a bone receives a low exposure, while a high exposure reaches the film under soft tissue areas of the subject. A consideration of film contrast must examine how the film responds to the difference in exposure produced by subject contrast. Film contrast depends on four factors:

1. Characteristic curve of the film.
2. Film density.
3. Screen or direct x-ray exposure.
4. Film processing.

Characteristic Curve

The shape of the characteristic curve tells us how much change in film density will occur as film exposure changes. The slope, or gradient, of the curve can be measured and expressed as a number. One such measurement is called **film gamma.** The gamma of a film is defined as the maximum slope of the characteristic curve, and is described by the formula:

$$\text{Gamma} = \frac{D_2 - D_1}{\log E_2 - \log E_1}$$

Figure 11–7   The gamma of an x-ray film

where D_2 and D_1 are the densities on the steepest part of the curve resulting from log relative exposures E_2 and E_1. Figure 11–7 shows an example of how film gamma is calculated. The gamma of x-ray films exposed with intensifying screens ranges from 2.0 to 3.5.

In radiology the concept of film gamma is of little value because, as illustrated in Figure 11–7, the maximum slope (steepest) portion of the characteristic curve is usually very short. We are interested in the slope of the curve over the entire range of useful radiographic densities (0.25 to 2.0). The slope (gradient) of a straight line joining two points of specified density on the characteristic curve is called the **average gradient.** The average gradient is usually calculated between density 0.25 and 2.0 above base and fog for radiographic films. Such a calculation is shown in Figure 11–8, which is the same curve from which gamma was calculated in Figure 11–7. In calculating average gradient, D_1 is always 0.25 and D_2 is 2.0; therefore, $D_2 - D_1$ is always 1.75. In Figure 11–8, log E_2 and E_1 are 1.4 and 0.85.

If the average gradient of the film used is greater than 1, the film will exaggerate subject contrast, and the higher the average gradient, the greater this exaggeration will be. A film with average gradient of 1 will not change subject contrast; a film with an average gradient of less than 1 will decrease subject contrast. Since contrast is very important in radiology, x-ray films all have an average gradient of greater than 1. For example, consider a radiograph of the hand (exposed with a screen-film combination) made with an x-ray beam of proper energy (kVp) to cause the bones to absorb four times as many photons as the soft tissue. This means that four times as many x-ray photons will reach the film under soft tissues as will reach the film under bone. The difference in log relative exposure, between bone and soft tissue, reaching the film under the hand, is 0.6 (log 4 = 0.6). If we assign a value of 1.5 as the log relative exposure in the soft tissue area (E_S), then the log relative exposure corresponding to the bones (E_B) is 0.9 (Figure 11–9). These two exposures will

Figure 11–8   The average gradient of an x-ray film

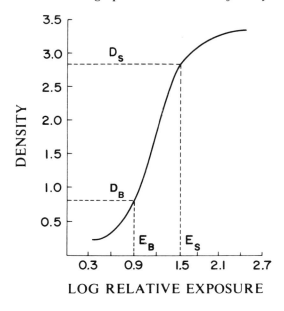

Figure 11–9   Film contrast amplifies subject contrast if the average gradient is greater than one

any one examination despite change in exposure time, milliamperes, or focus-film distance. However, all of these last mentioned factors will determine the actual value of the exposure, thereby determining the location of the exposure on the log relative exposure axis of the characteristic curve of the film. Let us consider an x-ray study of the abdomen in which the kVp chosen results in one area transmitting about 1.6 times more radiation than another. This means a log relative exposure difference of 0.2 (log 1.6 = 0.2). We will assume that the film used for this study has the characteristic curve depicted in Figure 11–10. If the factors of time, milliamperes, and focus-film distance (the inverse square law) are correct, the log relative exposures will produce film density falling along the steep portion of the characteristic curve. This will produce a density difference (radiographic contrast) of 0.6, or a difference in light transmission of 4:1 (antilog 0.6 = 4). However, if the exposure puts

produce film densities of 0.8 (bone density) and 2.8 (soft tissue density) on the hypothetical film's characteristic curve depicted in Figure 11–9. This is a density range of 2.0, corresponding to an overall brightness range of 100:1 when the film is transilluminated and viewed (100 is the antilog of 2.0). Thus, subject contrast resulting in an exposure range to the x-ray film of 4 to 1 has been exaggerated, or amplified, in the viewed radiograph into a brightness range (radiographic contrast) of 100 to 1.

Density

The slope of the characteristic curve (i.e., film contrast) changes with density. This is especially true in the toe and shoulder regions (Figure 11–5). Let us emphasize that the ratio of the difference in log relative exposure is determined by the kVp selected (such as the 4:1 ratio between soft tissue and bone in the example of the hand). If the kVp remains constant, this ratio will remain constant for

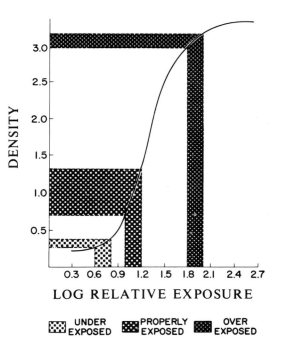

UNDER EXPOSED   PROPERLY EXPOSED   OVER EXPOSED

Figure 11–10   Incorrect exposures result in loss of contrast the developed densities on the toe of the curve, the film is underexposed (not enough mAs), and the density difference will fall to 0.13, or a difference in light transmission of 1.35 to 1 (antilog 0.13 = 1.35). Note that the exposure ratio has remained the same (i.e., log relative exposure difference of 0.2) because the kVp has not been changed. Similarly, overexposure, or too much mAs, will result in densities in the shoulder region of the characteristic curve of our hypothetical film-screen combination. As diagramed in Figure 11–10, this will result in a density difference (contrast) of 0.2, corresponding to a difference in light transmission of 1.59 to 1 (antilog 0.2 = 1.59). Exposures producing density at the level of 3 (0.1% of light transmitted) also produce less visible contrast under ordinary viewing conditions because the human eye has low sensitivity to contrast at low brightness levels. This is why a spotlight must be used to aid in viewing regions of high density.

Screen or Direct X-ray Exposure

If a film designed for exposure by light from intensifying screens is exposed to x rays directly, its characteristic curve has a considerably different shape than the curve obtained from exposure with screens. Remember, considerably more exposure (mAs) is required if no screens are used, since the intensification factor of screens may range from about 15 to 50 or more. Films exposed with par speed intensifying screens will require an x-ray exposure of approximately 1 mR to produce a density of 1; this value will rise to 30 mR or more with direct x-ray exposure.

At the same density, contrast is always lower for a film exposed to x rays only than for the same film exposed by light from intensifying screens. The reason for this difference in constrast is not precisely known. It probably is related to the complex manner in which the film emulsion responds to the energy of absorbed x-ray photons.

In addition, intensifying screens are relatively more sensitive than film to higher-energy x rays. The primary x-ray beam transmitted through the patient is of higher energy than the secondary, or scatter, radiation. Scatter radiation decreases contrast, as will be discussed in detail in Chapter 13. Since intensifying screens are relatively less sensitive to the lower energy of the scatter radiation, decrease in contrast will be minimized by screens. X-ray film, being more sensitive to lower-kVp x rays, may record the scatter radiation better than the higher-energy, information-containing primary beam. However, the variation in film sensitivity to x rays between 50 and 100 kVp is not very great and can usually be ignored in clinical radiology.

Stated another way, the average gradient of a double emulsion x-ray film will be greatest when the film is exposed with intensifying screens. Direct x-ray exposure will produce a lower average gradient. The photochemical reasons for this phenomenon are not known.

Film Processing (Development)

Increasing the time and/or temperature of development will, up to a point, increase the average gradient of a film (film speed is also increased). If development time is only 40% of normal, the gradient will be reduced to about 60% of maximum. However, fog will also be increased with increased development time or temperature, and fog decreases contrast. For these reasons, it is important to adhere to the manufacturer's standards in processing film. Automatic film-processing equipment has eliminated some of the problems associated with temperature of solutions and development time. To summarize, increasing the time or temperature of development will:

1. Increase average gradient (increase film contrast)
2. Increase film speed (increase density for a given exposure)
3. Increase fog (decrease film contrast)

Figure 11–11   Development time influences average gradient, speed, and fog

Figure 11–11 is a diagram of the effect of development time (or temperature) on average gradient, film speed, and fog.

Speed

The speed, or sensitivity, of an x-ray film is defined by the American Standards Association as the reciprocal of the exposure in roentgens required to produce a density of 1.0 above base and fog densities.

$$\text{Speed} = \frac{1}{\text{Roentgens}}$$

For example, if a film-screen combination required 1.2×10^{-3} R (1.2 milliroentgens) to produce a density of 1.0 above base and fog, its speed would be:

$$S = \frac{1}{.0012R} = \frac{833}{R} = 833 \text{ R}^{-1}$$

The average x-ray film used with intensifying screens has a speed of about 800. Similarly, a film exposed to x rays directly might require an exposure of 2.2×10^{-2} R (22 mR) for the same density, and its speed would be:

$$S = \frac{1}{.022R} = \frac{45}{R} = 45 \text{ R}^{-1}$$

The shape of the characteristic curve is controlled by film contrast; the film speed determines the location of the curve on the log exposure scale. Figure 11–12 shows the curves of two films which are identical

except that Film B is 0.3 log relative exposure units to the right of Film A. Both films will show identical film contrast, but Film B will require twice (antilog 0.3 = 2) as much

Figure 11–12   Film speed

Figure 11–13   Relative film speed varies with the density at which speed is measured

exposure (mAs) as Film A. Because the gradient of a characteristic curve varies with density, the relative speed between two films will be found to vary with the density at which speed is measured. For example, if a low-contrast and a high-contrast film are compared for speed, as in Figure 11–13, the relative speed between the two films might actually reverse with change in density. In our example, speed calculated at a density of 1.0 will show the low-contrast film (Film B) to be the fastest (i.e., Film B requires a lower log relative exposure to produce a density of 1.0 than Film A). At a density of 1.5 both films have the same speed, and above density 1.5 the higher-contrast Film A is faster than Film B. For medical x-ray films, relative film speed is usually compared at a density of 1.0 above base and fog.

Latitude

Unlike average gradient and speed, film latitude is not expressed in numerical terms. Latitude refers to the range of log relative exposure (mAs) which will produce density within the accepted range for diagnostic radiology (usually considered to be density 0.25 to 2.0). Let us consider two hypothetical films (Figure 11–14), one a high-contrast film (A) and one a lower-contrast film (B). If the density recorded on the film is to remain in the range of 0.25 to 2.0, Film A will be limited to a log relative exposure range of 0.75 to 1.42, or

a difference in log relative exposure of 0.67 corresponding to an actual ratio of 4.68 to 1 (antilog 0.67 = 4.68). Film B will remain in the designated density values over a range of log relative exposure from 0.85 to 2.35, or a difference in log exposure of 1.50 corresponding to an actual ratio of 31.6 to 1. Film B is said to have greater latitude than Film A in that it will accept a wider range of exposures. Notice that Film B has greater latitude but less film contrast. Generally speaking, **the latitude of a film varies inversely with film contrast.** There are two practical aspects to this concept of film latitude. For the technologist exposing a film, the film with more latitude makes the exposure less critical; if he has picked the proper kVp for adequate penetration, he has more room for error in his choice of exposure (mAs). Generally, the radiologist is interested in high contrast, which means films of less latitude. But there may be situations where a wide range of subject contrast (such as in the chest) must be recorded, and in such cases the film with the lower contrast but higher latitude may produce a radiograph in which many small changes in film exposures (i.e., subject contrast) can be recorded. Such lower-contrast but higher-latitude films are available to the radiologist. We will discuss another aspect of exposure latitude as it pertains to kVp and subject contrast in Chapter 13.

Double-emulsion Film

Films used for routine radiography have photosensitive emulsion coated on both sides of the base support. There is a physical and photographic reason for this. The emulsion is applied to the base in liquid form. When the emulsion dries, it shrinks to about one-tenth of its original volume. Most of the decrease in volume causes a decrease in thickness of the emulsion, but there is also a slight tendency to shrink in area. If emulsion were put on only one side of the base, shrinking of the emulsion would cause the film to curl toward the

Figure 11–14   Film B has greater latitude than Film A

emulsion side. An identical emulsion on each side of the base prevents this curling. The photographic advantage of a double emulsion is important only when the film is exposed with intensifying screens. We may assume each emulsion receives an identical exposure from each screen, for any filtering action of the front screen which might act to decrease the intensity of x rays reaching the back screen is so small as to be insignificant in clinical work. First, consider the case of a single emulsion film in a cassette, which receives two exposures, log E_1 and E_2, and responds with density D_1 and D_2. Film contrast for this exposure difference may be expressed:

$$\text{Contrast} = \frac{D_2 - D_1}{\log E_2 - \log E_1}$$

If this same exposure is now used to expose a double-emulsion film with light from intensifying screens, each emulsion will respond with density D_1 and D_2. When two films are superimposed, the resulting density is the sum of the densities of each film. Therefore, when the double-emulsion film is viewed, the densities of each emulsion are added, and the resulting total density will now be $D_1 + D_1 = 2D_1$ and $D_2 + D_2 = 2D_2$. The exposures E_2 and E_1 have not changed, but we have allowed two emulsions to respond to the exposure. The contrast which the eye now sees is:

$$\text{Contrast} = \frac{2D_2 - 2D_1}{\log E_2 - \log E_1} = \frac{2(D_2 - D_1)}{\log E_2 - \log E_1}$$

Since $\log E_2 - \log E_1$ is the same for each exposure, we may compare contrast without the $\log E_2 - \log E_1$ term:

Single Emulsion
Contrast = $D_2 - D_1$

Double Emulsion
Contrast = $2(D_2 - D_1)$

The double-emulsion film has produced twice the contrast of a single-emulsion film. Obviously, the overall density of the double emulsion is increased, resulting in increased film speed. For a film being exposed to x rays directly, a similar effect could be produced by making a single-emulsion film with a thicker emulsion. However, since light photons are easily absorbed by the emulsion, only the outer layer of the emulsion is affected by light from intensifying screens. This is one reason why x-ray film designed for exposure by light from two intensifying screens (in a cassette) has a thin emulsion on each side of the base, rather than a single thick emulsion.

EMULSION ABSORPTION

To expose an x-ray film with intensifying screens, it is necesary for the silver halide grains in the film to absorb the light emitted by the screen phosphor. The ability of the film grains to absorb light depends on the wavelength, or color, of the light. **Standard silver halide films absorb light in the ultra-violet, violet and blue regions of the visible spectrum.** Used with calcium tungstate or barium lead sulfate screens, such film worked well because these phosphors emitted light which was absorbed by natural silver halide, as shown in Figure 11–15. Notice that natural silver halide film does not absorb in the green and yellow portions of the visible spectrum, where much of the light from rare earth phosphors is emitted (Figure 11–17). You

Figure 11–15 The spectral emission of a barium lead sulfate and a calcium tungstate intensifying screen compared to the spectral sensitivity of natural silver halide. (not drawn to scale)

will recall that the peak wavelengths from rare earth screens, such as Kodak Lanex screens and 3 M Alpha screens, is produced by the terbium ion with about 60% of its energy at about 544 nm (green light). It is possible to extend the sensitivity of film to the green wavelengths by coating the silver halide grains with a thin layer of dye that absorbs the green light and then transfers this absorbed energy to the grain. Such green sensitive film is called **ortho** film. Similarly, the silver halide grain can be coated with a dye that absorbs red light, and this is called a **pan** film (panchromatic: sensitive to light of all colors). This is

illustrated in Figure 11–16. When rare earth screens are used, an appropriate green sensitive film should be used if one is to take advantage of all the light emitted by the screen. Such a combination is the Kodak Lanex screen and Ortho G film, illustrated in Figure 11–17.

Darkroom Safelight

The use of ortho films requires that the correct darkroom safelight be used. For many years an amber safelight (such as the Kodak Type 6B filter) has been used with blue-sensitive films. However, the amber safelight emits light to which ortho film is sensitive, and will produce "safelight fog" if used with such film. With ortho films a safelight filter shifted more toward the red is required (this will remove the green light to which ortho film is sensitive). Such a red safelight filter is the Kodak GS-1 filter. Figure 11–18 graphically illustrates the approximate sensitivity of regular silver halide film and ortho film, compared to the transmission of an amber (6B) and a red (GS-1) safelight filter.

Figure 11–16   Relative spectral sensitivity of natural silver halide, ortho and pan films

Print-thru

Print-thru, or crossover exposure, occurs when double emulsion films are used with two intensifying screens. **Print-thru**

Figure 11–17   Spectral emission of Kodak Lanex Regular screens and the spectral sensitivity of Kodak Ortho G film (the bars and curve are approximations used for illustration only, no attempt to achieve accuracy was made)

Figure 11–18   Spectral sensitivity of natural silver halide and ortho film compared to the transmission of an amber and a red safelight filter

refers to the fact that the light from one screen may pass through the emulsion nearest it and expose the film emulsion layer on the opposite side of the film. This "crossover" exposure contributes to image unsharpness (increased light diffusion) associated with use of intensifying screens. Print-thru is lowest with light in the ultraviolet region because light of this wavelength is more highly absorbed within the adjacent film emulsion. Print-thru, or crossover, is greater when green light systems are used.

Low-Dose Mammography

The Photo Products Department of the E.I. du Pont de Nemours & Co. has developed a film screen system designed specifically to provide the diagnostic clarity needed for mammography; this is marketed as the Lo-Dose system.[11] Perhaps a brief technical description of the Lo-Dose system will illustrate a practical application of some of the tedious details in the chapters dealing with films and screens.

The Lo-Dose system uses a single emulsion x-ray film, a single high-definition calcium tungstate intensifying screen, and a flexible vacuum cassette. The mammography screen is made with a calcium tungstate phosphor because its x-ray absorption in the energy range used in mammography (15 to 30 keV) is at least as high as other phosphors. The single screen phospher layer is 0.1 mm (.004 inches) thick and contains a yellow dye. Sharpness and resolution of the screen permit imaging calcifications as small as 0.1 mm, while x-ray absorption is high enough to allow minimum quantum noise (mottle) and maximum speed. The single emulsion x-ray film used with this screen eliminates parallax and print-thru as causes of unsharpness. Using the screen in the rear position, so that x rays pass through the film first, allows a small but perceptible gain in sharpness compared with the reverse position. Speed of the film is about half that of standard medium speed x-ray film; use of a faster film was found to cause a perceptible increase in quantum mottle. The use of a vacuum cassette insures intimate film-screen contact, eliminating another potential cause of unsharpness. This system will record a log exposure scale of 1.4 (i.e., an exposure range of 25:1), which is needed to visualize all breast tissue from the chest wall to the edge of the breast as well as abnormal soft tissue structures and calcifications. The density scale allows all detail in the breast image to be recorded at densities less than 3.0 to minimize the need for using high-intensity light to view the film. The exposure required with this system is about $1/7$ that required with direct x-ray exposure of high-speed industrial (single emulsion) films.

TRANSPARENCY VERSUS PRINT

Why are radiographs viewed as a transparency rather than as a print like an ordinary photograph? The density of a print is related to the amount of light reflected or absorbed by the paper. The density of the maximum black of most photographic printing papers is between 1.3 and 1.7. A few papers give density values as high as 2.0 (glossy-surface paper gives the highest maximum black). Obviously, such a limitation on maximum density would be intolerable in radiology where densities up to 2.0, and occasionally greater, are commonly encountered. This limitation is overcome by viewing the radiograph as a transparency which permits use of density ranges up to a maximum of 3.0 or more for diagnostic radiology films, and up to 6.0 for industrial x-ray use.

SUMMARY

The amount of blackening of an x-ray film is expressed by the term photographic density. The most useful range of density in diagnostic radiology is 0.25 to 2.0, although densities up to 3.0 are sometimes used.

Analysis of the characteristic curve of a

film provides information about the contrast, speed, and latitude of the film. Film contrast amplifies subject contrast if the average gradient of the film is greater than 1. Film contrast will vary with the amount of exposure (density), the way the film is exposed (intensifying screens or direct action of x rays), and the way the film is developed.

Double-emulsion films produce greater contrast than single-emulsion films (assuming light is used to expose the film).

X-ray film is viewed as a transparency because of the greater range of density available.

The film must be able to absorb the wavelength of light emitted by the intensifying screen. Some of the newer intensifying screen phosphors must be used with an appropriately sensitized (i.e., ortho) x-ray film.

REFERENCES

1. Bates, L. M.: Some Physical Factors Affecting Radiographic Image Quality: Their Theoretical Basis and Measurement. Public Health Service, Publication No. 999-RH-38, 1969.

2. Lawrence, D. J.: Kodak X-OMATIC and LANEX screens and Kodak films for medical radiography. Radiography Markets Division, Eastman Kodak Company File No. 5.03, June, 1976.

3. Meredith, W. J., and Massey, J. B.: *Fundamental Physics of Radiology.* Baltimore: Williams & Wilkins, 1968.

4. Ostrum, B. J., Becker, W., and Isard, H. J.: Low-dose mammography. Radiol. *109,* 323, 1973.

5. Presentation Script: "New Screen Technology." Prepared by Photo Products Department, E.I. du Pont de Nemours & Co.

6. Seeman, H. E.: *Physical and Photographic Principles of Medical Radiography.* New York: John Wiley and Sons, Inc., 1968.

7. Sensitometric Properties of X-ray Films. Rochester, N.Y.: Radiography Markets Division, Eastman Kodak Company.

8. Thompson, T. T.: Selecting medical x-ray film Part 1. Applied Radiol. *4,* 47, Sept./Oct., 1974.

9. ————: Selecting medical x-ray film Part II. Applied Radiol. *4,* 51, Nov./Dec., 1974.

10. Wayrynen, R. E.: Radiographic film. Contained in the syllabus of the 1975 AAPM Summer School "The Expanding Role of the Diagnostic Radiologic Physicist," Rice University, Houston, Texas. July 27–Aug. 1, 1975, p. 112.

11. Weiss, J. P., and Wayrynen, R. E.: Imaging system for low-dose mammography. J. Applied Photographic Engineering *2,* 7, 1976.

CHAPTER 12

Geometry of the Radiographic Image

We must briefly consider some of the factors of geometry and trigonometry which influence the quality of the image of a radiograph. We will only consider examples of x rays originating at the x-ray tube and directed at the patient (or test object) and an x-ray film. We will assume that any object placed in the x-ray beam will absorb all the x-ray photons that hit the object. This is a very unlikely situation, but it makes examples easier to draw and understand. Since x rays travel in straight lines, the x-ray beam can be drawn as a straight line that hits the object or the film. The fact that x rays are emitted in all directions from the target of the x-ray tube has been previously discussed. In our examples we will assume the ideal situation in which proper collimation has produced a beam which is perfectly cone shaped, and that the object is placed in the x-ray beam at a varying distance from the film. We will observe the beam from one side, so its shape can be drawn as a triangle, with the focal spot of the x-ray tube as the apex (origin of x rays) and the object or the film as the base of the triangle (Figure 12–1). In Figure 12–1, "h" represents the focal spot-object distance, and "H" the focal spot-film distance. This type of diagram will allow us to consider two triangles, one with the object as its base and the other with the film as its base (Figure 12–2). The two triangles have the same shape, but are of different sizes, and are known as **similar triangles. The sides and altitudes of similar triangles are proportional.** This means that, in Figure 12–2:

$$\frac{a}{A} = \frac{b}{B} = \frac{c}{C} = \frac{h}{H}$$

The altitude of a triangle is a perpendicular dropped from a vertex to the opposite side or to an extension of the opposite side.

By using simple line drawings to represent the conditions of our idealized x-ray object-film conditions, and applying the rule of similar triangles, it is possible to develop an understanding of the basic principles of magnification, distortion, and penumbra.

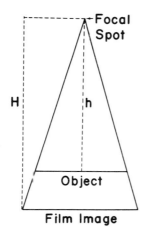

Figure 12–1 Schematic drawing of the relationship between an x-ray beam, the object being examined, and the image of the object on the film

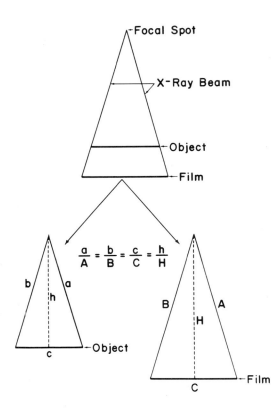

Figure 12–2 The proportional relationships of similar triangles

MAGNIFICATION

When an object is placed in the x-ray beam, it will cast a "shadow" on the film which will show some degree of enlargement. Since it is assumed that the object absorbs all the x rays that hit it, the developed film will show a clear area corresponding to the shape of the object, surrounded by blackened (exposed) film. If the object is round and flat, shaped like a coin, its magnified image will be round but larger than the coin. The image has been magnified, and the amount of magnification (M) can be measured as:

$$M = \frac{\text{Size of the Image}}{\text{Size of the Object}}$$

In the clinical situation the object may be a structure or foreign body within the patient which is not available for measure-

ment. But it is usually possible to determine the distance of the source of x rays (focal spot of the x-ray tube) from the film, as well as the distance of the object from the film, and the image size can be measured directly. By determining the degree of magnification, the true size of the object can be calculated. Refer to Figure 12–1, which shows a simple line drawing of an object placed some distance from the x-ray film, causing its image to be magnified by the diverging x-ray beam. The altitude of the large triangle (H) represents the distance from the focal spot of the x-ray tube to the film, often termed **focus-film distance.** The altitude of the smaller triangle (h) represents the distance from the focal spot to the object, or the **focus-object distance.** Since the sides and altitudes of similar triangles are proportional:

$$\frac{h}{H} = \frac{\text{OBJECT SIZE}}{\text{IMAGE SIZE}}$$

Since focus-film distance, image size, and focus-object distance can be measured directly, object size is easy to calculate. Notice that calculating simple magnification problems does not require that any formulas be learned. Consider a simple example. Using a 40-inch focus-film distance, the image of an object that is known to be 8 inches from the film measures 10 cm in length. What is the true length of the object, and how much magnification is present? Using Figure 12–1, we see that H = 40, h = 32 (40 − 8 = 32), and image size = 10 cm. Setting up the proportion:

$$\frac{40}{32} = \frac{10 \text{ cm}}{\text{OBJECT SIZE}}$$

Solving for object size:

$$\text{OBJECT SIZE} = \frac{(32)(10)}{40} = 8 \text{ cm}$$

$$\text{MAGNIFICATION} = \frac{\text{SIZE OF THE IMAGE}}{\text{SIZE OF THE OBJECT}} = \frac{10}{8} = 1.25$$

What if the object is not placed directly beneath the focal spot, but is displaced to one side so that the more oblique x rays are used to form an image? If the object is flat, and remains parallel to the film, magnification will be exactly the same for the object whether central or oblique x rays are used. Consider Figure 12–3, in which the coin is not directly beneath the x-ray tube, but is still parallel to the film. The altitude of the two triangles is exactly the same as it was when the object was directly under the focal spot (Figure 12–1) so the ratio of object to image size will be the same in each circumstance. In Figure 12–4, the three coins are parallel to, and the same distance

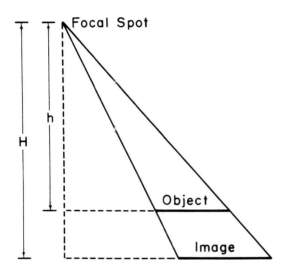

Figure 12–3 Magnification of an object by oblique rays

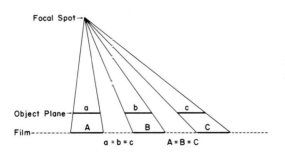

Figure 12–4 The magnification of three coins (a, b, c) all parallel to the film and the same distance above the film produces three round images (A, B, C) of equal size

above, the film. The image of each coin will be a circle, and all the circles will be the same size.

Under usual radiographical situations, magnification should be kept to a minimum. Two rules apply: (1) **Keep the object as close to the film as possible,** and (2) **Keep the focus-film distance as large as possible.**

Consider Figure 12–1 again. Since magnification is determined by the ratio of the altitude of the two triangles, we may write

$$\text{Magnification} = \frac{H}{h}$$

If $H/h = 1.0$, there is no magnification. The closer the object is to the film, the closer the magnitude of altitude h will approach the value of altitude H. An increase in focus-film distance (increasing H while leaving object-film distance unchanged) will also bring the ratio H/h closer to 1. To illustrate, assume an object is 6 inches from the film. What will be the magnification if the focus-film distance is (a) 40 inches, and (b) 72 inches? At 40 inches focus-film distance:

$$\frac{H}{h} = \frac{40}{34} = 1.18$$

At 72 inches focus-film distance:

$$\frac{H}{h} = \frac{72}{66} = 1.09$$

To review, magnification depends on two factors: (1) **object-film distance** and (2) **focus-film distance.**

DISTORTION

Distortion results from unequal magnification of different parts of the same object. Consider Figure 12–5 in which one coin (dashed line) is parallel to the film and the other coin (solid line AB) is tilted with respect to the plane of the film. The tilted coin undergoes distortion because of unequal magnification, side A is closer to the film than side B. The shape of the image of the tilted coin will be an ellipse, and its exact size and shape will vary with the amount of tilting.

Figure 12–5   Distortion of an object (line AB) which is not parallel to the film

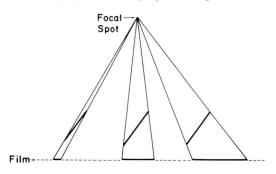

Figure 12–6   Distortion of the shape and size of the image of a tilted object depends upon the position of the object in the x-ray beam

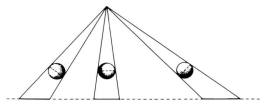

Figure 12–7   The size and shape of the image of a spherical object depends on the position of the object in relation to the central part of the x-ray beam

Distortion of the image of an object will be different in different parts of the x-ray beam. Figure 12–6 shows how distortion of the shape and size of three equally tilted coins will vary in different parts of the x-ray beam.

Distortion of thick objects occurs if they are not directly in the central part of the x-ray beam. Since different parts of thick objects are different distances from the x-ray film, each part will be magnified by a different amount. This will cause the shape of the image of most thick objects to be distorted. Only the part of a thick object which is parallel to the film will be un-distorted. Figure 12–7 illustrates the relative size and shape of the image of three spheres (such as steel ball bearings) which are in different parts of the x-ray beam. The sphere which lies in the center of the beam will exhibit a round (undistorted) magnified image. However, the image of each of the two laterally placed spheres will be an ellipse, because the x-ray beam "sees" a diameter of each of these spheres which is not parallel to the film. The x-ray beam "sees" a laterally placed spherical object in the same way it "sees" a round, flat object

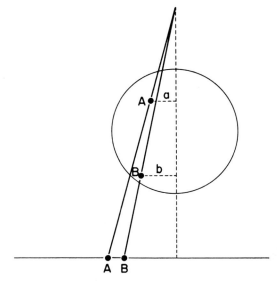

Figure 12–8   Distortion of position

(a coin), which is tilted with respect to the plane of the film. Notice the similarity between Figures 12–6 and 12–7.

Distortion of the relative position of the image of two objects may occur if the objects are at different distances from the film. For example, in Figure 12–8 two opaque objects, A and B, are present inside a circle. Object A is more medial than B, but A is farther from the film. The film image of object A will be lateral to the image of object B. This is because the distance between A and the midline (line a) has been magnified much more than has the distance between B and the central beam (line b). Distortion of position is minimal when the object is near the central part of the x-ray beam, and the object is placed as close to the film as possible.

PENUMBRA
From Latin **pene** (almost) and **umbra** (shadow)

Penumbra, often termed **edge gradient**, is defined as the region of partial illumination which surrounds the umbra, or complete shadow. In the discussion of magnification and distortion, it was assumed that the source of x rays (focal spot) was a point source. Actually, the focal spot is not a point. It has finite dimensions, usually ranging from 0.3 to 2.0 mm square. The focal spot acts as if it is composed of many point sources of x rays, with each point source forming its own image of an object. The edges of each of these images will not be in exactly the same spot on the film. In Figure 12–9 the edge of an object, as formed by two x-ray sources (A and B), which represent the opposite ends of a focal spot, is diagramed. The x rays must travel in a straight line from each point source to the film. Image edges A and B are not in the same place, and an image formed in this way has a fuzzy, or unsharp, margin. This zone of unsharpness is called **geometric unsharpness, penumbra,** or **edge gradient**, and represents the area where the margins caused by the many

"point sources" of x rays in the focal spot overlap. Figure 12–10 shows how the zone of penumbra is formed from an angled rotating anode; focal spot size has been

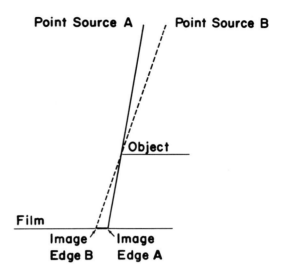

Figure 12–9   The focal spot acts as if it is composed of many point sources of x rays

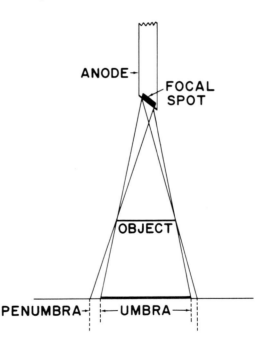

Figure 12–10   Penumbra (geometric unsharpness)

exaggerated. The region of complete image is called the **umbra,** which means shadow. These terms are used in astronomy to describe a solar eclipse, in which the umbra is the area of complete shadow within which a spectator can see no portion of the sun's disc, and the penumbra is the zone of partial shadow between the umbra and the full light. Notice that, as shown in Figure 12–10, the width of the penumbra is less on the anode side than on the cathode side of the x-ray tube. This effect can be used to achieve maximum sharpness by placing the object of greatest interest toward the anode side of the x-ray tube.

The width of blurring caused by penumbra can be calculated. Figure 12–11 shows the penumbra (P) caused by focal spot F (dimensions are exaggerated for illustration). Notice that two similar triangles are again formed, with the apex of each triangle at the object (labeled point X), the base of the upper triangle being the width of the focal spot and the base of the lower triangle being the width of the penumbra.

Since the sides and altitudes (H and h) of similar triangles are proportional, a simple proportion can be established between focal spot size (F), penumbra (P), focus-object distance (H), and object-film distance (h):

$$\frac{P}{F} = \frac{h}{H}$$

Using a 2-mm focal spot and focus-film distance of 40 inches, calculate the penumbra if the object is (a) 4 inches above the film and (b) 10 inches above the film. In case (a) focus-object distance (H) = 40 − 4 = 36 inches:

$$\frac{P}{2} = \frac{4}{36}$$

$$P = \frac{(4)\ (2)}{36}$$

$$P = 0.22\ \text{mm}$$

In case (b) H = 40 − 10 = 30 inches:

$$\frac{P}{2} = \frac{10}{30}$$

$$P = \frac{(2)\ (10)}{30}$$

$$P = 0.67\ \text{mm}$$

In case (b), if object-film distance remains 10 inches, but focus-film distance is increased to 72 inches, what will be the penumbra?

$$\frac{P}{2} = \frac{10}{62}$$

$$P = \frac{(2)\ (10)}{62}$$

$$P = 0.32\ \text{mm}$$

The importance of focal-spot size may be appreciated by substituting a focal-spot

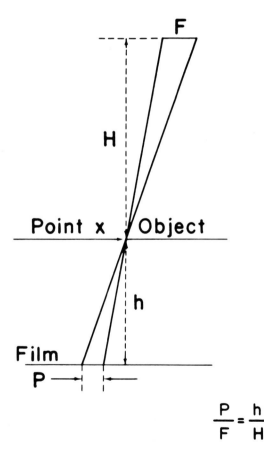

$$\frac{P}{F} = \frac{h}{H}$$

Figure 12–11 Calculation of the width of the zone of geometric unsharpness (penumbra) size of 1 mm in each of the preceding examples. The width of the penumbra will be one-half of that caused by a 2-mm focal spot. These situations illustrate the factors that will decrease penumbra:

(1) Put the object as close to the film as possible (make h small).
(2) Use as large a focus-object distance as possible (make H large).
(3) Use as small a focal spot as possible.

Notice that keeping the object as close to the film as possible, and using a long focus-film distance, also decreases magnification. The use of the magnification technique, which we will discuss in Chapter 20, causes an increase in geometric unsharpness.

MOTION UNSHARPNESS

Motion unsharpness is the term used to describe image unsharpness caused by motion of the examined object during the exposure. Object motion will produce the same type of image unsharpness as penumbra. Object motion may be minimized by immobilizing the patient or by using a short exposure time. Similar motion unsharpness will result if the focal spot moves during the exposure. X-ray tube motion is much less important than object motion, unless considerable magnification is present. The relationship between motion and magnification will be discussed in more detail in Chapter 20.

ABSORPTION UNSHARPNESS

Absorption unsharpness is caused by the way in which x rays are absorbed in the subject. This type of unsharpness arises from the gradual change in x-ray absorption across the boundary, or edge, of an object. To illustrate the meaning of absorption unsharpness, let us again assume that x rays originate from a point source (F). Figure 12–12 shows a truncated cone, a cube, and a sphere which all have the same thickness and are assumed to be made of the same material. The cone will show little absorption unsharpness since its

Figure 12–12 The origin of absorption unsharpness

edges are parallel to the diverging beam, and its edge will be sharply defined on the film. Upon inspection of Figure 12–12, it is apparent that the absorption of x rays by the cube will vary along the outer edge of its upper surface, with fewer x rays being absorbed along the sides, and more in the region of the lower corners. With the sphere, absorption unsharpness occurs across the entire image, with maximum x-ray absorption occurring only in the center. Absorption unsharpness produces a poorly defined margin in the image of most solid objects, because there is a gradual change in film density along the image edge. The cone shows high contrast (density difference) along its edge because there is a well defined line on the film where x-ray exposure changes from high (no absorption by the object) to low (high absorption by the object). But in the case of the cube and the sphere there is no abrupt change in the film exposure, only a gradual change, the magnitude of which depends on the shape of the object. The effect of absorption unsharpness is particularly important when the accurate measurement of small round or oval structures is necessary, as in coronary angiography. Since absorption unsharpness is caused by the shape of the object being examined, it will occur no matter how exacting the conditions of generating and recording the radiographic image. Perhaps the term "subject unsharpness" would be more accurate.

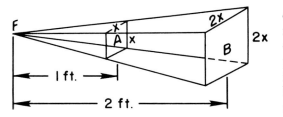

Figure 12–13 The inverse square law

INVERSE SQUARE LAW

X rays obey the physical laws of light. There is a well-known law of light propagation that states that the intensity of light falling on a flat surface from a point source is inversely proportional to the square of the distance from the point source. The principle is illustrated in Figure 12–13.

The number of x-ray photons emitted at the anode remains constant. At a distance of 1 foot, the diverging x-ray beam covers an area (A) represented by the square with each side of a dimension x, or an area of $x \cdot x = x^2$. At 2 feet, the diverging beam covers a square (B) in which each side is now twice as long as it was at 1 foot. The area covered by the beam at 2 feet is therefore $2x \cdot 2x = 4x^2$, which is 4 times the area at 1 foot. Since the intensity of the beam originating at the anode is constant, the intensity falling on square A must spread out over an area 4 times as large by the time it reaches square B. For example, assume that an x-ray tube has an output such that the intensity 1 foot from the tube is 144 units per square inch. At 2 feet, the 144 units are now divided between 4 square inches, or 36 units per square inch. Likewise, the intensity per square inch at 3 feet is:

$$\frac{144}{3^2} = \frac{144}{9} = 16 \text{ units per in}^2$$

and so forth. At 4 feet the intensity will be $(\frac{1}{4})^2$ or $\frac{1}{16}$ that at 1 foot.

A practical example will illustrate use of the inverse square law. Assume that an

exposure of 100 mAs (100 mA for 1 sec) is needed for a film of the abdomen using a 40-inch focus-film distance. Employing portable equipment, the maximum focus-film distance which can be obtained at the bedside is 30 inches. What mAs must be used to maintain the same radiographic density as that obtained at a 40-inch distance (kVp remains constant)? Since the intensities (mAs) of the x-ray beam at 40 and 30 inches are proportional to the squares of these distances:

$$\frac{100 \text{ mAs}}{X \text{ mAs}} = \frac{40^2}{30^2} = \frac{1600}{900}$$

$$X = \frac{(100)\ (900)}{1600} = 56.25 \text{ mAs}$$

The distance from the x-ray tube to the film should be kept as great as practical to minimize the geometric unsharpness caused by penumbra. This greater distance will increase the exposure (mAs) needed to maintain proper film density. Older techniques called for a 36-inch focus-film distance, but with x-ray tubes capable of increased output, a 40-inch distance is now routine. The increased mAs required in going from 36 to 40 inches is:

$$\frac{40^2}{36^2} = \frac{1600}{1296} = 1.23$$

or a 23% increase in mAs. As the output of x-ray tubes increases, techniques using up to 60-inch focus-film distance may become routine.

SUMMARY

Geometric factors that influence the quality of the radiographic image include magnification, distortion, penumbra, and motion. Absorption unsharpness produces a similar effect. Factors which will decrease unsharpness due to magnification, penumbra, and motion are:

MAGNIFICATION
1. Small object-film distance
2. Large focal spot-film distance

PENUMBRA
1. Small focal-spot size
2. Small object-film distance
3. Large focal spot-film distance

MOTION

1. Short exposure time
2. Maximum possible limitation of actual object motion

To minimize distortion, the object of interest should be kept parallel to the film and near the central portion of the x-ray beam, and magnification should be minimized.

The intensity of the x-ray beam varies inversely as the square of the distance from the x-ray tube.

REFERENCES

1. Bookstein, J. J., and Steck, W.: Effective focal-spot size. Radiol. *98*, 31, 1971.
2. Fuchs, A. W.: *Principles of Radiographic Exposure and Processing*. 2nd ed. Springfield, Charles C Thomas, 1958.
3. Meredith, W. J., and Ramsey, J. B.: *Fundamental Physics of Radiology*. Baltimore: Williams & Wilkins, 1968.
4. Method of focal spot image and measurements. Report of the International Commission on Radiological Units and Measurements. Radiol., *76*, 125, 1961; and Amer. J. Roentgen., *85*, 191, 1961.
5. Seeman, H. E.: *Physical and Photographic Principles of Medical Radiography*. New York: John Wiley and Sons, Inc., 1968.

CHAPTER 13

The Radiographic Image

The basic tool of diagnostic radiology is the radiographic image. The radiologist must be thoroughly familiar with the factors that govern the information content of these images. R. E. Wayrynen* suggests that the term **image clarity** be used to describe the visibility of diagnostically important detail in the radiograph. Two basic factors determine the clarity of the radiographic image: contrast and image quality.

IMAGE CLARITY

CONTRAST   IMAGE QUALITY

A discussion of image clarity is difficult because there are so many subjective factors involved. Many problems concerning image visibility are the result of the physiological and psychological reactions of the observer rather than the physical properties of the image. There is no well-defined relationship between the amount of information on a film and the accuracy of interpretation of the film. Many overlooked lesions are large and easy to see in retrospect. In this chapter the physical properties of contrast and image quality will be considered.

CONTRAST

The term **radiographic contrast** refers to the difference in density between areas

*Technical Manager, X-ray Markets, E. I. du Pont de Nemours & Co.

in the radiograph. Differing degrees of grayness, or contrast, allow us to "see" the information contained in the x-ray image. Radiographic contrast depends on three factors:

1. Subject contrast
2. Film contrast
3. Fog and scatter

Subject Contrast

Subject contrast, sometimes called **radiation contrast,** is the difference in x-ray intensity transmitted through one part of the subject compared to that through another part. In Figure 13–1, assume that a uniform beam of x rays strikes an object made up of a block of muscle (A) and a

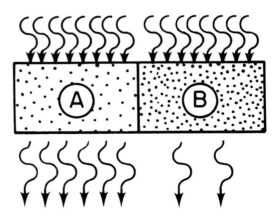

Figure 13–1 Equal thickness of muscle (A) and bone (B) do not equally attenuate an x-ray beam

161

block of bone (B) of equal thickness. Few x rays are transmitted through the bone, but most go through the muscle. The attenuated x-ray beam now contains many x rays in the area beneath muscle and few beneath bone; this difference of intensity in the beam caused by the object is subject contrast.

Obviously, the effect of subject contrast on the x-ray beam cannot be seen directly. But since the x-ray beam exposes the film, anything which attenuates the x-ray beam will similarly affect the radiographic image on the film. As has been previously discussed, variations in the intensity of the x-ray beam caused by subject contrast are greatly amplified by the film. Subject contrast is the result of the attenuation of the x-ray beam by the patient, and attenuation has been discussed in detail in Chapter 5. A brief review will emphasize the pertinent points.

Subject contrast depends upon:
1. Thickness difference
2. Density difference
3. Atomic number difference
4. Radiation quality (kVp)

Thickness Difference

If an x-ray beam is directed at two different thicknesses of the same material, the number of x rays transmitted through the thin part will be greater than the number transmitted through the thick part. This is a relatively simple but important factor contributing to subject contrast. If I_S is the intensity of the x-ray beam (I) transmitted through the thin (small) segment, and I_L the intensity through the thick (large) segment, subject contrast may be defined as (Figure 13–2):

$$\text{Subject Contrast} = \frac{I_S}{I_L}$$

Another less obvious cause of difference in tissue thickness is the presence of a gas-filled cavity. Since gas attenuates almost no x rays, the presence of a pocket of gas in a soft tissue mass has the same effect on the x-ray beam as decreasing the thick-

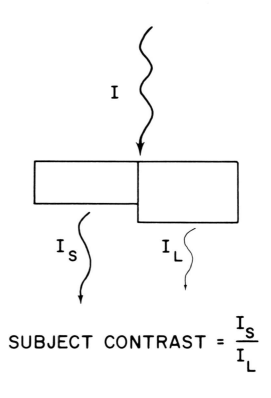

$$\text{SUBJECT CONTRAST} = \frac{I_S}{I_L}$$

Figure 13–2   Subject contrast

ness of the soft tissue mass. In ventriculography, the brain ventricles are visible because they are filled with air. The x-ray beam then "sees" the cross section of brain containing a gas-filled ventricle as being "thinner" than the adjacent solid brain substance.

Density Difference

The difference in density between body tissues is one of the most important factors in causing subject contrast. The greater the density (i.e., mass per unit volume) of a tissue, the greater is its ability to attenuate x rays. Consider ice and water. Since ice floats in water, it is less dense than water. Water is about 9% more dense than ice. Equal thicknesses of ice and water will demonstrate subject contrast to an x-ray beam because the water attenuates 9% more of the beam than the ice.

Atomic Number Difference

Subject contrast depends upon the relative difference in attenuation of the x-ray beam by different tissues in the body. In diagnostic radiology, attenuation of the x-ray beam by the photoelectric effect makes the most important contribution to subject contrast. Photoelectric absorption is increased in substances with high atomic numbers, especially when low-kVp x rays are used. The effective atomic numbers of bone, muscle (water), and fat are:

Bone	13.8
Muscle	7.4
Fat	5.9

Bone will attenuate many more x rays than muscle or fat, assuming equal thicknesses. Subject contrast between bone and muscle is high. Muscle and fat, with little difference in atomic number, show little difference in their ability to attenuate x rays by the photoelectric absorption process, and less difference by Compton reactions. Use of low kVp (below 30) x rays produces the greatest possible difference in photoelectric x-ray absorption between muscle and fat. Soft-tissue radiography, such as mammography, requires the use of low-kVp x rays because the small differences in atomic number between breast tissues produce no subject contrast unless maximum photoelectric effect is used.

Contrast Media

The use of contrast materials with high atomic numbers (53 for iodine and 56 for barium) gives high subject contrast. Photoelectric absorption of x rays in barium and iodine will be proportionally much greater than that in bone and tissue because of the large differences in atomic number.

Radiation Quality

The ability of an x-ray photon to penetrate tissue depends on its energy; high-kVp x rays have greater energy. Selecting the proper kVp is one of the most important matters to consider in choosing the proper exposure technique. If the kVp is too low, almost all the x rays are attenuated in the patient and never reach the film.

The kilovoltage selected has a great effect on subject contrast. Low kVp will produce high subject contrast, provided the kVp is high enough to adequately penetrate the part being examined.

Figure 13–3 Subject contrast varies with the kVp of the x-ray beam

In general terms, the reason low kVp produces greater subject (or radiation) contrast than high kVp can be explained by a simple example. In Figure 13–2, subject contrast was defined as $\frac{I_S}{I_L}$. Assume that 100 x rays of low kVp (such as 50 kVp) strike the object (Figure 13–3A). Most of these low-energy x rays are attenuated by the thick part, but quite a few can penetrate the thin part. Assume the numbers to be 25 (thick) and 40 (thin). By the definition of subject contrast:

$$\text{Subject Contrast} = \frac{40}{25} = 1.60$$

which states that the thin part transmits 60% more x rays than the thick part at 50 kVp. If the kVp is then increased to 80 (Figure 13–3B), more x rays will get through both the thick and thin parts. Both I_S and I_L will increase, but I_S will increase more than I_L, so the ratio $\frac{I_S}{I_L}$ becomes smaller, and subject contrast is decreased. Figure 13–3B assumes values of $I_S = 80$ and $I_L = 60$, giving subject contrast of $\frac{80}{60} = 1.33$, or only 33% difference in transmitted radiation intensity.

As a general rule, low kVp gives high subject contrast. This is often called **short-scale contrast** because everything is black or white on the film, with fewer shades of gray in between. High kVp gives lower subject contrast, called **long-scale contrast,** because there is a long scale of shades of gray between the lightest and the darkest portions of the image.

Exposure Latitude

A low-contrast film (shallow slope of the characteristic curve) has greater exposure latitude. That is, a wider range of mAs settings will produce proper film density, if the kVp is satisfactory. Similarly, kVp will also have an effect on exposure latitude. High-kVp techniques will allow a wider range of mAs settings (wide exposure latitude), but result in relatively less contrast. **Low-kVp techniques produce high subject contrast** because there is a large variation in the intensity of the transmitted x-ray beam in different parts of the patient. The x-ray film must then "decode" a range of exposure from low to high. This wide range of exposure (log relative exposure) must fall within the steep portion of the characteristic curve (Figure 13–4A).

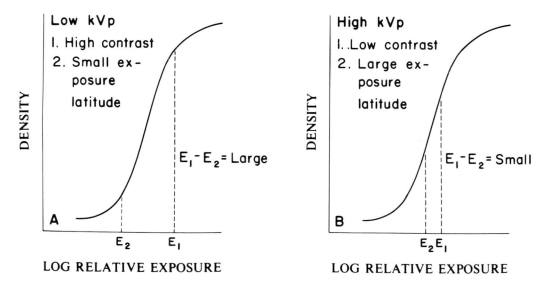

Figure 13–4   Exposure latitude varies with the kVp of the x-ray beam

When a low kVp is used, the mAs must be carefully selected. Figure 13–4A shows that if the exposure (mAs) is only a little too low, the low-exposure areas (i.e., under bone) will produce exposures in the toe area of the curve. Likewise, excessive mAs will rapidly move high-density exposures onto the shoulder of the curve. Both of these mistakes will decrease film contrast. High-kVp exposures produce less difference in intensity between areas of the attenuated x-ray beam; this is why **high kVp gives less subject contrast.** With a high-kVp technique, the film has to "decode" a smaller difference in log relative exposure between the low- and high-exposure areas. Figure 13–4B diagrams how a high-kVp technique (using the same object and film-screen system) will "use up" a much shorter portion of the steep portion of the film's characteristic curve. Using high kVp, the technologist has considerable room for error in the choice of mAs, because the exposure range can move up or down on the curve and still fall within the steep portion of the curve. To review: **kVp influences subject contrast** (exposure differences) **and exposure latitude; mAs controls film blackening** (density). Consider a specific example. A chest film (par-speed film-screen combination, 6-feet distance, no grid, exposed with factors of 70 kVp and 6.6 mAs [400 mA, 1/60 sec]) would result in a radiograph with high contrast. However, the exposure of 6.6 mAs is very critical at 70 kVp. An error of plus or minus 50% would probably produce a radiograph with a great deal of its density on the toe or shoulder of the film curve, resulting in an unacceptable loss of contrast. Another chest examination exposed at 100 kVp and about 3 mAs would result in a low-contrast radiograph, but changing the exposure (3 mAs) by a factor of plus or minus 100% would probably not reduce radiographic contrast. Obviously, fewer mAs, or more mAs, produces a lighter (less density), or darker (more density), radiograph, but the density range still falls on the steep portion of the film curve. At 100 kVp, the exposure can be varied considerably; this is termed **large exposure latitude.** At 70 kVp, the exposure must fall within a narrow range; i.e., there is small exposure latitude.

To make matters more complicated, kVp does have an effect on film blackening. This effect is approximately equal to the fourth power of the kVp. For example, if kVp is increased from 50 to 60, the change in film density (if mAs remains constant) will be about:

$$\frac{60^4}{50^4} = 2.07$$

Since kVp has doubled film density, mAs would have to be cut in half. An old rule says: "If you add 10 kVp, cut mAs in half." This holds true around 50 to 60 kVp, but kVp change has less effect on film density at higher ranges. For example, at 85 kVp, an increase of 15 kVp is required to double the film blackening power of the beam.

Subject contrast has been reviewed and seen to vary with the make-up of the subject (thickness, density, atomic number), the use of contrast material, and the kVp of the x-ray beam.

Film Contrast

Film contrast has been discussed as a photographic property of x-ray film. **X-ray film will significantly amplify subject contrast** provided the exposure (mAs) is correct (keep away from the toe and shoulder of the characteristic curve). Under good viewing conditions, a density difference of about 0.04 (difference in light transmission of 10%) can be seen.

Fog and Scatter

The effect of fog and scatter is to reduce radiographic contrast.

Scattered radiation is produced mainly as a result of **Compton** scattering. The amount of scatter radiation increases with increasing part thickness, field size, and energy of the x-ray beam (higher kVp). Scatter is minimized by collimation of the x-ray beam (use as small a field size as possible) and use of grids or air gaps. **Scatter radiation which reaches the x-ray film or film-screen combination produces unwanted density.**

Fog is strictly defined as those silver halide grains in the film emulsion which are developed even though they were not exposed by light or x rays. The amount of fog in an unexposed x-ray film can be demonstrated easily. Cut the unexposed film in half. Develop (fully process) one-half of the film and clear (fix, wash, and dry only) the other. The density difference between the two film halves represents the amount of fog present. **Fog produces unwanted film density, which lowers radiographic contrast.** Another type of unwanted film density may result from accidental exposure of film to light or x rays. This is usually also called "fog," or "exposure fog," and while the term is not absolutely correct, it has established itself by common usage. These two types of "fog" are different in origin, but both lower film contrast in the same manner.

True fog is increased by:
1. Improper film storage (high temperature or humidity).
2. Contaminated or exhausted developer solution.
3. Excessive time or temperature of development.
4. Use of high-speed film (highly sensitized grains).

Fog, "exposure fog," and scatter add density to the film. By knowing the magnitude of this density and the characteristic curve of the film, it is possible to calculate accurately the effect of the added density on radiographic contrast. Figure 13–5 shows how fog and scatter change the slope of the characteristic curve of a film (this is copied from a curve calculated by R. E. Wayrynen). Notice that the slope of the curve is decreased (contrast is decreased) most at lower levels of density. These are the densities most used in diagnostic radiology. In Figure 13–5 the gamma of

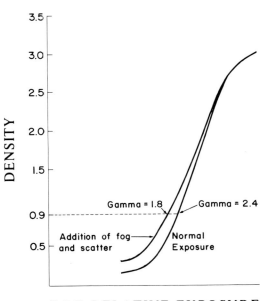

LOG RELATIVE EXPOSURE

Figure 13–5 Fog and scatter decrease radiographic contrast

the normal film, at a density of 0.9, is 2.4. When fog and scatter are added, the gamma drops to 1.8. At a density of 2.5, fog and scatter have no significant effect on the shape of the curve, but densities as high as 2.5 are seldom used in diagnostic radiology.

To repeat, fog and scatter are undesirable because they decrease radiographic contrast by decreasing film contrast.

IMAGE QUALITY

The second basic factor determining image clarity is image quality. The quality of the radiographic image may be defined as the ability of the film to record each point in the object as a point on the film. In radiology this point-for-point reproduction is never perfect, largely because of the diffusion of light by intensifying screens. There is no general agreement as to what should be included in a discussion of image quality. Our approach will involve almost no mathematics.

Image quality may be considered under the following headings:

Radiographic mottle
Sharpness
Resolution

Radiographic Mottle

If an x-ray film is mounted between intensifying screens and exposed to a uniform x-ray beam to produce a density of about 1.0, the resulting film will not show uniform density but will have an irregular, mottled appearance. This mottled appearance (due to small density differences) is easily detected by the unaided eye, and may be seen, if looked for, in any area of "uniform" density in a radiograph exposed with screens (for example, the area of a chest film not covered by the patient). This uneven texture, or mottle, seen on a film which "should" show perfectly uniform density is called **radiographic mottle.** Radiographic mottle has three components:

Only **quantum mottle** is of any importance in diagnostic radiology.

Film Graininess

Film graininess makes no contribution to the radiographic mottle observed in clinical radiology. Film graininess can be seen when the film is examined with a lens producing magnification of 5 to 10 diameters. With this magnification, the image is seen to be made up of a nonhomogeneous arrangement of silver grains in gelatin. Since a radiograph is almost never viewed at an enlargement of 5 diameters, film graininess is not seen.

Screen Mottle

Screen mottle has two components: **structure mottle** (not important) and **quantum mottle** (important). Structure mottle is caused by defects in the intensifying screen, such as varying thickness or physical imperfections in the phosphor layer. Such screen irregularities can occur, but the quality control used in screen manufacturing is so good that structure mottle may be dismissed as making no contribution to radiographic mottle.

Quantum mottle is the only important cause of radiographic mottle. **Quantum** refers to a discrete unit of energy, and, in this discussion, it may be considered the energy carried by one x-ray photon. An x-ray beam may be thought of as containing a certain number of x-ray photons, or an equivalent number of quanta.

By showing a pattern of mottle, or nonuniform density, the x-ray film is telling us that it has "seen" a nonuniform pattern of light on the surface of the intensifying screen. The nonuniform pattern of light on the screen is caused by fluctuations in the number of photons (or quanta) per square millimeter in the beam which arrived at the screen. What this means is that a "uniform" beam of x rays is not uniform at all. Suppose a "uniform" x-ray beam could be frozen in space and cut in cross-sections. If the number of x-ray photons per square millimeter were counted, it would be unlikely that any two square mm would contain exactly the same number of photons. The "uniform" beam is not uniform.

The actual number of x-ray photons per mm^2 obeys the law of probability, because the emission of x rays by the x-ray tube is a random event. The average number of photons per mm^2 can be calculated by adding the number in each mm^2 and dividing by the number of squares. It will then be found that the actual number in any square will almost never be the average value, but that all numbers will fall within a certain range (percent fluctuation) of the average. The law of probability says that the magnitude of this fluctuation is plus or minus the square root of the average number of photons per mm². For example, if an x-ray beam contains an average of 10,000 photons per mm², the number in any one square mm will fall in the range:

$$10,000 \pm \sqrt{10,000} = 10,000 \pm 100$$

or any mm² may be expected to contain between 9900 and 10,100 photons. In some of the squares (32%) the variation will be even greater than this.

The percent fluctuation in the actual number of photons per mm² becomes greater as the average number becomes smaller. If 100 photons are used, fluctuation will be $\pm \sqrt{100}$, or ± 10, giving a percent fluctuation of $\frac{10}{100}$, or 10%. Using 10,000 photons, fluctuation is ± 100, or a percent fluctuation of $\frac{100}{10,000}$ or 1%.

Quantum mottle is caused by the statistical fluctuation in the number of quanta per unit area absorbed by the intensifying screen. The fewer quanta (x-ray photons)

used, the greater will be the quantum mottle (more statistical fluctuation). Intensifying screens are used because they decrease the x-ray exposure (number of photons) needed to expose the x-ray film. Quantum mottle is seen when intensifying screens are used. Quantum mottle will be greater with high-kVp x rays because they produce a higher screen intensification factor.

The concept of quantum mottle is illustrated in Figure 13–6. The model consists of the cardboard top of a hatbox, small cardboard figures in the shape of a circle, square, and triangle placed in the hatbox top, and 1,000 pennies. The pennies represent x-ray quanta, and were dropped into the hatbox top in a completely random manner. Radiographs of the model were made after 10, 100, 500, and 1000 pennies had been dropped into the hatbox top. Notice that the radiograph of 10 pennies shows no information about the make-up of the model; 100 pennies show

Figure 13–6 The "pennies in the hatbox" model illustrating the concept of quantum mottle

that the box top is probably round; 500 pennies show three filling defects in a box top which is definitely round; and all 1000 pennies clearly define the shape of each filling defect. In other words, a lot of pennies (quanta) provided a lot of information about the model; fewer pennies provided less information; and too few pennies provided no useful information.

Quantum mottle is difficult to see unless a high-quality radiograph is produced. A film of high contrast and good quality will show visible quantum mottle. If film contrast and quality are poor, such as produced by poor film-screen contact, quantum mottle will not be visible. Thick intensifying screens may show less visible mottle on the film because of greater diffusion of light. A radiograph with poor visibility of image detail will also exhibit poor visibility of quantum mottle.

In summary, let us define radiographic mottle as the radiographic recording of the statistical fluctuations in a beam of x-ray photons.

Speed versus Noise

Radiographic mottle is often called **noise.** Allow us to repeat an important but poorly understood fact: **noise (quantum mottle) results from statistical fluctuation in the number of x-ray photons used (absorbed) by the intensifying screens to form the image.** With presently available films and screens it is possible to obtain a film-screen system so fast that noise makes the resulting image unsatisfactory except for a few special applications such as pelvimetry. Two basic premises must be remembered:

> High contrast images are
> SHARPNESS limited

> Low contrast images are
> NOISE limited

Since low constrast images comprise most diagnostically important information, noise may seriously compromise a radiograph.

The two ways to increase the speed of a film-screen radiographic system are obvious:

1. Use a faster screen.
2. Use a faster film.

The way the increase in speed affects system noise (quantum mottle) is not so obvious or easy to understand. Let us illustrate this difficulty by posing a question which experience has shown that almost everyone answers incorrectly. Assume two radiographs of an abdomen are made. Both exposures use the same medium speed x-ray film. The first exposure is made using par speed calcium tungstate screens. The second exposure is made using high speed calcium tungstate screens which are exactly twice as fast (i.e., require only half the mAs) as the par speed screens. Now for the question: which exposure (par speed or high speed screens) will produce the radiograph with the most noise (quantum mottle)? If you answer "the high speed system," you are wrong and in company with the majority of your

Par

20% ABSORPTION

Hi Plus

40% ABSORPTION

LESS PATIENT EXPOSURE
SAME NUMBER OF PHOTONS USED
SAME NOISE

Figure 13–7 Increasing speed by increasing the stopping power of the intensifying screen will not change noise colleagues. The correct answer: the noise is the same for both radiographs (the noise will be more difficult to see when the thick, fast screen is used because of more light diffusion, which causes decreased visibility of image detail). The rest of this section is an attempt to explain this relationship between noise and system speed, a concept made important in film-screen radiography by the introduction of non-calcium tungstate high speed intensifying screens and fast x-ray film.

Let us try to simplify the problem by stating that, with regard to noise, there are two ways to increase the speed (i.e., lower the x-ray dose to the patient) of a film-screen radiographic system:

1. Increase speed with no change in noise.
2. Increase speed and increase noise.

We need to examine each of these two methods in some detail.

1. **Increased speed with no change in noise can be done in two ways:**
    a. Increase phosphor layer thickness.
    b. Use a phosphor with a higher absorption coefficient for x rays.

Both these methods will increase the stopping power of the intensifying screen. Refer to Figure 13–7, which diagrams a par speed and a Hi Plus (twice the speed of par) DuPont calcium tungstate screen. If 10 x-ray photons arrive at the par screen, 2 photons are absorbed (assume 20% absorption). If one uses Hi Plus $CaWO_4$ screens, the screen will absorb 40% of the x-ray beam because it is thicker than a par screen. Thus, to cause the high speed screen to absorb 2 photons, we need only cause 5 photons to arrive at the screen (the amount of light produced per absorbed photon is the same in each screen). Since only half as many photons are required, exposure to the patient is cut in half and we speak of the Hi Plus screen as being twice as "fast" because we were able to decrease patient exposure by half (i.e., we cut the mAs in half). However, the only factor determining noise is: **THE**

NUMBER OF PHOTONS USED BY THE SCREEN. Both the par and Hi Plus $CaWO_4$ screens have **USED** the same number of photons. The faster screen has a thicker phosphor layer which absorbs a higher percentage of the x-ray beam. Stated another way: if the screen phosphor is the same, changes in screen speed will not result in any change in noise. This last statement has an exception: addition of a light absorbing dye to the screen phosphor layer will prevent some light from reaching the film. Because some light is lost, more photons must be absorbed by the screen to produce enough light to expose the film (i.e., use of dye in slow screens decreases noise). The price one must pay for increased speed in $CaWO_4$ screens is more **unsharpness** caused by light diffusion in the thicker phosphor layer. Thus, the choice of which $CaWO_4$ screen to use is a compromise of:

SHARPNESS vs. SPEED.

A phosphor with higher inherent absorption of x rays could give more speed without an increase in unsharpness (thicker screen not required) or noise (same x ray to light conversion efficiency as $CaWO_4$). The potential for this type of improvement is limited. Lead (atomic number 82) is the highest atomic number non-radioactive element. Tungsten (atomic number 74) is so close to lead that there is little room in the periodic table to discover phosphors with a higher atomic number. However, we have previously discussed how some of the new phosphors do gain some of their speed through higher inherent absorption of x rays by use of a favorably located K-absorption edge. Screen speed obtained in this manner is desirable because one then decreases patient exposure without any increase in noise or unsharpness.

2. **Increased speed with increased noise can be done in two ways:**
    a. Use a phosphor with a higher x ray to light conversion efficiency.
    b. Use a faster film.

Both of these processes will have identical effects on the noise content of the finished radiograph. The system cannot distinguish between a phosphor having a higher conversion efficiency and the use of a faster film. In each case the faster system will provide an image produced by use (absorption) of fewer photons in the screen with a corresponding increase in noise. This is illustrated in Figure 13–8, in which a par speed calcium tungstate screen (20% absorption of the x-ray beam) is compared to a rare earth screen (such as combined gadolinium oxysulfide and lanthanum oxysulfide) which also absorbs 20% of the x-ray beam but produces twice as much light per absorbed photon (in this example). Notice that the rare earth screen, by absorbing only one x-ray photon, has produced as much light as the $CaWO_4$ screen produced by absorbing two x-ray photons. It is this difference in photons absorbed by the screen that causes a change in the quantum noise (mottle). Similarly, if one uses identical screens but a film which is twice as fast, the faster film will be properly

exposed with half as much light, which the screen produces by absorbing half as many photons.

The new fast screen phosphors are faster than calcium tungstate because they:

1. Absorb (use) a larger percentage of the x-ray beam (no change in quantum noise).
2. Have a higher x ray to light conversion efficiency (with an increase in quantum noise).

It is possible to use a film-screen combination in which system quantum mottle (noise) will produce a perceptible decrease in the visibility of low contrast images on the radiograph. In choosing one of the non-calcium tungstate very fast screens one must reach a compromise between:

SPEED vs. NOISE.

Another way to look at quantum noise is to examine a terribly complex function called the **Wiener spectrum.** This may be thought of as the modulation transfer function (MTF) of the noise of an image, and we will briefly examine this concept after the discussion of MTF later in this chapter.

We will summarize the concept of quantum noise in film-screen radiography in outline form:

1. Increase speed with no change in noise.
   a. Increase phosphor layer thickness.
   b. Use a phosphor with a higher absorption coefficient for x rays.
2. Increase speed with increased noise.
   a. Use a phosphor with a higher x ray to light conversion efficiency.
   b. Use a faster film.

Sharpness

Sharpness is the ability of the x-ray film or film-screen system to define an edge. The inability of a film-screen system to record a sharp edge because of light diffu-

Calcium Tungstate

20%
ABSORPTION

Rare Earth

MORE LIGHT
PER
ABSORBED PHOTON

LESS PATIENT EXPOSURE
SMALLER NUMBER OF PHOTONS USED
MORE NOISE

Figure 13–8 Increasing speed by increasing the x-ray to light conversion efficiency of the phosphor will increase noise sion in the intensifying screen has been previously discussed. Sharpness and contrast are closely related in the subjective response they produce. An unsharp edge can be easily seen if contrast is high, but a sharp edge may be poorly visible if contrast is low.

Most of the causes of unsharpness have been previously discussed. We will review them briefly.

Geometric Unsharpness

Penumbra is minimized by using a small focal spot and keeping magnification as small as possible. If you understand why the term "edge gradient" (rather than penumbra) is now preferred, you really understand what geometric unsharpness means.

Motion Unsharpness

Subject motion can be minimized by using a short exposure time. Motion of the x-ray tube during the exposure will cause unsharpness, but it is not as important as motion of the object.

Absorption Unsharpness

Absorption unsharpness results because a patient is not made up of objects that have nice sharp edges. Absorption unsharpness is greatest for round or oval objects.

Screen Unsharpness

X-ray intensifying screens cause unsharp borders because of **light diffusion** in the screen phosphor layer. Good screen-film contact is essential.

Parallax Unsharpness

Parallax unsharpness is seen only with double-emulsion films. There is an image on each emulsion, and the images are separated by the width of the film base (.007 or .008 inches). When viewed from an angle, these two image edges will not overlap exactly. Parallax makes a negligible contribution to image unsharpness.

Total Unsharpness

In a radiographic image, all types of unsharpness are present. The proper method of calculating the total unsharpness is not known, but it is known that simple addition is not correct. For example, assume that total unsharpness equals:

$$U_T = \sqrt{U_g^2 + U_a^2 + U_m^2 + U_s^2}$$

where $U_T =$ total unsharpness
$U_g =$ geometric unsharpness
$U_a =$ absorption unsharpness
$U_m =$ motion unsharpness
$U_s =$ screen unsharpness

This formula is probably not correct, but will illustrate an important point. Assume an examination in which $U_g = 0.5$ mm, $U_a = 4$ mm, $U_m = 1$ mm, and $U_s = 0.6$ mm. What is total unsharpness?

$$U_T = \sqrt{(0.5)^2 + 4^2 + 1^2 + (0.6)^2} = 4.2 \text{ mm}$$

Notice that total unsharpness of 4.2 mm is largely determined by the single largest cause of unsharpness, which is 4 mm of absorption unsharpness in this example. If any unsharpness is significantly larger than the others, the largest cause of unsharpness almost completely controls total unsharpness. In our example absorption unsharpness of 4 mm is the most important. Decreasing U_g (smaller focal spot) or U_m (shorter exposure time) or U_s (detail screens) would not significantly improve image sharpness. Attempts to improve the image must be directed toward the factor most responsible for a poor image. Absorption unsharpness cannot be changed, but the unsharp image edge may be made more easily visible by increasing contrast. Therefore, by increasing contrast with a lower kVp technique, it is possible that actually increasing U_g (geometric unsharpness) and U_m (motion unsharpness) by using higher mAs (larger focal spot and longer exposure time) will produce a radiograph with better visibility of fine detail. The infinite variety of boundaries encountered in the patient compounds the problem of absorption unsharpness. No matter how good the geometrical conditions, absorption unsharpness may make exact delineation of the borders of small objects (such as opacified blood vessels) all but impossible.

Resolution

Imagine a photograph of a pastoral scene in which a barn and a windmill are depicted against the background of a dark blue sky. If the top edge of the roof of the barn is sharply outlined against the sky, the photograph has good sharpness. The term **sharpness** is used to describe the subjective response of crisp, or abrupt, edges (the objective correlate of sharpness is termed acutance). If each vane of the windmill is easily counted, the photograph has good resolution, or resolving power. Sharpness is the ability of an imaging system to record sharply defined margins, or abrupt edges. **Resolving power is the ability to record separate images of small objects which are placed very close together.** An imaging system may have the ability to record sharp edges, but be unable to resolve fine details. Another system may yield fuzzy, unsharp edges, but still be able to show much fine detail. Sharpness and resolving power are different, but they are related in the subjective response they produce.

Until recently, x-ray imaging systems were evaluated by their resolving power. For example, a par-speed intensifying screen might be described as having a resolving power of 8 lines per mm. Several methods of determining resolving power are used. One method uses a resolving power target made up of a series of parallel wires or lead strips, placed so that the space between each lead strip is equal to the width of the strip (Figure 13–9). In this system, a "line" actually means a line and a space, more appropriately termed a "line pair." For example, 4 lines per mm means that there are 4 lead strips or wires per mm, with each line $^1/_8$ mm wide and each space $^1/_8$ mm wide, so that each line pair is

Figure 13–9 A resolving power target consists of a series of lines and spaces

$^1/_4$ mm wide. A commonly used resolving power target is the Buckbee-Meers resolution plate which consists of line pairs varying from 1.0 to 9.6 per mm in 18 steps.[1]

A film-screen system is evaluated by how many line pairs per mm can be clearly seen in the developed radiograph. Another testing device uses a slit of adjustable width between two blocks of lead. After each x-ray exposure, this apparatus is moved across the film or film-screen combination a distance equal to the width of the slit, in this way producing a series of lines and spaces on the developed film.[6] All of these systems depend on an observer determining how many line pairs per mm he can see, and the number will vary among observers. It is argued that these measurements only evaluate the ability of the system to depict the image of a wire, or lead strip or slit, and do not necessarily pertain to the complex shapes and varying contrasts presented to a film-screen system (or fluoroscopic system) in clinical practice. Also, the resolving power only measures a limit. Knowing that a film-screen system will resolve 8 line pairs per mm tells us that it will not produce an image of 10 line pairs per mm, but says nothing about how good or bad a job it does at 2, 4, or 6 line pairs per mm.

The basic question to consider is: when the information in the x-ray image is transferred to the x-ray film (usually with light from intensifying screens), how much information is lost? The answer to this question is now being sought by evaluation of the line spread function and the modulation transfer function. The physics and mathematics involved in these determinations are highly complex. We hope to present the basic concepts in an understandable form without the use of any mathematics.

LINE SPREAD FUNCTION

The fact that light diffusion by intensifying screens causes blurred, or unsharp, image edges has been discussed. The line spread function provides a way to measure this effect.

The line spread function is determined as follows. A narrow slit is formed between two jaws made of metal highly opaque to x-rays, such as platinum. The width of the slit is usually 10 microns, and the metal jaws are about 2 mm thick. X rays passing through this slit are so severely collimated that they may be considered as a "line source" x-ray beam. The slit apparatus is placed in intimate contact with a film-screen system, and an exposure is made. Only the x rays passing through the 10-micron slit reach the intensifying screens. A perfect imaging system would produce an image of a line 10 microns wide on the developed film. However, because of light diffusion in the screens, the developed film will actually show density extending out for several hundred microns on each side. The photographic effect of the x-ray beam is spread over a total distance of 800, or more, microns (0.8 mm).[11] This technique provides a way to express the line spread function (LSF) numerically. Figure 13–10 shows line spread function graphs in which the relative density is shown to decrease with distance away from the 10-micron line source of x rays. Measuring film density over such a small area requires use of a microdensitometer which reads the density of an extremely small area of the film.

Notice on the hypothetical curves of Figure 13–10 (based on the work of Rossmann and Lubberts[11]) that the tailing off of image density is much more marked when high-speed screens are used than when medium-speed screens are used to produce the same density in the center. The shape of the curves in Figure 13–10 allows us to predict accurately that image boundaries will be less faithfully recorded when the image resulting from the use of high-speed screens is compared to that resulting from the use of slower screens. The less light diffusion, the sharper, or more abrupt, will be image edges. Sharper image edges allow imaging of finer detail in the radiograph.

Figure 13–10 Line spread function of medium-speed and fast screens. (Modified from Rossman and Lubberts)

The line spread function can also be used to measure the influence on the image of factors other than intensifying screens. These have included x-ray film, fluoroscopic screens, focal spots of x-ray tubes, x-ray image intensifiers, motion unsharpness, and scatter radiation.

The LSF of x-ray film exposed without screens (direct x-ray exposure) is difficult to measure. There is almost no diffusion of x rays and secondary electrons in the film, so the LSF is narrow. The grain size of an x-ray film may be as large as 2.0 microns. If an x-ray photon were to pass between two grains which were side by side, it might cause both grains to be developed, producing an image 4μ wide. The image of a line source x-ray beam exposing a film directly will be slightly broadened because of slight radiation diffusion and the finite size of the developed silver halide grains. However, image diffusion is so small that the LSF of film exposed to x rays is difficult to measure.

Is the determination of the line spread function of a screen-film system of any practical value? Through a series of complex mathematical manipulations the modulation transfer function of the screen-film system can be calculated from the line spread function, and the modulation transfer provides a way to measure the image quality which can be produced.

MODULATION TRANSFER FUNCTION

We have discussed how the clarity of the x-ray image is influenced by **contrast, sharpness,** and **resolution.** Each of these terms may be defined separately, but their complex interrelationships which ultimately determine image clarity are much more difficult to evaluate. The modulation transfer function is a concept that has been formulated to provide an objective measurement of the combined effects of sharpness and resolution. Let us consider the term modulation to mean a change in the amplitude (or intensity, or amount) of an information-carrying signal. Imagine a can which contains an unknown amount of thick oil. The oil is measured by pouring it into a graduated beaker. Some of the oil will stick to the sides of the can and escape detection. The information signal seen is the oil in the beaker. The amount of information (oil) seen is less than the total amount of information in the can; the signal has been modulated (changed) because some information was lost in the transfer of oil from the can to the beaker. If careful laboratory measurements determine that the can holds 500 ml of oil, but only 400 ml is measured, the information-detecting system used will detect $\frac{400}{500}$, or 0.8, of the total information. Similarly, the MTF is an attempt to measure the amount of information transferred from the invisible x-ray image to the detecting system (x-ray film, television image, etc.). The MTF represents a ratio between the information recorded and the total amount of information available, or

$$\text{MTF} = \frac{\text{Information Recorded}}{\text{Information Available}}.$$

Since recorded information can never be greater than available information, the MTF can never be greater than 1.

The MTF of a screen-film system is usually calculated from the corresponding line spread function by a complex mathematical operation termed "Fourier transformation." In practice, a computer may do the calculations from information it receives from the microdensitometer used to measure the densities making up the line spread function. A complete discussion of the specialized physics and mathematics involved in developing an MTF curve is far beyond the scope of this text, and most radiologists (including the authors) lack the specialized background necessary to understand such a treatment of the subject. We are indebted to R. E. Wayrynen for developing the following discussion of what the modulation transfer

Figure 13–11   Information is lost when the x-ray image of a resolving power target is recorded by a screen-film combination

function means, expressed in simple examples.

Consider a resolving power target (Figure 13–11). A radiograph of the target should produce a film with "square wave" changes in density, completely black in the area corresponding to the spaces and completely unexposed in areas corresponding to the metal strips, with abrupt density changes; i.e., sharp margins. Using a screen-film combination, the blackest black will have a density of about 3.0, and unexposed film will have a density of about 0.2 (base and fog densities). Because of light scattering by the screens, the actual radiograph will not show "square waves." The maximum density will be less than expected, "unexposed" areas of the film will react as if they had received exposure, and the transition from minimum to maximum density will be gradual, producing the "sine wave" density pattern expressed graphically in Figure 13–11. Light scattering causes density to be "shoveled off" the density peaks and "poured into" the valleys, causing a **decrease in image sharpness** (less abrupt image borders) and a **decrease in contrast** (density difference between the "peaks" and "valleys").

Now consider a resolving power target in which the widths of the opaque metal strips and the spaces become progressively smaller. The more line pairs per unit length, the greater the amount of information presented to the screen-film system. The amount of information is usually expressed as a certain number of line pairs per mm, or a certain number of cycles per mm, both being the same. Figure 13–12 is a diagram of what happens to the image of the resolving power target recorded by the screen-film combination as information content increases. The difference in density (contrast) on the developed film between areas of maximum exposure (under the spaces) and minimum exposure becomes less as information content increases. This is caused almost entirely by light scattering in the intensifying screens. Eventually, the screen-film system becomes unable to show any density difference between lines and spaces; this represents the limit of the resolving power of the system; i.e., the ability to record lines and spaces.

When an x-ray beam is directed onto a resolving power target, most of the x rays which encounter a space pass through the space, while those that encounter a metal

Figure 13–12   As the information content of a resolving power target increases, the ability of the screen-film system to record the x-ray image of the target decreases

Figure 13–13   The modulation transfer function of a screen-film system may be calculated by using a resolving power target

strip are absorbed. In the laboratory it is possible to measure the intensity of the x-ray beam under spaces (maximum exposure) and lead strips (minimum exposure). The intensity may be expressed in milliroentgens and represents the exposure received by the screen-film combination. A characteristic curve may be prepared in which the logarithm of the actual exposure (rather than relative exposure) is used to prepare the density-log E curve. On such a curve (Figure 13–13) the measured maximum (E_{max}) and minimum (E_{min}) exposures reaching the film are recorded. Then the exposed film is processed, and the developed maximum and minimum densities are carefully measured and plotted on the curve, shown as the obtained densities D'_{max} and D'_{min} in Figure 13–13. Notice that the maximum and minimum densities actually produced by the exposure are not the same as the densities expected from the measured exposures. The observed maximum density is less than predicted, and the observed minimum density is more than predicted. This is another way of graphically representing the effect of light scattering by the intensifying screens. Expressed another way, the film has acted as if it received a lower maximum exposure and a higher minimum exposure, as shown by the dotted lines in Figure 13–13.

The amplitude of the exposure input ($E_{max} - E_{min}$) to the film is known from actual measurement. The amplitude of the exposure "equivalent" output ($E'_{max} - E'_{min}$) has been calculated by knowing the characteristic curve of the film and measuring film density produced by the exposure. In addition, the width of the lines and spaces of the resolving power target are obviously known. Therefore, we may now calculate the modulation transfer function (MTF) of the screen-film system at a known frequency (lines per mm) as follows (Figure 13–13):

$$MTF = \frac{\text{exposure amplitude output}}{\text{exposure amplitude input}}$$

Using this rather laborious procedure, the MTF of a screen-film system could be calculated for 1, 2, 4, 6, 8, etc. line pairs per mm by using the appropriate resolving power target, measuring exposure input, and calculating the exposure "equivalent" output. A curve similar to Figure 13–14 would be developed, and this is the MTF curve of our hypothetical screen-film system. This curve tells us that at 1 line pair per mm the $\frac{\text{output}}{\text{input}}$ = about 0.8 (or 80%), which is good. At 4 line pairs per mm $\frac{\text{output}}{\text{input}}$ = about 0.3, and at 8 line pairs per mm it is about 0.1, or 10%. Remember, MTF curves are usually calculated from the line spread function, but the meaning of the MTF curve is easier to understand if it is discussed in terms of its derivation based on the use of resolving power targets.

How is an MTF curve useful? There are no "units" of MTF. It does not measure contrast or sharpness or resolution. For the clinical radiologist, MTF curves may be useful as a more accurate way to compare the imaging qualities of competing sys-

Figure 13–14   The modulation transfer function curve of a hypothetical screen-film system

tems, and pick the system which best suits his needs. Consider intensifying screens again. We have discussed the fact that resolving power measures only a limit. Assume Figure 13–14 is the MTF curve for a par-speed intensifying screen. The 10% response on the MTF curve corresponds roughly to the resolving power of the imaging system. In Figure 13–14 the 10% response is about 8 line pairs per mm, so this screen would have a resolving power of 8 lines (or line pairs) per mm. But the curve also allows us to compare the relative imaging properties of the screen at frequencies lower than the resolving power.

Now consider Figure 13–15 in which hypothetical MTF curves for two x-ray intensifying screens are shown: the differences in the curves are exaggerated for the purposes of illustration. Screen A has a resolving power (10% MTF) of 6 lines per mm, while the resolving power of Screen B is 14 line pairs per mm. From resolving power figures, Screen B is apparently a much better screen. However, the MTF curves show that at 4 lines per mm, Screen A has a response of 80%, while Screen B has fallen to 30%, and at 2 lines/mm the values are 90% and 50% respectively. Under normal viewing conditions the eye usually sees structures of a size corresponding to an information content between 2 and 4 line pairs per mm. For

routine radiography, the information recorded by Screen A will probably produce radiographs of greater diagnostic accuracy than those produced by Screen B. On the other hand, an attempt to record very small structures would require the use of Screen B. Obviously, the true difference in the characteristics and clinical applications of these screens can be appreciated only from a comparison of the respective MTF curves. Resolving power may be thought of as a single point on the MTF curves.

Modulation transfer function curves are being developed for all the imaging systems used in radiology, including screen-film systems, x-ray image amplifiers, cine and 70, 90 and 105 mm systems, and television viewing, including tape and disc image storage systems.

The MTF plays an important role in the evaluation of a complex imaging system. Consider, for example, a film-screen system which has a front screen, first film emulsion, film base, second film emulsion and back screen. In optical terms this is termed a cascaded system, or a series of cascaded imaging processes. In the chapter dealing with magnification radiography we will consider the film, the x-ray tube focal spot, the x-ray intensifying screens and the motion of the object being radiographed as four components in a cascaded system. Each of the components of a cascaded system has its own imaging properties, and it is often possible to express these properties in terms of the MTF of the particular component. Once the MTF of the components of a complex system are known, the total MTF of the entire system may be obtained by multiplying the MTFs of each of the components (this concept will be considered in some detail in the chapter on magnification). As an example, if one knows that, at an object frequency of 2 line pairs per mm, the MTF of x-ray film is 1.0 (i.e., the film is perfect), the MTF of the intensifying screens is 0.7 and the MTF of the focal spot of the x-ray tube is 0.8, then total system MTF will be $1.0 \times 0.7 \times 0.8 =$

Figure 13–15 Hypothetical MTF curves of two x-ray intensifying screens

0.56. The MTF concept allows each component of an imaging system to be studied so that the optimum system may be designed. Unfortunately, in diagnostic radiology it is difficult to objectively define the "optimum system" because the elements in a radiograph that allow one to arrive at a correct diagnosis are not easily defined. It is not correct to assume that by measuring the MTF for different imaging systems the radiologists can compare and decide what to buy. The ultimate practical use of MTF measurements to both radiologists and industry is still being evaluated.

NOISE AND THE WIENER SPECTRUM

We have previously introduced the concept of quantum mottle (or noise) caused by the fact that film-screen radiography is quantum limited (i.e., the radiograph may be formed with a relatively small number of x-ray photons). This noise may be apparent visually, and it can also be measured in the laboratory. The radiologist generally considers a radiograph made with average speed film and par speed screens as being pretty good. Such radiographs require that about 50,000 x-ray photons per square millimeter be absorbed by the screen to produce an average density of 1.0. In photography this would not be considered a good image, as a typical aerial photography film will use about twenty times as many photons to form its image.

One way to objectively describe noise is by the Wiener spectrum, sometimes called the power spectrum of noise. The mechanics of measuring radiographic mottle (noise) present difficult problems. In one method, the radiographic mottle is scanned by a microdensitometer, and the sampled density fluctuation is analyzed by a computer. Another method involves putting the "noisy" film into a type of microdensitometer in which it can be spun in a circle and illuminated from one side. The transmitted light is collected by a photo-multiplier behind a scanning aperture. The fluctuation in transmitted light intensity caused by radiographic mottle is converted to a voltage fluctuation in the photomultiplier tube. Electronic analysis of this voltage fluctuation performs what amounts to a Fourier analysis which can determine the frequency content in the noise pattern.

Let us consider for a moment what noise looks like on a microdensitometer scan. In previous discussions, we have assumed that such a scan across the image of a small object would produce a nice smooth scan of density change versus distance as shown in Figure 13–11. This is not a true picture of the situation. In Figure 13–16 A and B we show how a real microdensitometer scan across an image will appear. Assume identical screens are used, but in Figure 13–16 A a slow film (low noise) and in 13–16 B a fast film (high noise) is used. The small square aperture of the microdensitometer (i.e., 5 to 10 microns) will "see" the small, irregular density variations which constitute radiographic mottle, superimposed on the larger density change caused by the image of the object being radiographed. In fact, it is difficult to make accurate microdensitometer scans of noisy and unsharp images due to the presence of quantum mottle. Nice smooth

A. LOW NOISE

B. HIGH NOISE

Figure 13–16 Schematic depiction of a microdensitometer scan of the image of a blood vessel made with a low noise (A) and a high noise (B) imaging system microdensitometer scans of objects such as opacified blood vessels simply do not exist.

We must retreat for a moment and review the components of radiographic mottle. You will recall that there is both screen mottle (for practical purposes this is quantum mottle) and film graininess. While the eye does not normally see film grain, the microdensitometer is able to "see" the nonhomogeneous arrangement of clumps of silver in the gelatin. Thus, a microdensitometer will detect noise of two types:

1. Quantum mottle (statistical fluctuation of x-ray quanta absorbed in the screen).
2. Film grain (noise due to the inherent grain distribution in the film).

The Wiener spectrum is a measure of the total noise recorded by the film, **the sum of the grain noise and the quantum noise.** How does one distinguish film grain from screen mottle (quantum mottle)? This requires that two "flash" exposures of a film-screen system be made. The film in its cassette is simply placed under an x-ray tube and exposed at a reasonable kVp (one author uses 80 kVp) and low mAs so as to produce a density on the processed film of about 0.7. If the film and screen (or screens) are in intimate contact, the film will record quantum mottle resulting from the non-uniform absorption of x-ray quanta (and thus non-uniform production of light) in the screen, so the resulting noise will be made up of recorded quantum noise superimposed on the inherent film grain. To measure film grain alone a specially designed cassette is used. This cassette holds the screen (or screens) 13 or 14 mm away from the film, causing the individual light flashes (scintillations) from the screen to be blurred into a pattern of completely uniform illumination before the light reaches the film. In such a circumstance the film has been exposed with a truly uniform light source (i.e., quantum mottle has become undetectable in the light pattern by the time it reaches the

film), so any noise in the processed film must originate from inherent film grain. In all these experiments we assume (virtually always correctly) that the screens used are free of any structural defects that could produce noise.

Schematic representation of the Wiener spectrum of a film-screen system will depict (Figure 13–17):

1. Total system noise (quantum plus grain noise)
2. Film grain noise (grain noise)
3. Ability of the system to record the noise at increasing spatial frequency (recorded noise)

Notice in Figure 13–17 that the line depicting total (quantum plus grain) noise and grain noise are straight lines. This means that the amount of noise is the same at all spatial frequencies; this is termed white noise. Considering only noise, we may consider quantum mottle as the information input which we have asked the film-screen system to record. If the system were perfect, the amount of recorded quantum noise would be the same (white noise input) at all spatial frequencies. However, the MTF of the film-screen system limits the ability of the system to record information input, whether that information is the

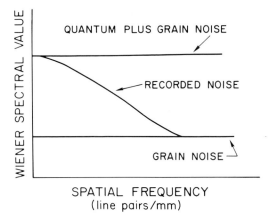

Figure 13–17 Schematic representation of the Wiener spectrum of a film-screen system

image of a skull, opacified blood vessel, or quantum mottle. The ability of the film-screen system to record noise decreases as the spatial frequency (line pairs per mm) increases, exactly as the ability of the system to record any image decreases with increasing spatial frequency. Depending on the MTF of the screen being used, a point is reached where quantum noise is no longer imaged, and at this point only inherent film grain remains for the micro-densitometer to detect (this might occur at about 6 to 10 line pairs per mm with typical screens). Let us not concern ourselves with a unit for measuring the Wiener spectrum, but be content to compare the position of a curve along the vertical axis to indicate more noise or less noise.

A couple of examples may make this topic easier to understand. Figure 13–18 shows the Wiener spectrum of radiographic mottle for two film-screen systems.

System A uses a sharp (thin) screen combined with a fast film. System B uses a less sharp (thicker) screen combined with a slower film. Notice that the inherent film grain white noise is greater for the fast film (i.e., larger clumps of silver more unevenly distributed in the gelatin) than the slow film. System A has an increased Wiener spectral noise value because fewer x-ray quanta were absorbed (i.e., the fast film required less light). The point where the total recorded noise curve merges with the film grain noise level indicates the relative MTF of each screen. The screen used in system A has the better MTF because it is able to record noise out to higher frequencies than system B. Without assigning any value units to the Wiener spectrum one may still derive a lot of information from these two curves (i.e., compare total noise, film graininess and system MTF).

Now consider Figure 13–19 which shows the Wiener spectral curves of three different screens used with the same film. Since systems A and B have the same total system noise at very low spatial frequency we can conclude that these two screens use the same number of x-ray quanta to expose the film. Likewise, since system A records noise at higher spatial frequencies, we

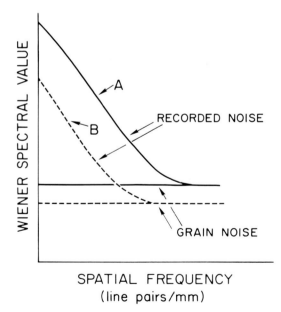

Figure 13–18 Schematic representation of the Wiener spectrum of a sharp screen combined with a fast film (A), and a less sharp screen combined with a slower film (B)

Figure 13–19 Schematic representation of the Wiener spectral curves of three different calcium tungstate intensifying screens used with the same film (see text)

know that screen A has a better MTF than screen B (probably because it is thinner). In fact, these two curves are similar to curves obtained with two par speed calcium tungstate screens made by different manufacturers.[20] Curve C represents a screen with significantly less total noise than the other two systems. This might be accomplished by using a less efficient screen phosphor (requiring absorption of more x-ray quanta to make an equal amount of light) or by use of the same phosphor and including a light absorbing dye in the phosphor layer. System C has a better MTF than the other systems because it records noise at a higher spatial frequency. This improved MTF might result from a thinner screen or from use of a dye in the screen to minimize light diffusion (acutance dye). This curve (C) is similar to a published Wiener spectral value curve of a detail calcium tungstate screen containing a yellow acutance dye to minimize light diffusion in the phosphor layer.[20]

As is true with MTF measurements, one finds it difficult to accurately define the ultimate use of Wiener spectral curves in diagnostic radiology. It is clear that new developments in design regarding system optics, noise and speed are offering the radiologist great flexibility in his choice of an imaging system. Unfortunately, this greater flexibility creates a problem of choice which requires greater understanding of the relation between system speed, noise and detail visibility.

SUMMARY

Image clarity is defined as the visibility of diagnostically important detail in the radiographic image. Image clarity is determined by contrast and image quality. Radiographic contrast depends on three factors: subject contrast, film contrast, and scatter radiation plus fog. Image quality is a difficult subject to discuss because there is no good definition of what actually constitutes diagnostically important detail. Quantum mottle interferes with the small-est perceptible contrast and is inversely proportional to the number of photons used to form an image. Sharpness is the ability of an imaging system to define a sharp edge. Resolving power is the ability of an imaging system to record separate images of small objects which are placed very close together. The line spread function, modulation transfer function, and Wiener spectrum are concepts to help develop a better understanding of the physical factors which control the information content of the radiographic image. We have attempted to introduce the fundamentals of LSF and MTF and Wiener spectrum in simple terms. The bibliography lists a number of excellent articles which explore these concepts in more detail.

REFERENCES

1. Bookstein, J. J., and Steck, W.: Effective focal spot size. Radiol. *98*, 31, 1971.
2. Cleare, H. M., Splettstosser, H. R., and Seeman, H. E.: An experimental study of the mottle produced by x-ray intensifying screens. Amer. J. Roentgen, *88*, 168, 1962.
3. Doi, K., and Rossman, K.: Measurement of optical and noise properties of screen-film systems in radiography. SPIE *56* (1975) MEDICAL X-RAY Photo-Optical Systems Evaluation.
4. Gopala Rao, U. V., and Bates, L. M.: The modulation transfer function of x-ray focal spots. Phys. Med. Biol. *14*, 93, 1968.
5. Holm, T.: Some aspects of radiographic information. Radiol. *83*, 319, 1964.
6. Morgan, R. H.: The frequency response function. Amer. J. Roentgen. *88*, 175, 1962.
7. Morgan, R. H., Bates, L. M., Gopala Rao, U. V., and Marinaro, A.: The frequency response characteristics of x-ray films and screens. Amer. J. Roentgen. *92*, 426, 1964.
8. Roesch, W. C., Mellins, H. Z., and Gregg, E. C.: Improvements in the radiological image: A report from the Radiation Study Section of the National Institutes of Health. Radiol. *97*, 442, 1970.
9. Rossman, K.: Image Quality. Contained in the syllabus of the proceedings of the AAPM 1971 Summer School, "Physics of Diagnostic Radiology" at Trinity University, San Antonio, Texas, July 12–17, 1971. USDHEW Publication No. (FDA) 74-8006, p. 220–281.
10. ———: Image-forming quality of radiographic screen-film systems: The line spread-function. Amer. J. Roentgen, *90*, 178, 1963.
11. ———: Image quality. Radiol. Clin. N. Amer. *7*, 419, 1969.

12. ———: Point spread-function, line spread-function and modulation transfer function. Radiol. *93*, 257, 1969.

13. Rossman, K., and Lubberts, G.: Some characteristics of the line spread-function and modulation transfer function of medical radiographic films and screen-film systems. Radiol. *86*, 235, 1966.

14. Rossman, K., and Sanderson, G.: Validity of the modulation transfer function of radiographic screen-film systems measured by the slit method. Phys. Med. Biol. *13*, 259, 1968.

15. Seeman, H. E.: Factors which influence image quality and speed of film-screen combinations (In) *Technological Needs for Reduction of Patient Dosage from Diagnostic Radiology* (M. L. Janower, ed.) Springfield: Charles C Thomas, 1963.

16. ———: Physical factors which determine roentgenographic contrast. Amer. J. Roentgen. *80*, 112, 1958.

17. ———: *Physical and Photographic Principles of Medical Radiography.* New York: John Wiley and Sons, Inc., 1968.

18. Strum, R. E., and Morgan, R. H.: Screen intensification systems and their limitations. Amer. J. Roentgen. *62*, 617, 1949.

19. Wagner, R. F., and Denny, E. W.: A primer on physical parameters affecting radiographic image quality. Contained in the syllabus of the joint BRH-ACR conference, "First Image Receptor Conference: Film/screen Combinations," at Arlington, Virginia, Nov. 13–15, 1975. HEW Publication (FDA) 77-8003, p. 35–58.

20. Wagner, R. F., and Weaver, K. E.: Prospects for x-ray exposure reduction using rare earth intensifying screens. Radiol. *118,* 183, 1976.

21. Wayrynen, R. E.: Personal communication.

CHAPTER 14

Fluoroscopy

X rays were discovered because of their ability to cause fluorescence, and the first x-ray image of a human part was observed fluoroscopically. Dr. Glasser in his book *Dr. W. C. Röntgen* recounts, "To test further the ability of lead to stop the rays, he selected a small lead piece, and in bringing it into position observed to his amazement, not only that the round dark shadow of the disc appeared on the screen, but that he actually could distinguish the outline of his thumb and finger, within which appeared darker shadows—the bones of his hand."[1]

During the years immediately following the discovery of x rays, film emulsions were of inferior quality and tube performance was unpredictable. Fluoroscopy was more reliable and probably more important than radiographic techniques. In the ensuing years equipment improved, and radiography moved to the forefront while fluoroscopy slipped to the subordinate role which it now maintains; i.e., principally for the study and detection of moving parts, and secondarily to position a part optimally to obtain better radiographs.

In recent years a large amount of accessory equipment has been developed to enhance and record the fluoroscopic image. These include x-ray image intensifiers, cine, television, and spot film cameras. However, in this chapter our discussion will be limited to conventional fluoroscopy.

THE FLUOROSCOPE

A fluoroscope has two essential components, an x-ray tube and a fluoroscopic screen. All of the other parts are designed either to protect the patient and operator from stray radiation or to facilitate the performance of an examination. The tube and screen are usually mounted at the opposite ends of a C-arm to maintain their alignment as shown in Figure 14–1. The operator moves the fluoroscopic screen over the patient, and the x-ray tube follows the screen beneath the tabletop. The only motion between the two occurs along a slip joint in the C-arm, which allows the screen to be raised and lowered to accommodate patients of various sizes.

A fluoroscopic x-ray tube is a standard rotating anode tube, the same as the ones used for radiography, but it is operated at a much lower tube current. Instead of the 100 to 1000 mA used in radiography, fluoroscopes are operated at currents ranging from 0.5 to 5.0 mA. The tube is equipped with shutters so that the operator can regulate the size and shape of the x-ray beam. The shutters are connected either electrically, or by cables, to lever arms mounted on the fluoroscopic screen. Permanent filtration equivalent to 2.5 mm of aluminum is recommended for fluoroscopy. The fluoroscopic screen is usually a Patterson type B-2, which produces light in the yellow-green band of the spectrum. A large quantity of radiation

LEAD GLASS
FLUORESCENT
SCREEN
SPOT FILM
SLOT
GRID

Figure 14–1   Fluoroscope

passes through the screen, and thus has easy access to the fluoroscopist. A lead-glass protective barrier is used to absorb this radiation (Figure 14–1) before it reaches the operator. The recommended thickness of the glass barrier in lead equivalents is as follows[2]:

Up to 100 kVp — 1.5 mm lead equivalent
100 to 125 kVp — 1.8 mm lead equivalent
Over 125 kVp — 2.0 mm lead equivalent

One of the principal reasons for employing fluoroscopy is to position a part optimally so as to isolate its image from obscuring shadows. Most fluoroscopes are equipped with a spot film device to record this image. To expose a spot film, the operator adjusts the field size and moves a film from a lead-shielded storage compartment into the fluoroscopic field. Usually, a small motor drives the film cassette into position in a slot between the fluoroscopic screen and the grid as shown in Figure 14–1. The fluoroscopic current automatically increases from approximately 3.0 mA to conventional radiographic levels (100 to 1000 mA) for the exposure. Most fluoroscopes are equipped with grids to absorb scatter radiation. Some units have specially designed shutters that automati-

cally adjust the x-ray beam to the exact size selected for a spot film.

A large variety of fluoroscopic tables have been designed to meet the needs of particular examinations. Two important safety factors are common to all of them. The first protects the patient—the x-ray tube target should be at least 18 inches below the tabletop. Exposure rates are measured at the tabletop, and they are excessively large if the tube is closer than 18 inches. Remember, the inverse square law is in effect during fluoroscopy, so the input side of the patient receives more radiation per unit area than the output side (disregarding the difference resulting from attenuation). The input dosage is unnecessarily large with short tube-tabletop distances. The tabletop exposure rate should not exceed 10 roentgens per minute, and with well-designed equipment, it should be considerably lower. The second safety factor applies only to tables that have a Bucky grid mechanism. Cassettes are slid into a tray beneath the grid through an opening in the side of the table. Most tables have a hinged lead strip that fills this opening when the grid is parked at either end of the table. If the opening is not shielded, scatter radiation originating from the undersurface of the tabletop has an unimpeded route to the fluoroscopist.

Another feature included in most systems, and required by law in many states, is a 5-minutes safety timer. It measures the accumulated fluoroscopic time during an examination and turns off the unit after 5 minutes. It is only a safety timer if it is coupled with good judgment on the part of the fluoroscopist, since it can be reset with little effort.

SCREEN ILLUMINATION

In 1941, at a meeting of the Radiologic Society of North America in Chicago, Dr. W. Edward Chamberlain[3] startled his audience when he announced that the light reflected from the piece of paper he was holding in his hand was 30,000 times brighter than the illumination of a fluoroscopic screen. Radiologists had always known that the fluoroscopic screen was poorly illuminated, but no one before Chamberlain had ever bothered to measure it. How can we see anything with so little light? The answer is found in the eye's amazing ability to adapt to low levels of illumination, which we will discuss later in this chapter.

The unit that is used to measure screen illumination is the millilambert, which is one-thousandth of a lambert. The definition of a **lambert** (the luminance of a perfectly diffusing surface emitting 1 lumen per square centimeter) is unimportant and meaningless to most radiologists. However, even if we do not understand the definition of a (milli)lambert, we can still appreciate the magnitude of its brightness from our everyday experiences. For example, most of our daylight hours are spent in an illumination of from 1 to 100 millilamberts.

The brightness of a fluoroscopic screen is only 0.01 to 0.001 millilambert,[3] depending upon the x-ray exposure factors and the density and thickness of the part being examined. This level may fall much lower during abdominal fluoroscopy of large patients. Radiographs of average density are illuminated by an x-ray viewbox to a brightness of approximately 10 millilamberts, which is 3 to 4 orders of magnitude brighter than the fluoroscopic screen. The fluoroscopic image is too poor to salvage by simply increasing exposure factors. Patient exposures of thousands of roentgens per minute are needed to bring the brightness of the fluoroscopic screen to ideal levels, clearly an intolerable situation. Fortunately, another system of light amplification has been developed, the x-ray image intensifier, which will be discussed in the next chapter.

VISUAL PHYSIOLOGY

Before progressing further with a discussion of fluoroscopy, we will digress and review visual physiology, especially as it relates to night vision. The illumination of the fluoroscopic screen is inadequate for daylight vision. It requires a completely different physiological mechanism, which we must understand, to utilize the small amount of available light as efficiently as possible.

The retina contains two different types of light receptors, rods and cones. The total number of receptors is about 135 million, of which only 7 million are cones. Their relative distribution is shown in Figure 14–2. Cones are concentrated in the fovea (150,000 per mm^2) and sparsely distributed over the remainder of the retina (4,000 to 6,000 per mm^2).[4] The fovea has no rods. All of the rest of the retina contains many more rods than cones. The greatest concentration of rods (160,000 per mm^2) occurs about 20° from the fovea. Cones function most efficiently in bright light, while rods function best with low levels of illumination. Daylight (cone) vision is called **photopic vision,** and night (rod) vision is called **scotopic vision.** The transition from one to the other is not sharply defined, and the overlap area is

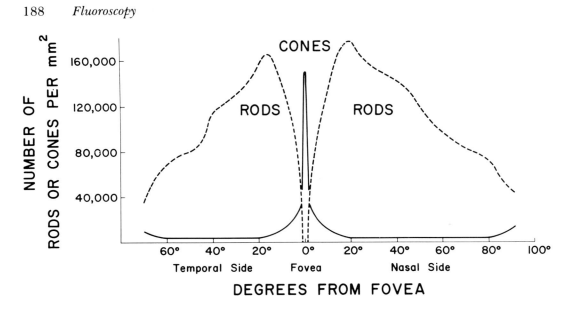

Figure 14–2   The distribution of rods and cones on the retina. (Adapted from Hartridge, H.: *Recent Advances in the Physiology of Vision*. Philadelphia; The Blakiston Co., 1950)

called **mesopic vision.** The fovea, with its dense concentration of cones, has the best photopic vision, but it is completely blind with low levels of illumination. Scotopic vision is entirely peripheral vision.

Dark Adaptation

Perhaps the most remarkable feature of the eye is its ability to adapt to a wide range of light intensities. Given sufficient time, the eye becomes more sensitive as the amount of light decreases, as shown in the dark adaptation curve in Figure 14–3. The curve was constructed by placing an observer in a completely darkened room, and periodically measuring the lowest detectable level of illumination. The eye adapts to the dark in two phases. The first phase represents the adaptation of cones. They adapt rapidly, but only to a minor degree, too little to be of any value to the fluoroscopist. The second phase of the dark adaptation curve represents the adaptation of rods, which is much slower and more pronounced than cone adaptation. The rods' sensitivity to dim light increases for ap-

proximately one hour, at which time it reaches a threshold, a point of maximum sensitivity. At this point, dark adaptation is complete and a longer period of darkness cannot further increase sensitivity. The threshold illumination for rods (i.e., the lowest detectable level of illumination) is

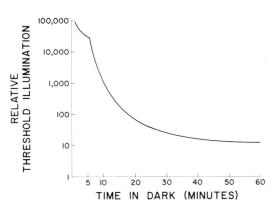

Figure 14–3 Dark adaptation curve. (Adapted from Davson, H.: *The Physiology of the Eye*. Boston; Little, Brown and Co., 1963)

about 0.000001 millilamberts,[3] which is well below the light level of a fluoroscopic screen (0.01 to 0.001 millilamberts). Rods are well suited for fluoroscopy, and in fact, they are the only detectors capable of functioning with so little light. The important point to remember about the dark adaptation curve is that it takes a full hour for the eyes to adapt completely. However, they are probably adequately adapted for fluoroscopy after 30 minutes.

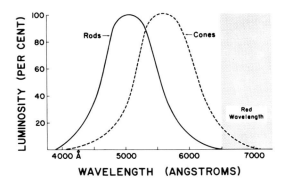

Figure 14–4 The sensitivity of rods and cones to various wavelengths. (Adapted from Davson, H.: *The Physiology of the Eye.* Boston: Little, Brown and Co., 1963)

Rods and cones are sensitive to different wavelengths of light as shown in Figure 14–4. Rods are most sensitive in the blue-green range (5000 Å), while cones have a peak sensitivity in the yellow-green range (5550 Å). Rods are blind to red light (6500 to 7500 Å), and cones are the only detectors capable of seeing red. This has a practical application in dark adaptation. Wearing red glasses, a fluoroscopist can adapt to the dark in ordinary room light. The red glasses transmit only red light, which does not affect the rods. The rods are shielded from all other wavelengths, and they adapt to the dark, while the cones see enough with the red light to permit ordinary activity.

Visual Acuity

Visual acuity is the ability of the eye to recognize the separation between multiple lines of equal width and spacing from a given viewing distance. It is usually measured in line pairs per millimeter (one line pair is a line and space of equal width). For example, the eye can easily resolve line pairs 1 mm thick from a distance of 20 cm. If the line pairs are made thinner and

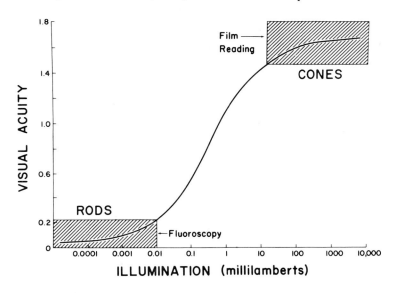

Figure 14–5 Visual acuity in line pairs for various wavelengths of light. (Adapted from Hecht, S.: The relationship between visual acuity and illumination. J. Gen. Physiol. *11,* 255, 1927)

closer together, or if the viewing distance is increased, eventually a point is reached where the eye can no longer resolve them. This point represents the visual acuity of the eye.

Visual acuity varies with illumination as shown in Figure 14–5. As the amount of light increases, visual acuity increases. At low levels of illumination, where rods are the only functioning receptors (scotopic vision), visual acuity is at its lowest level. As the amount of light increases, visual acuity improves until the illumination reaches the level required for photopic vision. At this point, visual acuity is near its maximum level and it is not significantly improved by more light. The visual acuity of cones is ten times greater than that of rods. Fluoroscopy resolution is limited by the visual acuity of the rods, and not by the resolution of the fluoroscopic screen. The screen usually displays more information than the eye can detect with scotopic vision.

Integration Time

The integration time of the eye is the time over which it can store information. An x-ray film can integrate over a long period of time; the eye cannot. The integration time of the eye is only 0.2 second.[5] This short time is a serious disadvantage during fluoroscopy, a disadvantage that is not shared by radiographic techniques. For example, if a radiographic image is too light, it can be darkened by lengthening the exposure time. If necessary, the exposure time can be increased to several seconds, and the film will gradually accumulate enough radiation to reach an optimum density. The eye cannot build a picture in this way. It can only integrate for 0.2 second, then it must begin over on a whole new picture. If the fluoroscopic image is not bright enough to be of good quality, it cannot be improved by prolonged observation. Nothing is gained by gazing at a fluoroscopic image for an extended period of time.

Two characteristics of rod (scotopic) vi-sion are worthy of special mention. First, rod vision is peripheral vision. Normally, we look directly at a point of interest, and the principal image is focused onto the retina at the fovea, which contains the greatest concentration of cones and maximum visual acuity. However, the fovea is blind to fluoroscopic levels of illumination since it contains no rods. The fluoroscopic image is seen best when the eyes look slightly to the side of the point of interest. Then the principal image is focused at the greatest concentration of rods, which is 20° to the side of the fovea. Second, rod vision is improved by motion. In fact, rods are incapable of holding a stationary image for a sustained period. If the gaze is fixed upon a stationary object, the peripheral visual field will gradually fade from view. Fluoroscopic vision is best when either the eyes or the fluoroscopic screen is kept moving continually.

STATISTICAL QUALITY OF THE FLUOROSCOPIC IMAGE

When we talk about fluoroscopic image quality, we must consider two different aspects of quality: the statistical quality of the image itself and the quality of the image that is actually perceived. A statistically superb image is of no value if the eye cannot capture it. In conventional fluoroscopy image quality is severely limited by the poor visual acuity of scotopic vision.

The fluoroscopic image exists at three different levels: (1) as an x-ray image; (2) as a light image on the fluoroscopic screen; and (3) as a light image on the retina of the eye. We will examine statistical quality (i.e., the number of photons making up the image) at each of these levels.

Compared to a standard roentgenogram, fluoroscopy begins with an inferior x-ray image. A simple way to demonstrate its inferiority is by comparing fluoroscopic and spot film exposure factors. No correction is needed for distance, grids, or other variables since they are the same for both systems. The following exposure factors were used in our department for abdominal fluoroscopy of a fairly large patient:

	SPOT FILM	FLUOROSCOPY
kVp	85	85
mA	150	3
Time (sec)	0.4	0.2*
mAs	60	0.6
Ratio	**100**	**1**

A fluoroscopic time (*) of 0.2 seconds, the integration time of the eye, is used for the comparison. The number of mAs (product of milliamperes and seconds) is proportional to the total number of photons involved in the two techniques. The ratio is 100 to 1; i.e., the x-ray image contains 100 times as many photons as the fluoroscopic image. Even if 150 mA is used for fluoroscopy, image quality is still inferior, because the spot film can integrate over a longer period of time.

One last point about the comparison between fluoroscopy and spot films is worth mentioning, even though it is not related to our present discussion. With the factors given above, each spot film results in a 60 mAs exposure to the patient, which is equivalent to 20 seconds of fluoroscopic time. With very large patients and long exposure times, one spot film may be equal to more than a minute of fluoroscopic time. We do not mean to condemn spot films, but merely to point out their cost in exposure to both the patient and the fluoroscopist.

Sturm and Morgan[6] measured the number of photons in each link of the fluoroscopic chain; their results are summarized in Figure 14–6. The numbers are for abdominal fluoroscopy, and of course they will vary depending upon the thickness and density of the patient. Their reference point was 1 square millimeter of fluoroscopic screen; i.e., the number of x-ray photons directed at, and the number of light photons emitted from, 1 mm^2 of screen. The x-ray tube delivers 5,000,000 photons per second, and 99% of them are

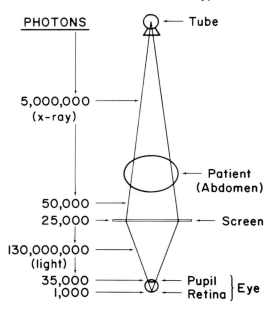

Figure 14–6 The number of x-ray and light photons per sq. millimeter of fluoroscopic screen per second. (Adapted from the measurements of Sturm, R.E., and Morgan, R.H.: Screen intensification systems and their limitations. Amer. J. Roentgen. *62*, 613, 1949)

absorbed in the patient. One-half of the remaining 50,000 photons pass through the screen, and contribute nothing to image formation. Approximately 25,000 photons are absorbed by the screen.

Each x-ray photon produces many light photons, so the 25,000 x-ray photons are swelled to 130,000,000 light photons, easily enough to produce a good image if the eye could capture them. The eye is the weakest link in the chain. It defines the lowest level of photon flux. From a viewing distance of 20 cm, only one photon out of approximately 100,000 is absorbed by the retina, and the rest are lost. From each millimeter of screen, only about 1000 photons reach the retina each second. Two factors are responsible for this tremendous loss. The first and most important is the narrow angle subtended by the eye from a viewing distance of 20 cm. Each millimeter of the fluoroscopic screen is like a tiny light bulb. It sends out light photons in all directions, and they obey the inverse square law. The only ones that enter the eye are those falling on an area 20 cm away that is the size of the pupil (50 mm²). The second reason for the loss of photons is absorption in the conducting system of the eye (cornea, lens, vitreous, and aqueous) and incomplete absorption by the retina. The eye does not transmit all of the photons that enter the pupil, and the retina does not absorb all of the photons it receives. Perhaps, these are defense measures to protect the retina from the damaging effects of bright light.

In summary, photons are lost from the x-ray beam by attenuation in the patient and transmission through the fluoroscopic screen. Their numbers are greatly increased in the conversion from x-ray to light photons, but unfortunately most of these never reach the retina. They are lost either by diffusion according to the inverse square law or within the eye itself. Only about 1000 photons are absorbed by the retina each second. By the standards of the eye, a second is a long time. It can only integrate for 0.2 second, so its image is made up of the photons that it can gather in 0.2 second which, in this example, represents only 200 photons.

Statistical fluctuations in the number of photons in the x-ray beam are more important in fluoroscopy than they are in radiography, because the total numbers are smaller in fluoroscopy. The production of x rays is a random process. The x-ray beam is not perfectly uniform in two adjacent areas, nor is it identical in the same area from one instant to the next. The same is true of light photons from the fluoroscopic screen. The number of photons fluctuates according to the law of statistics; i.e., the square root of the total number generated. We can examine the importance of statistical fluctuations by comparing two x-ray (or light) beams. Let us suppose that the first beam has 100

photons, and the second, being more intense, has 10,000 photons. Their square roots are:

Beam I	Beam II
$\sqrt{100} = 10;$	$\sqrt{10,000} = 100$

It appears that the statistical fluctuations are greater in the more intense beam, but in actual fact, the opposite is true. The percentage fluctuation is what is important, and not the absolute numbers. We can compare percentages by dividing the square root by the total intensity and multiplying by 100:

Beam I	Beam II
$\frac{10}{100} \times 100 = 10\%;$	$\frac{100}{10,000} \times 100 = 1\%$

As you can see, the less intense beam fluctuates considerably more than the more intense beam.

The number of light photons absorbed on the retina of the eye will also show statistical fluctuations. In the example above, with 200 photons per square millimeter of fluoroscopic screen, the statistical fluctuation is the square root of 200, or ±14. At one instant 214 photons may make up an image, the next instant only 186. Variations of this magnitude can completely obscure an image, especially if the inherent contrast is low.

SUMMARY

A fluoroscope has only two essential components: an x-ray tube and a fluorescent screen, and they are usually mounted on a C-arm to maintain their alignment. The following safety features are recommended: 2.5 mm aluminum equivalent of permanent filtration, shutters to regulate field size, lead glass to absorb radiation transmitted through the screen, and an 18-inch minimum distance between the x-ray target and the tabletop. The exposure dose at the tabletop should not exceed 10 roentgens per minute.

The illumination of a fluoroscopic screen is only 1/10,000 as bright as that used to view average density radiographs. The screen illumination is such that the fluoroscopic image can only be seen with night (scotopic) vision with its associated diminished visual acuity and the inconvenience of dark adaptation. The statistical quality of the fluoroscopic image is poor to begin with, since it is composed of a relatively small number of photons, and its quality is further reduced by the eye's inability to gather the light photons that are available. The whole problem is compounded by scotopic vision, a physiologically inferior viewing system. The result is an image that is too poor to be salvaged by increasing exposure factors, and the only way to improve its quality significantly is by a system of light amplification, the image intensifier, which we will discuss in the next chapter.

1. Glasser, O.: *Dr. W. C. Röntgen.* Springfield: Charles C Thomas, 1945.
2. *Medical X-Ray and Gamma-Ray Protection for Energies up to 10 MeV.* Washington, D.C.: National Council on Radiation Protection and Measurements Report No. 33, 1968.
3. Chamberlain, W.E.: Fluoroscopes and fluoroscopy. Radiol. *38*, 383, 1942.
4. Last, R.J.: *Eugene Wolff's Anatomy of the Eye and Orbit.* 6th ed., Philadelphia: W.B. Saunders Co., 1968.
5. Davson, H.: *The Physiology of the Eye.* Boston; Little, Brown and Co., 1963.
6. Sturm, R.E., and Morgan, R.H.: Screen intensification systems and their limitations. Amer. J. Roentgen. *62*, 613, 1949.

CHAPTER 15

X-ray Image Intensifiers

Conventional fluoroscopy has two serious limitations: a statistically inferior image and too little light for photopic (daylight) vision. Radiologists have always been aware of these limitations, but there was nothing they could do to improve the situation. They had to wait for a major technological breakthrough. In the early 1950s, after a wait of more than 50 years, the breakthrough came with the development of the x-ray image intensifier. The image intensifier has revolutionized fluoroscopy. Its image is bright enough for scotopic vision and small enough to be conveniently coupled to cine, television, or spot film cameras.

IMAGE INTENSIFIER DESIGN

The components of an x-ray image intensifier are shown in Figure 15–1. The tube itself is an evacuated glass envelope, a vacuum tube, which contains four basic elements:

1. Input phosphor and photocathode.
2. Electrostatic focusing lens.
3. Accelerating anode.
4. Output phosphor.

After an x-ray beam passes through the patient, it enters the image intensifier tube. The input fluorescent screen absorbs x-ray photons and converts their energy into light photons. The light photons strike the photocathode causing it to emit photoelectrons. These electrons are immediately drawn away from the photocathode by the

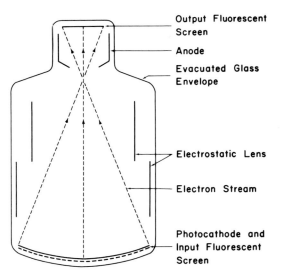

Figure 15–1   X-ray image intensifier tube

high potential difference between it and the accelerating anode. As the electrons flow from the cathode toward the anode, they are focused by an electrostatic lens, which guides them to the output fluorescent screen without distorting their geometric configuration. The electrons strike the output screen, which emits the light photons that carry the fluoroscopic image to the eye of the observer. In the intensifier tube, the image is carried first by x-ray photons, then by light photons, next by electrons, and finally by light photons.

1. First generation image intensifiers had silver activated zinc cadmium sulfide crystals (ZnS—CdS: Ag) in the **input fluorescent screen.** Second generation intensifiers have cesium iodide (CsI) input screens. We will compare the relative merits of the two later in the chapter. The screen must be in intimate contact with the photocathode so that the system does not lose resolution. Figure 15–2A shows the arrangement of the input screen and photocathode. They are separated by a thin transparent layer, which prevents the fluorescent screen from reacting chemically with the photocathode. Remember that these layers are thin, only a small fraction of a millimeter, and little information is lost as the image is transferred from the screen to the photocathode.

The **photocathode** is a photoemissive metal (usually a combination of antimony and cesium compounds). When light from the fluorescent screen strikes the photo-

cathode, it emits photoelectrons in numbers proportional to the brightness of the screen.

Besides functioning as a photoemissive surface, the photocathode also serves as the cathode of the image tube. It is usually kept at ground potential.

2. The **electrostatic focusing lens** is made up of a series of positively charged electrodes that are usually plated onto the inside surface of the glass envelope. These electrodes focus the electron beam as it flows from the photocathode toward the output phosphor. Electron focusing inverts the image. Each point on the input phosphor is focused to a specific point on the opposite side of the output phosphor. For undistorted focusing, all photoelectrons must travel the same distance. The distance between corresponding points in the image on two phosphors is equalized by curving the input phosphor. The image on the output phosphor is reduced in size,

Figure 15–2 A, Input phosphor and photocathode; B, output phosphor of an image intensifier

which is one of the principal reasons why it is brighter, a point to which we will return later.

3. The **accelerating anode** is located in the neck of the image tube, as shown in Figure 15–1. Its function is to draw electrons from the photocathode and accelerate them toward the output screen. The anode has a positive potential of 25,000 volts (25 kV), so it accelerates electrons to a tremendous velocity.

4. The **output fluorescent screen** of all image intensifiers is silver activated zinc cadmium sulfide, the same material used in first generation input phosphors; but the crystal size and layer thickness is reduced to maintain resolution in the minified image. Since the electrons are greatly accelerated, they emit more light photons from the output screen than were originally present at the input screen. The number of light photons is increased approximately 50 fold. The fluoroscopist observes this brighter image through a viewing system, usually a series of mirrors or a television camera.

A thin layer of aluminum is plated onto the fluorescent screen (Figure 15–2B) to prevent light from moving retrograde through the tube and activating the photocathode. The aluminum layer is very thin, and high-energy photoelectrons easily pass through it en route to the output screen. This layer also serves as a ground to remove spent electrons from the image tube. If they were not removed, they would

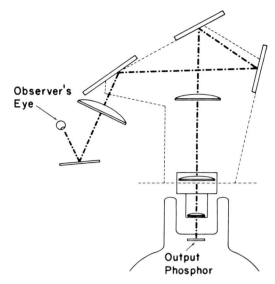

Figure 15–4 Mirror optical system of an image intensifier

accumulate on the output phosphor and build up a negative charge.

The glass tube of the image intensifier is enclosed in a lead-lined metal container which is mounted on the C-arm of the fluoroscope in place of the conventional fluoroscopic screen. The lead lining protects the operator from stray radiation, and a lead-glass window over the output phosphor absorbs radiation that passes through the intensifier.

The output screen is optically coupled to a viewing system by means of a tandem lens (Figure 15–3). The image is viewed either directly through a series of lenses and mirrors, or indirectly through closed-circuit television. A movable mirror, mounted at a 45° angle between the tandem lenses, allows the operator to switch recording and viewing modes. If the mirror is semitransparent, so that some light is transmitted and the rest reflected, the image can be monitored during cine-fluorography.

A mirror optical system is shown in Figure 15–4. As you can see, light travels a

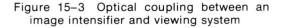

Figure 15–3 Optical coupling between an image intensifier and viewing system

long distance and it is reflected and focused several times. This results in a considerable loss of photons, which is the main disadvantage of any mirror system. The mirror image is only visible in a small viewing angle. If the operator moves his head a few degrees to one side, the image is lost. His freedom of movement is limited by the mirror, making it difficult, if not impossible, to palpate the patient. Also, only one observer can view the image, which is a serious disadvantage in training beginning fluoroscopists.

BRIGHTNESS GAIN

Two methods are used to evaluate the brightness gain of image intensifiers. The first compares the luminance of an intensifier output screen to a Patterson type B-2 fluoroscopy screen when both are exposed to the same quantity of radiation. The brightness gain is the ratio of the two illuminations.

$$\text{Brightness gain} = \frac{\text{Intensifier luminance}}{\text{Patterson B-2 luminance}}$$

If the image intensifier is 1000 times brighter, the brightness gain is 1000. The concept is easy to understand and was readily accepted by radiologists. However, Patterson type B-2 fluoroscopic screens vary from one batch to another and deteriorate at an unpredictable rate with time, so brightness gain measurements are not reproducible. Because of this lack of reproducibility, the International Commission on Radiologic Units and Measurements (ICRU) recommended a second method of evaluation, called the conversion factor,[1] to supersede the older brightness gain method. The conversion factor is a ratio of the luminance of the output phosphor to the input exposure rate.

$$\text{Conversion factor} = \frac{\text{candelas/m}^2}{\text{milli roentgens/sec}}$$

Output screen luminance is measured in candelas (defined as the luminous intensity, in the perpendicular direction, of a surface of a 1/600,000 m^2 of a black body at the temperature of freezing platinum under a pressure of 101,325 Newtons/m^2 . . . ridiculous to remember). Radiation quality and output luminance are explicitly defined, so the method is accurate and reproducible.

The brightness gain of an image intensifier comes from two completely unrelated sources. They are called minification gain and flux gain. We will discuss them separately.

Minification Gain

The brightness gain from minification is produced by a reduction in image size. The quantity of the gain depends upon the relative areas of the input and output screens. Since the size of an intensifier is usually indicated by its diameter, it is more convenient to express minification gain in terms of diameter.

$$\text{Minification gain} = \left(\frac{d_I}{d_o}\right)^2$$

d_I = diameter of input screen
d_o = diameter of output screen

Most x-ray image intensifiers have an input screen from 5 to 9 inches in diameter and an output screen approximately 1 inch in diameter. With a 1-inch output screen, the minification gain is simply the square of the diameter of the input screen; i.e., a 9-inch intensifier has a gain of 81.

The brightness gain from minification does not improve the statistical quality of the fluoroscopic image. The same number of light photons make up the image regardless of the size of the output screen. For example, a 6-inch intensifier with a 2-inch output phosphor has a minification gain of 9 ($6^2 \div 2^2 = 36 \div 4 = 9$), while the same intensifier with a 1-inch output phosphor has a gain of 36. However, the total light output of both units is exactly the same, so the same number of photons make up both images. The photons are compressed together on the smaller screen and the image is brighter, but its statistical quality is not improved.

Theoretically, brightness can be increased indefinitely by minification. A 9-inch intensifier with a $1/16$-inch output screen would have a brightness gain from minification alone of over 20,000. However, excess minification produces a very small image, which has a definite disadvantage. Before the image can be viewed, it must be greatly magnified, which also magnifies the fluoroscopic crystals in the output screen, resulting in a precipitous drop in resolution.

Flux Gain

Flux gain increases the brightness of the fluoroscopic image by a factor of approximately 50. For each light photon from the input screen, 50 light photons are emitted by the output screen. In simplified terms, you can think of one light photon from the input screen ejecting one electron from the photocathode. The electron is accelerated to the opposite end of the tube, gaining enough energy to produce 50 light photons at the output screen.

The total brightness gain of an image intensifier is the product of minification and flux gains.

Brightness gain = minification gain × flux gain

For example, with a flux gain of 50 and a minification gain of 81 (9-inch intensifier with a 1-inch output screen) the total brightness gain is 4050 (50 × 81). In general, brightness gains from modern image intensifiers are always over 1000 and frequently as high as 6000.

CESIUM IODIDE IMAGE INTENSIFIERS

Image quality is dramatically better with cesium iodide input screens than it was with the older zinc cadmium sulfide screens. Two physical characteristics of cesium iodide make it superior: (1) a greater packing density and (2) a more favorable effective atomic number. Cesium iodide can be vacuum deposited and requires no inert binder, so more active material can be packed into a given space.

The packing density of cesium iodide is 3 times greater than zinc cadmium sulfide. Phosphor thicknesses have been reduced comparably from approximately 0.3 mm with zinc cadmium sulfide to 0.1 mm with cesium iodide. The principal advantage of the thinner phosphor layer is improved resolution.

Ideally, for maximum photoelectric absorption, the K-absorption edge of a phosphor should be as close to the energy of the x-ray beam as possible, provided the energy of the edge does not exceed that of the beam. An obvious problem arises in attempting to accomplish this ideal. Beam energy is a spectrum, a whole array of energies, while the K-edge is a single point, or at most, several points depending upon the number of absorbers in the phosphor. The mean energy of an x-ray beam is approximately one-third of its peak energy depending somewhat on the energy level and filtration. Most adult fluoroscopy is done at a peak energy of from 100 to 120 kVp, which is a mean energy between 33 and 40 keV. Table 15–1 shows the K-edges of elements used as phosphors in various types of screens. The energy of the K-edge of cadmium (26.7 keV) is quite good, but its chemical mates, zinc (9.7 keV) and sul-

Table 15–1 Atomic Number and K-absorption Edge of Elements Commonly Used in Intensifying Screens

ELEMENT	ATOMIC NUMBER	K-ABSORPTION EDGE (keV)
Sulfur	16	2.5
Calcium	20	4.0
Zinc	30	9.7
Selenium	34	12.7
Yttrium	39	17.0
Cadmium	48	26.7
Iodine	53	33.2
Cesium	55	36.0
Lanthanum	57	39.0
Gadolinium	64	50.2
Tungsten	74	69.5

fur (2.5 keV) are far from ideal. The K-edges of cesium (36 keV) and iodine (33.2 keV) are almost perfect. The more appropriate atomic numbers of cesium and iodine give these screens a substantial advantage over zinc cadmium sulfide. Cesium iodide input screens absorb approximately two-thirds of the incident beam as opposed to less than one-third for zinc cadmium sulfide, even though the cesium iodide screen is only one-third as thick.

IMAGE QUALITY

In evaluating image quality with image intensifiers, we must evaluate the same two factors that we considered with conventional fluoroscopy. The first is the statistical quality of the image, and the second is the adequacy of the light level for photopic (cone) vision. If an intensifier does nothing but brighten the image to the level where it can be seen with photopic vision, it has accomplished a great deal. Remember, photopic visual acuity is 10 times better than scotopic visual acuity. A brightness gain of approximately 1000 will satisfy the light requirements for photopic vision. All modern image intensifiers easily reach this level. The brighter image has several secondary benefits. Dark adaptation is unnecessary. The lights can be turned on in the fluoroscopic room, which relieves patient apprehension and simplifies the examination, especially in children. The image is also bright enough for safe cinefluorography.

Statistical Image Quality (Quantum Mottle)

The number of absorbed x-ray photons determines the highest possible statistical quality of an imaging system. No form of intensification can improve the image above the statistical level of the absorbed photons. The overall statistical quality of a system is determined by the lowest point, called the **quantum sink.** The quantum sink determines the amount of quantum mottle that we see in the final image. The low point is analogous to the weakest link in a chain. For the same reason that a chain cannot be stronger than its weakest link, the statistical quality of an image cannot be higher than its lowest point. In an image intensifier system, the quantum sink may be either at the input phosphor or retina of the eye, depending upon the efficiency of optical coupling. If the low point is at the input phosphor, quality can be improved only by the absorption of more x-ray photons. With a mirror optical system, a large number of photons are lost through repeated reflections and the low point is at the retina. In this case, statistical quality can be improved, i.e. the quantum sink raised, by a higher x-ray-to-light conversion efficiency, but quality can never be raised above that of the absorbed photons.

The number of absorbed photons can be increased in two ways: (1) by increasing the number of photons in the incident beam and (2) by capturing a higher percentage of the incident photons. Cesium iodide image tubes capture a greater percentage of the incident beam than either conventional fluoroscopic screens or older intensifiers, so statistical quality is superior for any given level of exposure. Statistical fluctuations manifest themselves in the radiographic image as quantum mottle—a sort of grainy appearance. The visibility of mottle is determined by the resolution and contrast levels of the system. Mottle is more visible in a high resolution, high contrast image. As we shall see momentarily, cesium iodide image tubes improve both resolution and contrast, so in evaluating overall image quality opposing forces are at work. For any given level of exposure, the image is statistically superior, but the mottle that is present is easier to see and therefore more distracting.

The mottle level can be adjusted with image intensifiers by changing exposure factors. Increasing exposures increases the number of absorbed photons, which decreases statistical fluctuations. If the image

Figure 15–5 Effect of a diaphragm on the brightness of an imaging system

intensifier is used with a cine or spot film camera, where increasing the exposure may overexpose the film, an iris-type diaphragm can be incorporated into the optical system to decrease the light output reaching the film. In Figure 15–5, the exposure/frame is 2 times greater in B than in A, but both films are exposed to the same density. Balanced film densities are maintained because the diaphragm intercepts half of the light from the output phosphor in B. At first glance, it looks like the diaphragm cuts the size of the image in half, but such is not the case. The light shown in the optical system all arises from a single point, the center of the output phosphor, and the diaphragm intercepts half of the light from this point. The same effect occurs for every point on the output phosphor. The net result of doubling the exposure and halving the light output is an image of unchanged brightness, but improved statistical quality.

While image intensifiers were in a developmental stage, it was felt that one of their principal advantages would be greatly reduced patient exposures. However, even before the first image intensifier was perfected, Sturm and Morgan[2] pointed out an important fact. The number of photons in the x-ray image cannot be decreased indefinitely. Eventually a point is reached where there are not enough photons to produce an image. The fluoroscopic x-ray image is close to that point. A large decrease in the number of x-ray photons would cause a serious de-

terioration of image quality. In actual practice, image intensifiers have not significantly decreased patient exposures. Most radiologists are using 2 to 5 mA for adult abdominal fluoroscopy, which is approximately the same as pre-intensifier levels.

Contrast

Contrast can be determined in a variety of ways and there is no universal agreement as to which is best. The following is a description of the simplest method. A ¼-inch thick lead disc is placed over the center of the input screen. Disc size is selected to cover 10% of the screen, i.e. a 0.9-inch diameter disc is used for a 9-inch image intensifier. The input phosphor, with the disc in place, is exposed to a specified quantity of radiation and brightness is measured at the output phosphor. Contrast is the brightness ratio of the periphery to the center of the output screen. Defined in this way, contrast ratios range from approximately 7:1 to 10:1 depending upon the manufacturer. Contrast is definitely better with cesium iodide tubes than it was with the older zinc cadium sulfide tubes.

Two factors tend to diminish contrast in image intensifiers. First, the input screen does not absorb all of the photons in the x-ray beam. Some are transmitted through the intensifier tube, and a few are eventually absorbed by the output screen. These transmitted photons contribute to the illumination of the output phosphor but not to image formation. They produce a background of fog that reduces image contrast in the same way that scattered x-ray photons produce fog and reduce contrast in a radiographic image. The second reason for reduced contrast in an image intensifier is retrograde light flow from the output screen. Most retrograde light flow is blocked by a thin layer of aluminum on the back of the screen. However, the aluminum layer must be extremely thin, or it would absorb the electrons that convey the fluoroscopic image. Some light photons penetrate through the aluminum, pass back through the image tube, and activate the photocathode. The cathode emits photoelectrons, and their distribution bears no relationship to the principal image. These electrons produce "fog" and further reduce image contrast.

Resolution

The resolution of zinc cadmium sulfide image tubes is 1 to 2 line pairs per millimeter (1p/mm), which is a little less than the resolution of a conventional fluoroscopic screen. The apparent improvement that the fluoroscopist observes is entirely from the increased visual acuity of photopic vision. The resolution of cesium iodide image tubes is approximately 4 1p/mm, a dramatic improvement over zinc cadmium sulfide. The individual CsI crystals are somewhat aligned and the phosphor layer is thinner, both contributing to improved resolution.

The resolution of an imaging system is usually expressed in terms of its modulation transfer function (MTF). At any given frequency (number of line pairs/mm), the MTF is a specific number which is always less than one. The overall MTF of the system is the product of the component parts. We can use the following series of fractions to demonstrate the effect of the components.

$$.9 \times .1 = .09$$
$$.8 \times .2 = .16$$
$$.7 \times .3 = .21$$
$$.6 \times .4 = .24$$
$$.5 \times .5 = .25$$

If the numbers were added instead of multiplied, they would all be equal. However, when they are multiplied, the largest product is obtained when both numbers are equal (i.e. 0.5 × 0.5). If the numbers are a great deal different, their product is much closer to the size of the smaller number. Modulation transfer functions behave in exactly the same way. If the MTF of the glass envelope of an image

intensifier is 0.9 and the input phosphor 0.1, at a frequency of 3 1p/mm, their combined MTF is 0.09. Trying to develop a better glass envelope would be a foolish investment. The maximum effort should be directed at improving the input phosphor which is obviously the weaker link in this chain.

Figure 15–6 shows MTF curves for a hypothetical image intensifier. The product of all of the component curves yields the curve for the overall system. In this example, the performance of the input and output phosphors are very similar. In older (zinc cadmium sulfide) tubes, the MTF of the input screen was less than the MTF of the output screen. Research and development was directed at input phosphors, and now, thanks to cesium iodide, the two are close. The resolution requirements of the output screen are dependent upon the size and resolving power of the input screen. A 9 inch input screen with a resolution of 4 1p/mm, presents a total of 914 1p to the output screen (9 in. × 25.4 mm/in. × 4 1p/mm = 914 1p). A 15 mm output screen, a fairly common size, has to handle 61 1p/mm (914 ÷ 15 mm = 61 1p/mm). A 15 mm output screen with a 6 inch input screen only has to resolve 41 1p/mm (6 × 25.4 × 4 ÷ 15 = 41). Because of this difference, the weakest link in the

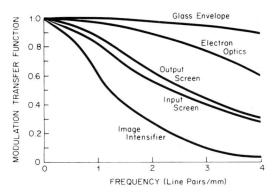

Figure 15–6 Modulation transfer function for an image intensifier and its component parts

system may shift from the input phosphor with a 6 inch tube to the output phosphor with a 9 inch tube.

Distortion

In the present state of development, electron focusing is not uniform across the entire width of an image intensifier. Electrons at the center of the unit are more accurately focused than those at the periphery. Peripheral electrons tend to flare out from an ideal course. The result is unequal magnification, which produces peripheral distortion. The amount of distortion is always greater with large intensifiers, because the further an electron is from the center of the intensifier, the more difficult it is to focus. Figure 15–7 shows a cine image of a coarse wire screen taken with a 9-inch intensifier. As you can see, the wires curve out at the periphery. Generally this distortion does not hamper routine fluoroscopy, but it may make it difficult to evaluate straight lines; for example, in the reduction of a fracture.

Unequal magnification also causes unequal illumination. The center of the output screen is brighter than the periphery, as shown in Figure 15–7. The peripheral image is displayed over a larger area of the output screen, and thus its brightness gain

from minification is less than that in the center. A fall off in brightness at the periphery of an image is called **vignetting.** Unequal focusing has another effect on image quality; i.e., resolution is better in the center of the screen.

In summary, the center of the image intensifier screen has better resolution, a brighter image, and less geometric distortion. It follows logically that a small image intensifier, which encompasses only the central, more accurately focused electrons, produces a better-quality image than a large unit.

DUAL-FIELD IMAGE INTENSIFIERS

Dual-field, or triple field, image intensifiers attempt to resolve the conflicts between image size and quality. They can be operated in several modes, including a 4.5-inch, a 6-inch, or a 9-inch mode. The 9-inch mode is used when it is necessary to view large anatomic areas. When size is unimportant, the 4.5 or 6-inch mode is used because of their better image quality.

Field size is changed by applying a simple electronic principle; i.e., the higher the voltage on the electrostatic focusing lens, the more the electron beam is focused. Figure 15–8 shows this principle applied to a dual-field image intensifier. In the 9-inch

Figure 15–7 Test film of a wire screen (35-mm cine frame) from a 9-inch image intensifier. (Courtesy of Harold Alsobrook, R. T.)

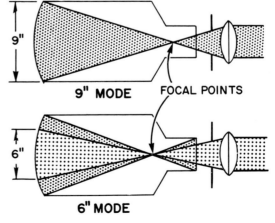

Figure 15–8 Dual-field image intensifier

mode, the electrostatic focusing voltage is decreased. The electrons focus to a point, or cross, close to the output phosphor and the final image is actually smaller than the phosphor. In the 6-inch mode, the electrostatic focusing voltage is increased, and the electrons focus farther away from the output phosphor. After the electrons cross, they diverge, so the image on the output phosphor is larger than it is in the 9-inch mode. The optical system is preset to cover only the format, or size, of the smaller image of the 9-inch mode. In the 6-inch mode, the optical system "sees" only the central portion of the image; i.e., the part derived from the central 6 inches of the input phosphor. Since this image is less minified, it appears to be magnified when it is viewed through a television monitor or a series of mirrors. The physical size of the input and output screens is the same in both modes. The only thing that changes is the size of the output image. Obviously, the 6-inch and 9-inch modes have different minification gains. Exposure factors are automatically increased when the unit is used in the 6-inch mode to compensate for the decreased brightness from minification.

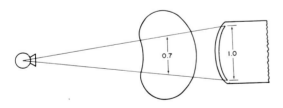

Figure 15–9   Reduction of fluoroscopic field size by an image intensifier

While we are discussing intensifier size, there is another point to consider. A 9-inch image intensifier does not encompass a 9-inch field in the patient. The x-ray image is magnified by divergence of the beam, as shown in Figure 15–9. The intensifier sees a much smaller field than its size would imply, which is an important point to consider when ordering a unit to perform a particular function.

SUMMARY

An x-ray image intensifier is an electronic vacuum tube consisting of an input phosphor and photocathode, electrostatic focusing lens, accelerating anode, and output phosphor. It converts an x-ray image into a light image, then to an electron image, and finally, back to a light image of diminished size and increased brightness. Electron acceleration produces a flux gain and size reduction produces a minification gain. The total brightness gain is the product of the gains from flux and minification. Image intensifiers make their most important contribution by increasing screen illumination to the level required for photopic (cone) vision with its superior visual acuity. They have made dark adaptation a thing of the past and cinefluorography a safe procedure. Lastly, they have brought the television camera into the fluoroscopic room and opened up a whole new world of electronic communication.

REFERENCES

1. Methods of Evaluating Radiological Equipment and Materials. ICRU Handbook 89. National Bureau of Standards, Washington, D. C., 1963.
2. Sturm, R. E., and Morgan, R. H.: Screen intensification systems and their limitations. Amer. J. Roentgen. *62*, 613, 1949.

CHAPTER 16

Cinefluorography

Cinefluorography is the process of recording fluoroscopic images on movie (cine) film. Before the invention of the image intensifier, cinefluorography required excessively large patient exposures, so it was never widely accepted for clinical radiography. Patient exposures were large for two reasons. First, optical coupling was inefficient, because the cine camera had to be placed a long distance from the fluoroscopic screen to encompass its large size. Most of the available light was lost due to the inverse square law, and only a small percentage reached the camera. Second, screen illumination was not bright enough to expose the film without increasing the x-ray exposure factors, which meant more radiation. Thus, because patient exposures were intolerably high, cine techniques were relegated to animal experiments and a few research projects.

The birth of safe, clinically applicable cinefluorography came in the early 1950s after the invention of the image intensifier, which solved the problems which had frustrated earlier attempts. Its image was bright enough to expose the film without exposing the patient excessively, and the image was small enough to couple efficiently to a cine camera.

Two film sizes are currently being used for cinefluorography, 16 and 35 mm. In the United States, 98% of all cine is done on 35 mm film; and 95% of all cine studies involve the heart. Therefore, our major emphasis will be on 35 mm cardiac cinefluorography.

The basic components of a modern cinefluorography system are as follows:

1. Camera
2. Image intensifier
3. Optical system
4. X-ray photon image
5. Radiographic equipment
6. Film
7. Processor
8. Projector

These components can be likened to a length of chain, all tied closely together and all limited by the weakest link. For optimum results, at the lowest possible cost in both dollars and patient exposure, the links should all be of equal strength. Occasionally, an expensive generator is coupled to an expensive image intensifier and then the film is developed in an inexpensive processor of inferior quality. The results are usually unsatisfactory.

Each of the eight basic components in the cinefluorographic system will be discussed separately in the order listed above. Most of our recommendations are taken from the Report of Inter-Society Commission for Heart Disease Resources.[1]

CINE CAMERA

Cinefluorography is married to the motion picture industry. We are stuck with their horizontal rectangular format, even though it is not well-suited to our needs.

16 mm FILM

35 mm FILM

7.5 x 10.3 mm

18 mm x 24 mm

Figure 16–1 Film formats as defined by the apertures of 16 mm and 35 mm cameras

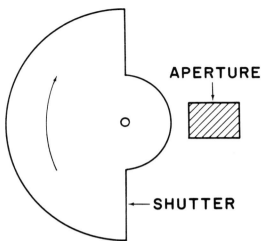

APERTURE

SHUTTER

Figure 16–2 Cine camera shutter

PRESSURE PLATE

PULLDOWN ARM

SUPPLY REEL

TAKEUP REEL

Figure 16–3 Cine camera

All cine cameras are commercial movie cameras with a few minor modifications. Two film sizes are available, 16 and 35 mm. The basic components of the camera are a lens, iris diaphragm, shutter, aperture, pressure plate, pulldown arm, and film-transport mechanism. The lens and iris diaphragm will be discussed in more detail later in the chapter.

Light enters the camera through the lens and is restricted by the **aperture,** a rectangular opening in the front of the camera. The size and shape of the aperture define the configuration of the image reaching the film. Figure 16–1 shows the image sizes as defined by the apertures of 16- and 35-mm cameras. Apertures for 35 mm film are usually 18 × 24 mm.

The **shutter** is a rotating disc with a sector cut out of its periphery as shown in Figure 16–2. It is located in front of the aperture. As the shutter rotates, it interrupts light flow into the camera. The size of the shutter opening is expressed as the number of degrees in the cut-out portion of the sector. Openings of 160° to 180° are usually employed for cinefluorography. While the shutter is closed, the **pulldown arm** (Figure 16–3) advances the film to the correct position for the next exposure. The **pressure plate** holds the film against the camera aperture so that it is located in the proper image plane.

An electric-drive motor advances the film from the supply reel past the aperture to the takeup reel. A meter attached to the supply reel indicates the amount of unexposed film in the camera. The x-ray pulses and shutter opening are synchronized by an electrical signal from the drive motor. The framing frequency, or number of frames per second, is usually a divisible or multiple of 60; i.e., 7½, 15, 30, 60 or 120.

The combination of the framing frequency and shutter opening determines the amount of time available for both the exposure and pulldown. For example, with a 180° shutter opening and 60 frames per second, the time available for both the exposure and pulldown is $1/120$ sec. At slower framing frequencies, both are longer. With a smaller shutter opening, the available exposure time is shorter than the pulldown time.

Framing

The output phosphor of the image intensifier and the camera aperture have different shapes, so a portion of either the image or film frame must be discarded. The term "framing" refers to the utilization of the available area on the film as shown in Figure 16–4. The Report of the Inter-Society Commission for Heart Disease Resources[1] classifies the various degrees of framing for 35-mm film as follows:

1. **Underframing:** The maximum dimension of the fluoroscopic image is shorter than the smallest dimension of the frame (not illustrated in Figure 16–4). Underframing is due to a faulty optical system and should be avoided.

2. **Exact Framing:** The diameter of the circular intensifier image and shorter dimension of the film (18 mm) are the same. No part of the image is lost, but only 58% of the cine frame is used. Exact framing is recommended when the long axis of the part being examined is vertically oriented, such as the esophagus. It is not generally recommended for cardiac cinefluorography.

3. **Overframing:** The diameter of the circular image is greater than the shortest dimension of the film, so part of the image is lost.

a. **Mean Diameter Framing:** The diameter of the circular image is halfway between the largest and smallest dimensions of the film ($24 + 18 = 42 \div 2 = 21$ mm); 73% of the film area is used and only 4% of the image is wasted.

b. **Equal Area Framing:** The area of the circular image, both within and outside the picture frame, is equal to the area of the rectangular frame (not shown in Figure 16–4); 87% of the film area is used and 15% of the image is wasted. This is the framing type recommended by the International Commission on Radiation Units and Measurements.[2] The diameter of the fluoroscopic image is 23.5 mm, which is

FRAMING MODE	EXACT FRAMING	MEAN DIAMETER FRAMING	MAXIMUM HORIZONTAL FRAMING	SUBTOTAL OVER-FRAMING	TOTAL OVER-FRAMING
ILLUSTRATION	18 mm / 18 mm / 24 mm	21 mm	24 mm	27 mm	30 mm
FILM AREA USED	58 %	73 %	88 %	96 %	100 %
IMAGE AREA UNUSED	0 %	4 %	16 %	28 %	39 %
RELATIVE IMAGE SIZE	1.0	1.17	1.33	1.50	1.67

Figure 16–4 Framing methods (modified from Table 5 of the Report of the Inter-Society Commission for Heart Disease Resources[1])

almost identical to the diameter of the image from maximum horizontal framing.

c. **Maximum Horizontal Framing:** The diameter of the circular image and width of the rectangular field are identical (24 mm). Approximately 12% of the film area is unused and 16% of the image is wasted.

d. **Subtotal Overframing:** The diameter of the circular image is midway between the image diameter for maximum horizontal framing and total overframing (24 + 30 = 54 ÷ 2 = 27 mm); 90% of the film area is used and 28% of the image is wasted.

e. **Total Overframing:** The diameter of the circular image is equal to the diagonal measurement of the rectangular aperture (30 mm). All of the film is used but 39% of the image is wasted.

Framing and Patient Exposure

The x-ray beam should be restricted to coincide with the framing method. Figure 16–4 shows the percentage of the potential image area that is unused by the various framing methods. If the beam is not correspondingly restricted, these areas of the patient are exposed but the image is never recorded. The problem is actually more complex than Figure 16–4 implies. Most fluoroscopic installations have rectangular field collimators. Figure 16–5 shows the problem diagrammatically. The cine frame is rectangular with a 4:3 ratio of the horizontal and vertical sides (i.e. 24 × 18 mm), the image intensifier is round and the x-ray field is either square or rectangular. With this arrangement of shapes, a portion of either the x-ray field or the image intensifier must be wasted with all framing methods except total overframing. With all other framing methods, some portion of the recorded image is lost.

Two examples, one with exact framing and the other with total overframing, will demonstrate the potential magnitude of the patient overexposure. In both examples, we will assume that the x-ray field is square and that its sides are tangential to the input phosphor of the image intensifier as shown in Figure 16–5. With exact framing, none of the image is wasted but the x-ray field is 1.3 times (25 ÷ 20 = 1.3) as large as the image intensifier. The patient exposure (in terms of area) is comparably greater. The only solution is a circular field collimator. The second example, total overframing, poses a potentially greater exposure hazard. If the x-ray field is restricted so its sides are tangential to the image intensifier, a common practice, the exposed patient area is 2.1 times (25 ÷ 12 = 2.1) greater than the recorded area. In this case, the solution is simple— restrict the x-ray beam to the recorded area and not to the image intensifier. With

Figure 16–5   Comparison of field shapes for the cine frame, image intensifier, and x-ray field

all other framing methods, the magnitude of the problem is intermediate between these two extremes, but the solution is more complex in that it demands dual collimation, i.e. both circular and rectangular field collimation.

Framing and Image Size

Framing determines the size of objects in the cine image. Figure 16–6 compares image sizes for exact framing, total overframing, and exaggerated total (plus) overframing. The fluoroscopic image is shown on the left, the recorded, or cine image on the right. The size of the fluoroscopic image is determined by the size of the anatomic part, shown here as an arrow. The size of the comparable cine image is determined by the type of framing, which in turn is determined by the degree of magnification in the optical system. The optical system can be used to record all, or only a small portion of the output phosphor. When the lens zooms in on a small area of the phosphor, the image enlarges as shown on the right side of Figure 16–6. In theory, exaggerated overframing could be used to magnify the image indefinitely, but other considerations, which will be discussed in Chapter 20, intervene to destroy image quality and make exaggerated overframing impractical. It is only shown here to illustrate the principle and is not recommended for routine clinical use.

Figure 16–4 indicates the relative image sizes for the various types of framing using exact framing as the norm. Image size increases as the degree of framing increases up to a maximum of 1.67 times for total overframing. Greater degrees of overframing are not recommended for routine clinical use.

Framing and Image Intensifier Size

The size of the object recorded on cine film decreases as the size of the image intensifier increases. This may seem like a paradox at first glance, but the explanation is quite simple and is shown diagrammatically in Figure 16–7. The illustration shows three different size image intensifiers (A, B and C), all recording the same object (arrow) with the same degree of radiographic magnification, with the same framing format, and on the same size film. With the 4½ inch intensifier (A), the image of the arrow fills the cine frame; with the 9 inch intensifier (C), the image is only half as

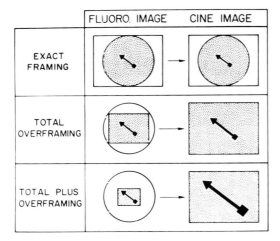

Figure 16–6 Overframing enlarges the x-ray image

Figure 16–7 Image sizes for various size image intensifiers

large; and with the 6 inch unit (B), the image is intermediate in size. The loss in image size with the larger intensifier can be at least partially recouped with overframing (D).

Framing Recommendations

The following framing recommendations are made by the Inter-Society Commission for Heart Disease Resources.[1] "Exact framing is not recommended for angiocardiography. For many angiocardiographic studies mean diameter overframing will provide moderate magnification without serious loss of field size. Maximum horizontal overframing provides more magnification and is desirable for coronary arteriography. More severe overframing can be used with large intensifiers to produce intermediate formats and with small intensifiers for coronary arteriography when marked magnification is desired and panning is not objectionable. When dual mode intensifiers are used, consideration must be given to the effect overframing will have on each mode."

IMAGE INTENSIFIER

Image intensifiers are described in detail in Chapter 15. We will only review those points that are especially important, or unique to cinefluorography. The newer cesium iodide tubes have dramatically improved the cine image. They are far superior to the older zinc-cadmium sulfide tubes. Cesium iodide tubes are superior for three reasons: (1) improved quantum detection, (2) better resolution, and (3) better contrast. The improved quantum detection results from a greater packing density (more active material per unit thickness) and a better match between the K-absorption edge of both the cesium and iodine atoms and the mean energy of the x-ray beam. Resolution is better because light diffusion is less in the phosphorescent layer. Diffusion is inherently less in cesium iodide image tubes and this advantage is accentuated by the fact that the phosphor

layer is thinner than in zinc-cadmium sulfide tubes. Resolution is also better because of improvement in the photocathode, electron optics and output phosphor. The contrast improvement is largely related to increased quantum detection, i.e. fewer photons pass through the input phosphor to reach the output phosphor and thus reduce contrast.

The energy conversion factor (Chapter 15, page 197), an expression of the quantity of light produced per absorbed photon, is lower with cesium-iodide image intensifiers than with the older zinc-cadmium sulfide tubes, but this is not of major importance. A higher conversion factor does not improve the statistical quality of the image. Instead, statistical quality deteriorates and quantum mottle becomes more of a problem. Quantum mottle is discussed in more detail later in this chapter. If the conversion factor is too high, some of the light gain must be discarded. This is accomplished with an aperture (diaphragm with a small hole) between the two tandem lenses (see Figure 15–5, page 200). Discarding some of the light results in higher patient exposures, but produces a statistically better image.

The optimum size image intensifier for cinefluorography is the smallest one that will accomplish the job. A 15 to 17 cm intensifier (approximately 6 inches) is appropriate for coronary arteriography and most pediatric angiography. Larger dual or triple mode units are recommended for adult angiography. In general, a single mode unit can outperform a dual mode intensifier of any given size. The advantage of the dual mode is versatility.

Image Intensifier Performance

The resolution, contrast and brightness of the image intensifier should be checked at least every three months. Resolution should not be less than: (1) 3.5 line pairs per millimeter (1p/mm) for 15 to 17 cm intensifiers or (2) 2.5 1p/mm for larger multiple mode units. Resolution is measured at the face of the input phosphor with a lead line pair phantom at 50 kVp. The test is done at normal working distances without any other absorber in the path of the x-ray beam.

No generally accepted method is available for measuring contrast. One simple method employs a ¼-inch thick lead disc cut into a circle whose surface area is 10% of the area of the input phosphor. The disc is positioned over the center of the input phosphor and the phosphor and disc are exposed to 20 mR/min at 65 kVp. The output phosphor brightness is measured over the disc and adjacent uncovered screen. Tube contrast is a ratio of the two brightnesses. This type of contrast measurement is quite variable. For older tubes, it usually falls between 1:6 and 1:7. Newer tubes have a contrast ratio of about 1:12. Tube contrast measurements of this sort are a useful way of following the performance of any particular unit.

The conversion factor is used to measure image intensifier brightness. Conversion factors should be over 75 for 15 to 17 cm image intensifiers and over 100 for 22 to 23 cm tubes. Brightness and contrast both deteriorate with time at a rate of about 10% per year.

Wavelength of Light from the Output Phosphor

The output phosphor of both the older and newer image intensifiers is P20, zinc cadmium sulfide-silver activated (ZnCdS:Ag). It emits at a peak wavelength of 550 nanometers (nm) which is in the yellow-green part of the spectrum. About one-half of the output phosphor's light falls in a rather narrow range of 550 ± 25 nm (5500 angstroms) as shown in Figure 16–8. Cine film must be selected to accommodate these wavelengths. Only orthochromatic and panchromatic films make a suitable accommodation. Orthochromatic films are sensitive to wavelengths in the violet, blue, green and yellow portion of the spectrum. Panchromatic films are sensitive to the entire spectrum, including orange and red.

OPTICAL SYSTEM

The optical system performs the seemingly simple task of conveying an image from the image intensifier, through a tandem lens (2 lenses separated by a beam-splitting mirror), to the cine film. In this era of advanced technology, you would not think this would be a difficult task. A technology that has produced an instrument as complex as an image intensifier should have no problem with the design of a few pieces of glass. However, the optical system is more complex than it appears to be at first glance, and its design affects the performance of the entire cine system.

Characteristics of a Lens

Before we discuss the optical coupling between the image intensifier and cine film, we must first review several important characteristics of lenses. These are as follows:

1. Focal length
2. Magnification
3. Relative aperture
4. Depth of focus
5. Depth of field
6. Resolution

WAVELENGTH OF LIGHT FROM OUTPUT PHOSPHOR OF IMAGE INTENSIFIER (nanometers)

Figure 16–8 Wavelength of the light from output phosphor of image intensifier

7. Vignetting
8. Chromatic aberrations
9. Spherical aberrations

Focal Length

The **optical axis** of a lens is an imaginary line passing perpendicular to the plane of a lens and through its geometric center. When a parallel bundle of light, for instance light from the sun, passes through a biconvex lens, all of its rays except the central one are bent toward the optical axis (Figure 16–9). Rays at the periphery are deviated more than those near the center, and the central ray passes through in a straight line. They all converge at a point, which is called the **focal point.** The **focal length** of a lens is the distance between the focal point and the center of the lens. Note in Figure 16–9 that a lens has two focal points (F), one on each side, equidistant from the central plane of the lens. Since light can pass through a lens in either direction, it follows logically that a ray passing through a focal point on one side will emerge on the opposite side in a course parallel to the optical axis.

Magnification

Magnification is defined as the ratio of image size to object size.

$$\text{Magnification} = \frac{\text{Image size}}{\text{Object size}}$$

The image may be larger, smaller or equal to the object, so magnification can be greater than, equal to, or less than 1. If magnification is less than 1, the image is actually minified, or reduced in size. The degree of magnification depends upon three factors: (1) object distance, (2) image distance and (3) focal length. The impor-

OBJECTS   IMAGES

Figure 16–10   Magnification

tance of each factor is demonstrated in Figure 16–10. The objects are to the left of the lens, and their images are to the right. The images form at the image or focal plane, which is determined by the intersections of two or more light rays originating from the same point. One of the two rays shown in the illustration passes through the near focal point and emerges parallel to the optical axis; the other ray begins parallel to the optical axis and emerges in a course that passes through the far focal point.

The relative size of the object and image for a particular lens depends upon the object distance. If the object is located at a distance of two focal lengths from the lens (Figure 16–10 A), the object and image are equal in size. If the object is at a shorter distance, the image is larger. The same focal length lens is shown in both (A) and (B), but the image is twice as large in (B) because of the shorter object distance.

Figure 16–10 B also shows the important relationship between the image distance and object distance. As the illustration is labeled, the image is magnified two times. However, by simply reversing the light direction, or in this case the object and image labels in the drawing, the magnification changes to 0.5.

Figure 16–9   Focal point (F) of a lens

The third factor that affects magnification is the focal length of a lens. In Figure 16–10 B and C, the object distance is the same for both lenses. However, the image is more magnified in (C) because the lens has a longer focal length. For a particular object distance, the degree of magnification is directly proportional to the focal length, i.e. the longer the focal length, the greater the magnification. The focal length is a characteristic of the lens itself. It is the only factor affecting magnification that cannot be changed.

Relative Aperture (Speed)

Relative aperture refers to the speed of a lens, which is probably its most important characteristic. If you find it difficult to think of a lens as being fast, perhaps it will help to think in terms of how fast it can gather enough light to expose a film. Then the concept is easily understood; i.e. a fast lens is one that produces a fast (short) exposure.

The speed of a lens is determined by its ability to concentrate light at the image plane. Concentration refers to light intensity per unit area, and depends upon both the total quantity of available light and the area over which it is distributed. The total quantity of light is determined by the size of a lens, and the area of distribution by the lens' focal length. A lens is like a window. More light flows through a large window than a small one, and the same thing is true for a lens; i.e., a large lens gathers more light than a small one. Focal length is important because it (along with the object distance) determines the degree of magnification, and therefore, the area of the image. A lens with a short focal length causes less magnification, and produces a smaller image than one with a long focal length (assuming equal object distances). Therefore, the available light is more concentrated by a lens with a short focal length. In summary, a fast lens is one with a large diameter (to gather more light) and a short focal length (to concentrate the light into a small area).

The relative aperture (speed) of a lens is indicated by an "f" number, usually written as f/4 or f/8. The lower the f-number the faster the lens. The f-number is determined by dividing the focal length of a lens by its diameter:

$$\text{f-number} = \frac{\text{focal length}}{\text{diameter}}$$

Figure 16–11 shows the relationships between lens diameter, focal length, and relative aperture. As you can seen, focal length and diameter are independent of each other. A large and small lens can both have the same focal length, but they will have different f-numbers. Also, two lenses can have the same f-number and have different diameters and focal lengths.

F-numbers are expressed in the following standard series: 0.70, 1.0, 1.4, 2.0, 2.8, 4.0, 5.6, 8.0, 11, 16, etc. Each lower numbered f-stop allows twice as much light to reach the image plane as the next higher f-number in the series. An f/2.8 lens, then, is twice as fast as an f/4.0 lens and four times as fast as an f/5.6 lens. You can also compare the relative speed of two lenses by comparing the square of their f-numbers. This is occasionally necessary, because many f-numbers fall between the ones in the standard series. The arithmetic is simple. For example, a 16-mm cine camera

Figure 16–11   Relationship between relative aperture (f-number), focal length and lens diameter

might have an f/0.9 lens and 35-mm cameras an f/1.8 lens. Comparing the squares of their f-numbers:

$$\frac{(1.8)^2}{(0.9)^2} = \frac{3.24}{0.81} = 4$$

Thus this 16-mm camera lens is four times as fast as the 35-mm camera lens.

Depth of Field and Depth of Focus

Depth of field and depth of focus are closely related so we will discuss them together. Depth of focus refers to the range of distances over which the image is in sharp, or relatively sharp focus. Depth of field is the range of distances within which objects are in sharp, or relatively sharp focus. They are both similar, but one refers to the object plane (depth of field) and the other to the image plane (depth of focus). Theoretically, for any given object distance, a lens only forms an image at a specific distance from its center (i.e., at the image plane), and the image is out of focus at all other distances. Actually, the image plane is not sharply defined, and there is a range of distances within which the image is reasonably well focused. The same is true for the object plane. Both the depth of field and depth of focus are dependent upon the f-number of the lens. The greater the f-number (slower the lens), the greater the depth of field and focus. As we shall see later, both can be improved by an iris diaphragm which decreases the functional size of the lens. Depth of field is relatively unimportant in cine fluorography because the object (output phosphor image) is flat. However, depth of focus is important, and cine camera lenses must be accurately positioned in order to maintain the resolution of the system.

Resolution

The overall resolution of an imaging system is determined by the performance of its individual components. The component with the poorest resolution limits the entire system. In cinefluorography, the image intensifier is the limiting factor, since it has the poorest resolution. A well-designed lens system can easily outperform an image intensifier, so optical coupling can be achieved without a significant reduction in the resolving power of the system.

Vignetting

Vignetting is a decrease in light intensity at the periphery of an image. We first met this phenomenon when we discussed image intensifiers. The cause of vignetting is different with a lens, but the result is the same. Figure 16–12 shows the cause of vignetting. In the illustration, the center of the output phosphor of the image inten-

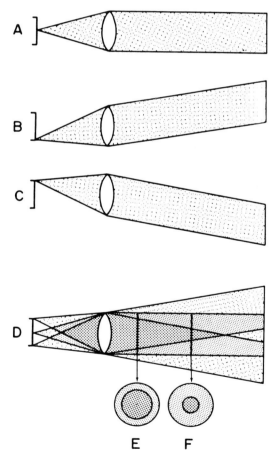

Figure 16–12 Vignetting

sifier is located at the focal point of the lens. (Later we will see that the first cine lens is positioned in this manner.) The upper three illustrations show bundles of parallel light rays originating from the center, bottom, and top of the output phosphor. The bundle of parallel light rays from the center of the phosphor (A) is also parallel to the optical axis of the lens. Light from the bottom (B) and top (C) of the phosphor is in a parallel bundle, but the bundle is directed along a course oblique to the optical axis. When the three bundles are added together (D), they produce a central triangle of intense illumination surrounded by areas of lesser illumination. The illustration only shows a two-dimensional presentation of a three-dimensional light beam. The intensely illuminated central triangle is actually a cone. Cross-sections through the center of the beam are shown in (E) and (F). The size of the maximally illuminated area is larger in (E) because the cross-section is closer to the lens. Vignetting is least pronounced close to the lens and increases as the distance from the lens increases.

Spherical and Chromatic Aberrations

A spherical aberration is caused by the inability of a lens to bring a monochromatic bundle of light from all parts of the lens to a point focus. A chromatic aberration is caused by the inability of a lens to bring a white light (which is polychromatic) to sharp focus. These two aberrations are inherent in all lenses. Optical engineers have minimized the aberrations through good design, but the problem can never be completely eliminated.

Figure 16–13 shows both aberrations schematically. In A, a narrow beam of white light is refracted into its individual components by a prism. Each color, or wavelength, is refracted to a different degree. White light enters the prism and a rainbow of colors emerges. A curved lens behaves in much the same way in that different wavelengths are refracted dif-

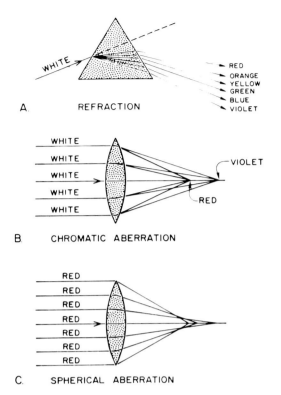

Figure 16–13   Refraction (A), chromatic (B) and spherical (C) aberrations

ferently. Figure 16–13 B shows the red and violet components of a white (polychromatic) light beam. These two colors are focused to two different points. All other colors (wavelengths) fall between red and violet. The result is a fuzzy image with poor resolution and contrast. Figure 16–13 C shows a spherical aberration. All of the incident light has the same wavelength, i.e. it is monochromatic (red in the illustration). Because of the curved surface of the lens, refraction is never perfectly balanced at the center and periphery. Even though the light is monochromatic, it is still not brought to point focus. Peripheral refraction is greater than central refraction, so the periphery of the lens has a shorter focal length than the center. The result is a more fuzzy, lower resolution, lower contrast image than an image formed by a lens that has been corrected for spherical aberration.

Auxiliary Apertures

The effective f-number of a lens can be changed without changing either the focal length or diameter of the lens. The f-number is changed by interposing an iris diaphragm next to the lens as shown in Figure 16–14. The same lens is shown in both A and B. Its diameter (maximum aperture) and focal length are both 5 cm, so its f-number is 1 (A). When an opaque object with a 1-cm hole (iris diaphragm) is placed next to the lens (B), the f-number changes to 5. The technique of changing f-numbers with a diaphragm is familiar to all photographers. All but the cheapest cameras are equipped with variable diaphragms.

At first glance, the diaphragm appears to restrict the size of the field and block out a part of the picture. Such is not the case. All of the light shown in Figure 16–14 A and B originates from one point in the center of the arrow. A similar light bundle could be drawn for any other point. Therefore, the brightness of the image is decreased but its size is not affected. The brightness in the illustration decreases by a factor of 25:

$$\frac{1^2}{5^2} = \frac{1}{25}$$

Placing a small aperture in the light beam produces four desirable effects:

1. Contrast improves
2. Resolution improves
3. Spherical aberrations decrease
4. Depth of field and depth of focus increase

As a general rule, most lenses perform best at about 2 f-stops above their maximum opening, i.e. an f/2 lens usually functions best at f/4 (f/2; f/2.8; f/4—the second f-stop). If the aperture is made small, in the f/16 to f/32 range, resolution and contrast begin to deteriorate somewhat due to diffraction. Therefore, small apertures should be avoided for cinefluorography. Photographers use these small apertures when a maximum depth of field is needed for esthetic purposes; but a great depth of field is of little value to a radiologist who is recording a nearly flat image.

Lens Selection for Cinefluorography

Now that we have discussed some of the characteristics of lenses, we can look into the design of the optical system for a cine camera. In order to make a lens with high resolution and minimum vignetting, several optical elements are used for each lens, sometimes as many as nine pieces of glass. As you can imagine, the design of such a lens is extremely complex, and it is usually carried out with the aid of a computer. However, even though the lens is made up of many elements, it still has an f-number and focal length of its own.

Figure 16–15 shows a simplified cinefluorographic lens system. The lenses are

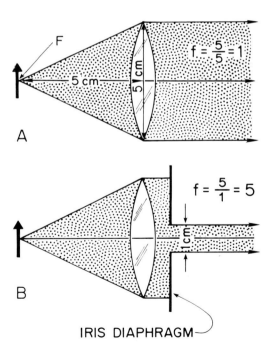

Figure 16–14 Changing the relative aperture with an iris diaphragm

COLLECTOR LENS

CAMERA LENS

MIRROR

OUTPUT PHOSPHOR

CINE FILM

IRIS DIAPHRAGM

Figure 16–15 Schematic cinefluorographic optical system

depicted as single pieces of glass, but each is actually made up of several elements. A large diameter **collector** lens receives the fluoroscopic image from the output phosphor of the image intensifier and collimates the image for the camera lens. The phosphor is positioned at the focal plane of the lens, so the image is transmitted by parallel bundles of light. A smaller diameter **camera lens** receives this light bundle and refocuses it into an image on the cine film. Since the light is transmitted from one lens to the other in a parallel bundle, the amount of separation between the lenses does not affect focusing. However, it does affect vignetting, which produces a serious problem for the lens designer. There are three ways to diminish vignetting:

1. Make the first lens large to increase the size of the cone that is relatively free of vignetting.
2. Make the second lens small so it fits inside the vignetting free cone.
3. Place the second lens close to the first lens in the larger portion of the cone of maximal illuminations.

The final design of the optical system is always a compromise. A certain amount of vignetting is tolerated. The first lens is always as large as possible (and large lenses are expensive); the second lens is always smaller than the first; and the two lenses are placed as close together as the beam-

splitting mirror allows. The mirror deflects a small amount of light (approximately 10%) to a television camera or mirror optical system for image monitoring. Optical coupling would be more efficient if the beam-splitting mirror could be discarded, but at the present time no other system permits simultaneous image monitoring and recording.

Focal Length of the Camera Lens

In our previous discussion we pointed out that focal length and object distance determine the degree of magnification. The object distance for cinefluorographic lenses is always the same as their focal lengths. The lenses are purposely positioned with their image planes (output phosphor and cine film) at their focal points. This arrangement accommodates a beam-splitting mirror, since the image is transferred from one lens to the other in a parallel bundle.

Figure 16–16 shows the relationship between the focal length of the two lenses and size of the output phosphor and cine images. The tandem lenses can be pictured as a pinhole positioned at the junction, or crossover of two similar triangles. When any three factors are known, the fourth can be calculated by setting up proportional triangles.

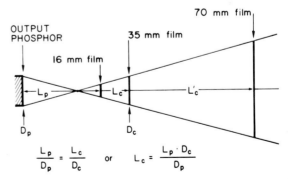

OUTPUT PHOSPHOR

16 mm film

35 mm film

70 mm film

L_p L_c L'_c

D_p D_c

$$\frac{L_p}{D_p} = \frac{L_c}{D_c} \quad \text{or} \quad L_c = \frac{L_p \cdot D_c}{D_p}$$

Figure 16–16 Relationship between focal length and image sizes for cinefluorographic lenses

$$L_c = \frac{L_p \cdot D_c}{D_p}$$

L_c = focal length of camera lens
L_p = focal length of phosphor (collector) lens
D_c = diameter of camera (cine) image
D_p = diameter of output phosphor image

For example, a representative size for an output phosphor is 18 mm and a common focal length for an output phosphor (collector) lens is 65 mm with a 9 inch image intensifier. If we decide to use total overframing, the diameter of the 35-mm cine image will be 30 mm. The focal length of the camera lens should be:

$$L_c = \frac{L_p \cdot D_c}{D_p} = \frac{65 \times 30}{18} = 108 \text{ mm}$$

If we had selected exact framing for the same system, the focal length of the camera lens should be:

$$L_c = \frac{L_p \cdot D_c}{D_p} = \frac{65 \cdot 18}{18} = 65 \text{ mm}$$

The focal lengths for camera lenses for 35-mm cinefluorography are usually between 80 and 135 mm, depending upon the framing mode selected. Once a particular lens has been selected, it can only be changed at considerable expense. Zoom lenses, usually of lesser quality, have variable focal lengths but are not generally available for cine systems, consequently, the framing mode should be chosen with great care.

Speed of the Optical System

A cine optical system is designed to be as fast as reasonable cost and modern technology permit. Collector lenses are exceedingly fast, usually f/0.75. To limit vignetting, the diameter of the camera lens is only one-half as large as the collecting lens. Once the size of the output phosphor, speed of the collector lens, and framing mode have been established, the speed of the system is determined by the maximum aperture, or f-number, of the camera lens. As the focal length of the camera lens is increased to cover larger framing formats, the brightness of the cine image will decrease, unless the f-number (iris diaphragm) is also changed. If the f-number is changed, the brightness change is ½ or 2 times for each f-stop, depending on whether the iris aperture is made smaller or larger.

Earlier image intensifying tubes used a P20 input phosphor (zinc cadmium sulfide: silver activated). The light intensity was somewhat limited. Consequently, a fast lens and film combination was required to obtain an adequate exposure. The introduction of cesium iodide: sodium activated as an input phosphor increased light intensity by a magnitude of about five times. Consequently, selecting the fastest lensfilm combination is no longer an absolute necessity. A fast lens is still important to allow stopping down at least two f-stops to permit exposure conditions within the critical resolution of the lens. This optimizes the performance of the lens. As long as the film selected can be exposed within this critical resolution range, film speed is of relatively small importance. The main advantage of slower films is a finer grained emulsion.

Regardless of the lens-film combination, a 20 μR/frame input dosage is necessary to minimize quantum mottle.[1]

THE X-RAY PHOTON IMAGE

The first prerequisite for optimum cinefluorography is a good x-ray photon image. This is the image that exists in space after the x-ray beam has traversed the patient and before the beam reaches the image intensifier. Scatter radiation should be minimized by beam restrictors (collimators) and a radiographic grid. Assuming scatter radiation is at a minimum, four other factors affect the quality of the x-ray photon image:

1. Quantum mottle
2. Motion unsharpness
3. Geometric unsharpness
4. Contrast

Quantum Mottle

Quantum mottle is caused by statistical fluctuations in the number of x-ray quanta (photons) absorbed by the input phosphor. The mottle does not become visible until an image is produced, but the statistical fluctuations exist prior to absorption of the photons by the input phosphor.

There must be a certain minimum number of photons to produce a statistically satisfactory image. This minimum, for either 16- or 35-mm film, is 20 μR per frame[1] when viewed at 24 or more frames per second. At lower viewing rates, larger exposures are recommended. Exposures of less than 20 μR per frame generate too much quantum mottle to produce a satisfactory image.

Figure 16–17 shows that the "graininess" on a cine film is due primarily to quantum mottle rather than film graininess. The two pictures in the illustration were both made with the same 35-mm film (Kodak CRS Film), the same coarse (1 cm) wire screen, the same magnification, and the same processing system. The only difference between the two films is in the manner in which they were exposed. Film A was exposed by the output phosphor of a 9-inch image intensifier, so it is a picture of a radiographic image. Film B is an ordinary light photograph taken with a 35-mm camera. The mottled appearance of the x-ray image (A) is from random statistical fluctuations in the number of x-ray photons, which is quantum mottle by

Figure 16–17   Quantum mottle: (A) x-ray image; (B) light image

definition. Regardless of the film size, the amount of quantum mottle depends upon the number of photons comprising the x-ray image. An image composed of a large number of x-ray photons has less quantum mottle (statistical fluctuation), and it is a better-quality image (smoother or more uniform in appearance) than one composed of only a small number of photons.

When a cinefluorography system exhibits quantum mottle, the best way to eliminate the mottle is to increase the mAs (milliampere-seconds). This will increase the number of x-ray photons absorbed by the input phosphor, which is the primary method for decreasing quantum mottle. Increasing the number of absorbed quanta will also increase the overall density of the processed film. Film density can then be decreased by decreasing the kilovoltage, which will also increase contrast. Greater contrast is usually desirable. Another way to compensate for increased mAs is to use a smaller opening in the iris diaphragm, i.e., a higher f-number.

Motion Unsharpness

Each cine film is a separate picture, exposed with its own individual pulse of radiation. The length of the pulse should be kept as short as possible to stop patient motion without seriously compromising other factors important to image quality. The other important quality factors are contrast and quantum mottle. Exposures of 3 to 5 milliseconds (ms) are recommended. Exposure times can be reduced in several ways—higher kVp, more mA, a faster lens, a faster film, etc. In general, all of these, except more mA, tend to produce more quantum mottle and/or less contrast. For example, halving the exposure with a faster film halves the number of photons in the x-ray image and thus increases quantum mottle. Increasing the kilovoltage shortens the exposure, but increases quantum mottle and reduces contrast. With current technology, the heat tolerance of the x-ray tube makes it impractical to produce repetitive exposures below the 3 to 5 ms range.

Geometric Unsharpness

Geometric unsharpness is caused by magnification and the finite size of the focal spot (penumbra). Focal spot sizes for cinefluorography should be as small as practical. An 0.6 mm focal spot is recommended for most situations; 1.0 mm is recommended for large patients and 0.3 mm for magnification radiography. Industry standards (self-imposed) allow for a 50% tolerance in focal spot sizes. An 0.6 mm focal spot may actually be 0.9 mm and still meet industrial standards. As we shall see later (Chapter 20), this size may increase by more than two times under peak load. Cine tubes should be special-ordered with actual (based on pinhole or star pattern radiographs), rather than nominal focal spot sizes requested. Manufacturers will meet these requirements at an additional cost.

Magnification is minimized by keeping the image intensifier as close to the patient as possible, and by using a long target-table top distance. The minimum recommended separation between the x-ray target and patient support (table top) is 55 cm.

Contrast

The overall contrast of the cine image is determined by many factors, the first of which is the kVp of the x-ray beam. Optimum contrast is obtained with a voltage between 60 and 90 kVp. Lower voltages (below 60 kVp) subject the patient to excess radiation, while higher voltages produce too little contrast and too much quantum mottle. In general, kVp's on the low side of the range are preferred. The higher side of the range should be reserved for large patients. The film type, processing and viewing conditions also affect image contrast. These factors will be discussed in more detail later.

X-RAY APPARATUS

Many angiocardiographic labs are designed for both serial filming and cinefluorography. The energy demands for cine are generally less than those for serial filming, so the serial filming dictates the energy requirements for the room. The following recommendations pertain to a lab designated exclusively for cinefluorography. They are taken from the Report of the Inter-Society Commission for Heart Disease Resources.[1]

Generator

A 3-phase, 12-pulse, or constant potential generator is recommended. The current (mA) output rating should be three times the cine pulse output to minimize voltage fluctuations during exposures. A 700 to 1000 mA, 100 kVp generator is recommended unless the transformer design insures stable voltages and currents during pulsing (low impedance). In this case, a 500 mA generator will suffice. Pulsing and brightness controls are essential and they will be discussed in more detail after we describe the x-ray tube.

X-ray Tubes

The instantaneous exposure tolerances of an x-ray tube are determined by the (1) size of the focal spot, (2) diameter of the anode, (3) anode angle, and (4) the rotational speed of the anode. The maximum continuous output is determined by (1) the anode's capacity to store heat and (2) the ability of the anode and housing to dissipate heat into the environment. Individual cine exposures are small by conventional radiographic standards, but they may be repeated 60 times a second for several seconds, so total heat loading is very large. A tube with the following characteristics is recommended for routine 35-mm cardiac cinefluorography.

Focal spot size	0.6 mm
Heat rating	60 kW
Anode diameter	100 mm
Target angle	6°–12°
Cooling	Circulatory liquid
Rotational velocity	10,000 rpm

The optimum target angle is dictated by the size of the image intensifier and distance between the intensifier and x-ray target. Small anode angles (6°) have greater x-ray output so they are recommended with small image intensifiers where the field size is not compromised by the heel effect. A 0.3-mm focal spot should be used for magnification techniques and 1.0 mm size is acceptable for large patients or where ultrashort exposures are mandatory.

The X-ray Exposure

The timing and intensity of the x-ray exposure are controlled during cinefluorography by two electrical signals that originate from within the cine system. One signal coordinates the x-ray exposure with the open time of the camera shutter (synchronization), and the other maintains a constant level of intensifier illumination by varying the exposure factors for areas of different thickness or density.

Synchronization

When cinefluorographic equipment was in the embryonic stages of its development, x rays were generated continuously throughout a filming sequence, and the patient was needlessly irradiated when the camera shutter was closed. These continuous exposures had two serious disadvantages: patient exposures were large, and they shortened the life expectancy of the x-ray tube. In all modern cinefluorographic systems, the x-ray output is intermittent, and the exposure is synchronized with the open time of the camera shutter. Synchronization is controlled by an electrical signal from commutators and brushes of the camera motor. After the motor opens the shutter and advances the film, it signals the generator to make an exposure.

Earlier in the chapter, we mentioned that the framing frequency is always a multiple, or fraction, of 60 (7½, 15, 30, 60, 120). The choice of the number 60 was not an arbitrary decision. Thirty-five years ago

Figure 16–18 Synchronization locked into two different phases of full-wave rectified radiation

when the decision was made, all x-ray circuits in this country operated on 60-cycle alternating current, usually with full-wave rectification. X rays were generated in 120 short bursts each second. Operating the camera shutters at the same frequency as the x-ray pulses insured a uniform exposure for each frame, regardless of what part of the cycle synchronization locked into. Figure 16–18 shows synchronization locked into the beginning (A) and middle (B) of the x-ray cycle. In each case, the exposures are exactly the same from frame-to-frame. The examples shown are for 60 frames per second (f/s), but the results are the same from other frequencies provided they are multiples of 60. With a framing frequency out of phase with the electrical supply, consecutive frames would be exposed to a slightly different portion of the x-ray cycle. Some frames would receive more radiation than others, depending upon whether they are exposed by the peaks or valleys of the radiation output.

Pulsed Radiation

The newer cinefluorographic units deliver x rays with a completely different wave form than that used for conventional fluoroscopy. Instead of the high ripple pulsations usually generated with full-wave rectification, the x rays are generated in short, intense bursts, called pulses. This is

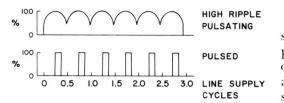

Figure 16–19 Comparison of high ripple pulsations (full-wave rectification) and cine pulses

achieved with either thyratron or grid-controlled x-ray tubes, both of which allow instantaneous on-off switching of the x-ray pulse. Only the central, high-voltage portion of the electrical cycle is used to generate x rays, and the rest of the cycle is discarded. Figure 16–19 shows the wave form from pulsed radiation along with that from full-wave rectification for comparison. The nomenclature is a little confusing, because both wave forms show pulsations. However, cine pulses have a wave form that is square, which is completely different from the rounded wave form of full-wave rectification. A single pulse is used with 3 phase generators. The beginning and termination of the pulse are square, like those shown in Figure 16–19. The length of the pulse is determined by the time required to expose the film. Its height is constant except for ripple pulsations.

The output phosphor of an image intensifier has a certain amount of inherent persistence which produces an **afterglow** of illumination following the cessation of an x-ray pulse. If synchronization of the shutter opening and x-ray pulse is perfectly timed, the light from afterglow can be utilized for part of the total film exposure with a comparable reduction in the patient's x-ray exposure. Figure 16–20 shows an ideally synchronized cine exposure. The x-ray pulse occurs immediately after the shutter opens, afterglow falls entirely within the open time, and no radiation is generated while the shutter is closed.

Afterglow should not persist beyond its frame of origin. If it is carried into the next frame, the persistent image will be different from the new image; and quality will deteriorate. With pulsed radiation, the only function of the camera shutter is to prevent afterglow from reaching the film during its transport time. If an image intensifier discarded an image the instant the burst of radiation terminated, merely pulsing the radiation would be an entirely adequate way of controlling the exposure, and the shutter would be superfluous. The shutter does not control the film exposure in the examples shown in Figure 16–20. Even if the shutter remained open perma-

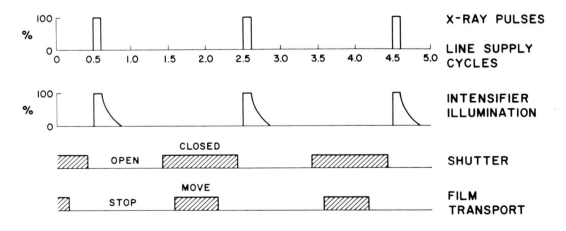

Figure 16–20 Coordination between the x-ray pulse, afterglow and film transport

nently, the film could be transported without impairing image quality, since the intensifier has already discarded its image. However, the framing frequency in the illustration is only 30 f/s. At higher frequencies (60 or more f/s) afterglow may persist into the film-transport time, and the shutter intercepts it before it reaches the film, thus performing an important function.

Brightness Control

The brightness of the intensifier image changes constantly as the fluoroscope is moved from one area of the patient to another, and as contrast material enters and leaves the fluoroscopic field. Since cine film does not have enough exposure latitude to encompass the varying intensities coming from the patient, a method of brightness control is needed in order to ensure proper film density. This is managed in one of two ways, either by measuring the current flowing across the image intensifier or by measuring the brightness of the output phosphor. In both systems, a signal is sent back to the x-ray generator to regulate the intensity of the x-ray pulse. Three basic methods for brightness stabilization are in current use: (1) variable voltage (kVp), (2) variable tube current (mA) and (3) variable pulse width (exposure time).

(1) **Variable voltage (kVp):** A motor driven autotransformer in the primary circuit varies the kVp in response to brightness sensing electrodes in either the image intensifier or optical system. This method has the advantage of covering a very wide range of patient thickness. It has three disadvantages: (1) it is relatively slow; (2) if kVp's get too high, contrast decreases; (3) when the kVp goes up, the number of absorbed photons goes down and quantum mottle becomes a problem. The method works well with a large (30 to 50 kW) generator. Then the mA and time can be set near optimum levels and the kilovoltage only has to make minor adjustments.

(2) **Variable tube current:** With this method the exposure time (pulse width) and voltage are preselected and brightness is regulated by varying the mA. The method only works well with large generators (30 to 50 kW) and it should not be used with generators smaller than 30 kW. A variable tube current has three disadvantages: (1) the response time is slow; (2) it requires considerable expertise to operate satisfactorily; and (3) the brightness range is quite limited. It works best when combined with a variable voltage.

(3) **Variable pulse width (time):** In this system the mA is set at the maximum heat tolerance level, the kVp is optimized, and the timer regulates the exposure. The system suffers from the same shortcomings as variable tube current. It has the advantage of a near instantaneous response time (0.1 ms). Each cine frame can be separately photo-timed.

All three systems work best with large generators (30 to 50 kW) and all three require considerable operator experience. The optimum method is a combination of variable kVp and variable time, coupled to a large generator. The kilovoltage is set for optimum contrast, brightness is controlled by varying the exposure time, and if the upper limit of the exposure time is reached, the kVp is automically raised to provide full exposure control. The system offers the advantages of simplicity and a rapid response time.

All brightness regulators are like photo-timers. They function empirically and must be adjusted by trial and error until the image brightness meets the requirements of the particular film-processor system.

Monitoring the Cine Examination

In order for the radiologist to conduct a cine examination, he must be able to monitor the cine image. The beam-splitting mirror reflects approximately 10% of the light from the image intensifier for monitoring purposes. While this percentage is small, it must be remembered that the exposure factors and brightness of the intensifier phosphor are greatly increased during cinefluorography, and the monitoring image brightness is not much different than that used for routine fluoroscopy. At low framing frequencies, the image flickers because the x rays are pulsed, but flicker does not interfere with monitoring. The reflected light can be viewed in one of two ways: either directly with a mirror optical system, or indirectly through closed-circuit television.

CINE FILM

The characteristics of radiographic film were discussed in detail in Chapters 10 and 11, so we will only review a few features especially pertinent to cinefluorography. The film is only one component in a complex system. However, when the image is unsatisfactory, the film is often incorrectly blamed. For example, if contrast is too high, the first inclination is to switch to a lower contrast film. A better choice would be to evaluate the **system contrast,** correct the deficiencies that exist, and then reassess the problem. System contrast is determined by the contrast of the individual components; the more important ones will be discussed next.

(1) **Radiographic contrast** depends upon kVp, patient thickness, scatter radiation, contrast materials, etc.

(2) **Image intensifier contrast** deteriorates with time. This is especially noticeable in the older zinc-cadmium sulfide tubes.

(3) **Optical system contrast** deteriorates with larger lens openings. Apertures should be used to bring the f-number of the system within the critical resolution of the lens, usually two f-stops above the maximum aperture.

(4) **Processing** is one of the most important factors influencing system contrast. Processing time, temperature, agitation and replenishment are the critical elements of processing that affect film contrast.

(5) **Viewing conditions** have a profound effect upon image contrast. A brightly lit room diminishes contrast. A dirty lens, an inadequately bright bulb or a dirty screen also diminishes contrast.

(6) **Inherent film contrast** is the last link in the chain. A high-, medium- or low-contrast film should not be chosen until all other factors in the imaging system have been optimized. Then, the inherent contrast of the film should be used to fine tune the total system contrast using the processing recommendations of the manufacturer.

Types of Cine Film

Table 16–1 shows representative films that are recommended for cinefluorography. Important characteristics to consider are speed and contrast. In general, faster films tend to be grainier than slow films. The graininess of a fast film may contribute to the "noise" seen in the projected image. However, this contribution is usually minor relative to the increase in quantum mottle that occurs with faster films. Quantum mottle increases because fewer x-ray photons are needed to produce an image.

Film should not be selected until all the components of the system have been evaluated. A film should then be chosen to have the appropriate contrast for the system. This film should be as slow as the exposure factors permit. After the film is selected, it should be tested on a phantom and processed as recommended. The phantom tests should include a series of exposures made with different size iris diaphragm openings (f-numbers). This f-stop series will allow the selection of the proper aperture to match the film density with the other established parameters. The processed films should be analyzed in a projector to duplicate the viewing conditions that will exist for later clinical studies. A patient should not be examined until

Table 16–1.   Representative 35-mm Cinefluorographic Films*

KODAK FILM	DEVELOPMENT TIME (SECONDS)	RELATIVE SPEED†	AVERAGE GRADIENT‡	BASE
CFX	90	100	1.5	acetate
CFA	30	40	1.6	polyester
CFS	60	30	1.7	polyester
CFH	60	30	2.1	acetate
CFR	90	15	1.2	acetate

*These negative films were processed in a KODAK Sensitometric Processor, Model C, with maximum agitation. Processing chemicals were KODAK Liquid X-ray Developer and Replenisher at 86°F (30°C) and KODAK *RP* X-OMAT Fixer and Replenisher. A sensitometric exposure of 1/50 second was used. A KODAK WRATTEN Filter No. 34 was used to simulate a P20 phosphor.

†KODAK CFX Film arbitrarily assigned a relative speed of 100 in the 86°F, 90-second process; speed measured at 0.85 density above gross fog.

‡Average gradient: Slope of line connecting 0.15 and 1.50 density above gross fog.

NOTE: Since these data have been obtained under ideal conditions, without the introduction of the many variables of cinefluorography, they can be used only as a starting point.

the system has been thoroughly analyzed by phantom studies.

PROCESSING

Improper processing and excessive quantum mottle are the two most important factors that degrade cine image quality. We have already discussed quantum mottle. Now, we will discuss processing. The first rule is that a cine lab should have its own cine film processor. Automatic processors designed for motion picture processing are preferable since they are designed to rigidly control the factors that regulate cine film quality.

Good cine processors are expensive. Between 2 and 3% of the total cinefluorographic laboratory costs should be dedicated to the processor. [Between 2 and 3% of $500,000 (1977 cost of a modern laboratory) is between $10,000 and $15,000.] Many desirable features of cine processors are presented in the Report of the Inter-Society Commission for Heart Disease Resources.[1]

Processing should be kept in the hands of skilled professionals and not turned over to the least skilled and lowest paid

member of the angiographic team. The following six factors are involved in successful processing.

(1) **Temperature Control:** Temperature is a critical element in cine processing. Ideally, developer temperature should be controlled to ±0.25° Fahrenheit (±0.14° Celsius)—variations of greater than ±0.5° (±0.28°C) are unacceptable. Other temperatures should be kept within 1 or 2° F of their recommended values.

(2) **Machine Speed:** Processing time is controlled by the film transport speed. The actual transport speed, not that shown on the controls, should not exceed ±5% of the speed required for acceptable processing.

(3) **Agitation:** Good agitation is desirable. Agitation must be uniform throughout the developer tank, but especially at the beginning of the cycle. Uneven agitation causes mottle and irregular streaks. Proper agitation (1) helps produce the film's inherent speed and contrast, (2) insures uniform processing from frame-to-frame, and (3) prevents exhaustion products of development from inducing artifacts.

(4) **Replenishment:** Both the developer and fixer must be replenished to assure

optimum processing. Recommended replenishment rates should be obtained from the manufacturer and followed as starting points. Replenishment should accomplish the following three objectives: (1) restore the used developer and fixer agents to maintain the sensitometric characteristics of the film, (2) dilute the solutions to prevent the buildup of reaction products, and (3) maintain the solutions at the proper level in the tanks. Improper replenishment of the developer will affect film density, contrast, and fog. Overreplenishment of the fixer is wasteful. Underreplenishment may affect washing, drying, and the storage life of the processed film. Too high a developer temperature produces the same effect as overreplenishing; while too low a temperature is comparable to underreplenishing.

(5) **Filtration:** Particulate matter from the developing and fixing solutions tends to cling to film during processing. These particles produce minus density spots on the film. They are then greatly magnified when the film is projected. A filter should be used to remove particles larger than 25 microns (μ).

(6) **Film Drying:** Relative humidity and temperature are the most important factors in film drying. They control the physical characteristics of the film. Insufficient drying leaves the film soft and tacky. Overdrying causes excess curl and brittleness. In general, film should be dried at the lowest temperature consistent with adequate drying and in relation to the ambient relative humidity. Most processors are set for 125° F. If the film does not have the proper physical characteristics, it may break or jam in the projector.

Quality Control

Cine processors should be monitored on a daily basis to ensure consistency of performance. Records should be kept of solution temperatures, developer immersion times, developer and fixer replenishment rates and solution changes. When an an-

giographic suite is first installed, a complete H & D curve should be plotted to serve as a standard for future comparisons. These curves should be reconstructed whenever any component in the processing system is changed or whenever a spot check of daily performance falls outside accepted norms.

The heart of a quality control program is a short pre-exposed film strip, similar to the one shown in Figure 16–21. The film strip was exposed to precisely controlled steps of increasing light intensity by an instrument called a **sensitometer.** Several manufacturers produce commercial units designed specifically for this purpose. They all vary somewhat in design. The one that was used to expose the strips shown in the illustration is a DuPont Cine Sensitometer. With this unit, the film is only exposed on the emulsion side. Sensitometers for x-ray film expose from both sides because x-ray film has a double emulsion. The light source in the cine sensitometer is green to match the yellow-green light of the intensifier output phosphor. The exposure is made through a step wedge of neutral density filters. Successive steps in the filter differ in density by the square

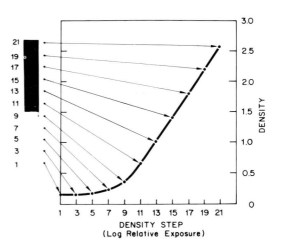

Figure 16–21 Characteristic (H & D) curve of a typical cine film

root of 2. Thus, every other step (i.e. 2 steps) doubles, or halves (depending upon the direction) the quantity of light reaching the film. The log relative exposure difference between every other step is 0.3 and the total range of exposure is 3.

The density of the steps in the test film is read with a densitometer and plotted on graph paper to construct an H & D curve like the ones shown in Figures 16–21 and 22. Both of these illustrations show the same curve, but the numbers on the x-axes have been changed from density steps in Figure 16–21 to log relative exposures in Figure 16–22. The average gradient of the film was determined by first selecting two points on the H & D curve and then by connecting these points with a straight line as shown in Figure 16–22. Densities of 0.15 and 1.5 above gross fog were used to define the points. The gross fog density was 0.16. Densities of 0.31 (0.15 + 0.16) and 1.66 (1.5 + 0.16) were used to define the average gradient which turned out to be 1.13 on our test film. This value is quite low compared to x-ray film, but the Inter-Society Commission[1] recommends a low average gradient for cine film. Log relative exposures and average gradients are described in more detail in Chapter 11.

The construction of H & D curves is too time-consuming to use as a daily check of system performance. Lawrence has described a much quicker and more practical method.[3] Instead of measuring the density of the whole film strip, he only measures a few preselected steps. The density of these steps quantitates three important film characteristics: (1) gross fog, (2) speed and (3) contrast. Gross fog is the density of an unexposed portion of the film (step 1 on the film strip). The density of the unexposed film is the sum of base fog (the density of the film base plus emulsion) and processor or darkroom fog. Film speed (called the **speed index** by Lawrence) is the density of one preselected step. Film contrast (called the **contrast index**) is the difference in the density between two preselected steps. These three parameters are then plotted on a **processor control chart** like the one shown in Figure 16–23. The density of step 13 was used for the speed index in this chart; the contrast index was the difference in density between steps 14 and 10. Upper and lower limits were then set to define the range of acceptable variation.

If any parameter slips out of the acceptable range, an investigation is undertaken to determine the cause. The first step is always to repeat the test, i.e. expose another film strip and repeat the measurements. If the error persists, then a systematic search is begun, guided in part by the particular parameter(s) that has changed. For example, suppose that gross fog and the speed index go up, and the contrast index goes down. Gross fog is not particularly sensitive to changes in replenishment rates or developer temperature. Consequently a light leak is a more likely cause for the problem. One common source of a light leak is a defective safe light (x-ray film safe lights are unsatisfactory for cine film). If the gross fog in our

Figure 16–22   Average gradients of the film shown in Figure 16–21

Figure 16–23 Processing control chart

example had been normal and the speed index had risen while the contrast fell, then an error in replenishment or developer temperature would have been a more likely cause.

PROJECTORS

Projectors have not kept pace with the other components in the cine system, at least not for 35-mm film. No 35-mm projector has all of the features that are desirable for image review. Only two, the Tage Arno (Copenhagen, Denmark) and Vanguard XR-35 (Vanguard Instrument Company, Melville, New York) projectors are in common usage. Other commercial units are either prohibitively expensive or poorly designed for cinefluorography.

Projectors have three functioning components: (1) a film transport mechanism, (2) a light source and condenser optics and (3) an imaging optics. The film transport mechanism should conveniently accept large rolls of any standard polyester or acetate-based film, have a continuously variable forward and reverse transport at frame rates from 1 to 50 frames/sec, and not damage the film with repeated viewing. The transport should also be quiet, flickerless and hold the film motionless for single framing. The condenser optics focus the filament of the light source into the aperture of the projection lens. The condenser has a heat absorbing glass to reduce the heat of the projector beam so as not to burn the film. The imaging optics projects and focuses the cine image onto the built-in screen or to a small conference room screen. The optical system should produce a bright, high contrast, critically focused image with uniform resolution across the entire width of the image. The projector lamp should also have a variable brightness control.

FRAMING FREQUENCY

The optimum framing frequency for a cine examination should be determined by the speed of the physiological motion being recorded. The exposures should be frequent enough to record only a slight difference between consecutive frames. Too few pictures produces a jerky motion, and too many needlessly irradiate the patient. For example, 7.5 frames/sec (f/s) is adequate for the stomach and duodenum, while 30 to 60 f/s is required for coronary angiography.

A cine film should be projected at a speed of at least 16 f/s in order for the eye to perceive a smoothly flowing motion. If the film was recorded at a slower frequency, the image will appear to be moving faster than it actually is; if recording was faster, motion will be slowed down. In either case, the picture will flow smoothly. If the projector is operated at a frequency of less than 16 f/s, the eye recognizes individual cine frames, and it cannot integrate from one frame to the next. The result is the kind of jerky motion usually associated with old Charlie Chaplin movies.

Stop-Action versus Motion Pictures

With pulsed radiation individual cine frames are exposed by a single, short-duration pulse, short enough to stop most physiological motion. Each frame contains a sharp image that is ideal for stop-action viewing, i.e., for examining the frames individually. However, these sharp images do not necessarily produce the best motion pictures. In fact, some degree of blurring is desirable to help convey the sense of motion.

Most cinefluorographic films are viewed as both stop-action and motion pictures. As a general rule, blurring distracts more from stop-action pictures than sharp images do from motion pictures, which is why cinefluorographic exposures are as short as possible. The quality of a cine image may be improved by showing it as a motion picture, because of an averaging

out of quantum mottle. Fortunately, the eye does not "see" the individual frames of a motion picture. Instead, the eye sees several frames. It integrates these images, adds them together, and smooths out the information voids left by quantum mottle. The resulting movie image is visually superior to the image of any individual frame. When cine film is projected at lower than 24 f/s, the number of integrated frames is too small to significantly improve image quality. If the film is meant to be shown at fewer than 24 f/s, it may be necessary to increase the x-ray exposure above the recommended 20 μR/f, to compensate for the resulting loss in image quality.

Flicker

Flicker is a completely different and more difficult problem to eliminate than jerky motion. Flicker persists up to approximately 50 f/s, while jerky motion is eliminated at 16 f/s. Physiologists measure the eye's ability to detect flicker by rotating a partial disc, similar to the camera shutter, in front of a light source. The eye recognizes individual flashes up to approximately 50 per second, depending upon the brightness of the light. At higher flash frequencies, the light appears to be continuous, and flicker disappears. For example, an ordinary incandescent lamp flickers 120 times/sec with alternating current, but the eye perceives a continuous light. Radiologists usually accept flicker, and it does not seriously interfere with perception. Interestingly, the movie industry has devised an ingenious method of eliminating flicker. The projector shutter is run two times as fast as the film, and each frame is shown twice. Since movie film is normally made at 24 f/s, by showing each frame twice, the number of light pulses is increased to 48, which is sufficient to eliminate flicker.

PATIENT EXPOSURES

The amount of radiation that a patient receives during a cinefluoroscopic examination depends upon many factors (mA, kVp, distance, patient thickness, grids, intensifier size, camera f-number, processing, etc.), but the following three are more important than the others:

1. Synchronization
2. Framing frequency
3. F-number of the optical system

Fortunately, all modern equipment is synchronized, which decreases patient exposures by at least 50%. The framing frequency is usually dictated by the nature of the examination, but it is fairly obvious that the more frames that are exposed per second, the greater the patient's exposure. Filming should be performed within the critical resolution of the cine lens. This is generally about two f-numbers smaller than the maximum lens aperture.

The Inter-Society Commission for Heart Disease Resources[1] recommends a minimum exposure of 20 μR/f, measured at the front of the image intensifier. Before we can compare the recommended exposures with those in the literature, we must have comparable units of measurement. Since skin (or tabletop) exposure rates are usually reported in the literature, we will convert the 20 μR/f into skin exposures. For an example, we will consider a 60 f/s cine examination of the heart. Assuming the patient to be large, up to 99% of the initial beam may be absorbed by the patient and grid, or lost via the inverse square law. Thus, the skin exposure is 100 times as large as the image intensifier exposure.

The patient receives a per frame exposure of:

$$100 \times 20 \ \mu\text{R/f} = 2000 \ \mu\text{R/f (or 2 mR/f)}$$

This 2 mR/f skin exposure can be converted to mR/min by multiplying it by the number of f/s and sec/min:

$$2 \ \text{mR/f} \times 60 \ \text{f/s} \times 60 \ \text{s/m} = 7200 \ \text{mR/min}$$

In this example, the patient's skin received an exposure of 7.2 R/min at 60 f/s. If the framing frequency was halved, the exposure would also be halved to 3.6 R/min.

Table 16–2 shows some of the exposure rates reported in the literature. They are generally higher than the examples above. However, all of these exposures were measured during the era of zinc cadmium sulfide image intensifiers. We would anticipate that the exposures would be lower with cesium iodide image tubes.

SPOT FILM CAMERAS

Spot film cameras are almost identical to cine cameras. Film sizes are larger and framing rates slower, but optical coupling is the same with tandem lenses and a beam-splitting mirror. Spot film cameras require a lens with a longer focal length to cover the larger film formats. Four sizes are commercially available at the present time—70-, 90- and 105-mm roll film and 100-mm cut film. The optimum size is a matter of personal preference, but everyone agrees that the image must be large enough to view without magnification.

Table 16–2. Exposure Rates for Cinefluorography

AUTHOR	YEAR	ANATOMIC AREA	FILM SIZE (mm)	FRAMES PER SECOND	EXPOSURE RATE (R/min.)
Feddema	1960	Stomach	35	16	6–20
Speyer	1960	Stomach	16	16	7–45
Tristan	1960	Esophagus	35	15	21
Chérigie	1961	Stomach	16	25	20–25
Nunnally	1970	Heart	35	60	28–64

Summarized from Kaude, J.: Integral dose in 35 mm cinefluorography of the gastrointestinal tract. Acta Radiol. (Diagn.) (Stockholm) 7:1970, 1968.

Spot film cameras are used in two different clinical settings. Initially, their use was limited to gastrointestinal fluoroscopy, because the resolution and contrast of the older zinc-cadmium sulfide image tubes were inadequate for more intricate structures. GI barium studies did not require a high resolution imaging system and the barium provided excellent inherent contrast. In this setting, spot film cameras were merely used as a substitute for conventional spot films. After cesium iodide image tubes were developed, a second application became apparent. Spot film cameras could be used for serial filming in various kinds of angiography. The limiting factor in this application is the relatively small size of the image intensifier compared to cut film changers. The problem can be partially offset by panning, i.e. moving the image tube during the procedure to increase the area of coverage.

Advantages and Disadvantages of Spot Film Cameras

The principal advantage of spot film cameras over direct filming methods is a substantial reduction in patient exposure. A rough idea of the degree of reduction is shown in Table 16–3. The recommended per frame exposure for spot film cameras is 100 microroentgens (μR). The exposure for a comparable serial film is 300 μR—three times as much. The disadvantages, and other advantages of spot film cameras relate to convenience, economics, and the clinical setting. For gastroenterology, cameras are more convenient than conventional spot films. The film does not have to be changed between exposures, and the delay between the initiation and completion of an exposure is shorter because no cassette has to be moved into position for a spot film camera. The only part that moves to start an exposure is the small beam-splitting mirror. Exposure times are shorter so motion is less likely to be a problem. Also, films can be taken more rapidly. Most commercial units are designed to function at a maximum framing frequency of 6 to 12 frames/second.

The **advantages** of spot film cameras for serial angiography are as follows:
1. Reduction in procedure time.
2. Ease of performance.
3. Constant monitoring of the images during the performance of a study.
4. Reduced patient exposure.
5. Shorter exposure times.
6. Reduced equipment wear.
7. Cheaper film and processing.
8. Reduced film storage problems.

The **disadvantages** of spot film cameras for serial angiography are as follows:
1. Limited film coverage which prevents application in certain areas. For example, in peripheral angiography each extremity must be studied separately.
2. More experience is required to learn panning techniques.
3. Medical personnel in the angiography suite receive additional radiation exposure.

Table 16–3. Recommended per Frame (or Film) Exposures for Various Imaging Systems[1]

IMAGING SYSTEM	FILM SIZE	EXPOSURE/FRAME
Cinefluorography	16–35 mm	20 μR
Spot film camera	70–105 mm	100 μR
Serial radiography	35 × 35 cm (14 × 14 inch)	300 μR

4. Not applicable to studies of some neoplasms because of the reduced resolution of the image intensifier.

Framing Methods

Spot film cameras have a square image which simplifies framing compared to cinefluorography. Remember, cine film has a 4 × 3 (24 × 18 mm) format and the image can be framed to either film dimension. Only four framing formats are recommended for spot film cameras compared to six (or more) for cine film. The four formats are shown in Figure 16–24 and summarized as follows:

1. **Exact framing.** The entire circular intensifier image is included in the useable square film frame. The word **useable** refers to the fact that a part of the film is lost to the transport system, i.e. perforations along the edge of the film. The exact amount depends upon the film size and design of the transport system and varies somewhat from one manufacturer to another. With exact framing, no part of the image is lost, but 21% of the film is wasted.

2. **Equal area framing.** The area of the intensifier image is equal to the useable square film area. Approximately 9% of both the image and film are lost.

3. **Mean diameter framing.** The diame-

ter of the intensifier is equal to the mean of the transverse and diagonal dimensions of the useful square film area; 16% of the image is lost but only 4% of the film is unused.

4. **Total overframing.** The diameter of the image intensifier is equal to the diagonal dimension of the useful square film area. The entire film is used, but 36% of the image is unused.

The optimum framing format depends upon several factors: (1) the size of the image intensifier, (2) the size of the film, and (3) the clinical application for which the imaging system is intended. For any given system, the size of the recorded image enlarges as the diameter of the format increases. This is shown diagrammatically in Figure 16–24. Note in the illustration that the arrow increases in size as the framing format increases. For this reason, more overframing is recommended for small formats (70 mm) than for larger formats (105 mm). In general, exact framing is not recommended for any clinical application. It is especially undesirable for 70 mm film, because the final image is too small. Total overframing is not recommended except possibly for 70-mm film where maximum magnification is desirable. Either equal area or mean diameter framing are recommended for most clini-

FRAMING MODE	EXACT FRAMING	EQUAL AREA FRAMING	MEAN DIAMETER FRAMING	TOTAL OVERFRAMING
ILLUSTRATION				
FILM AREA USED	79%	91%	96%	100%
IMAGE AREA UNUSED	0%	9%	16%	36%
RELATIVE IMAGE SIZE	1.0	1.13	1.21	1.41

Figure 16–24 Framing formats for spot film cameras

cal situations.[1] Total overframing is impractical with larger film sizes (100 and 105 mm) because the required focal length of the camera lens becomes prohibitively long. As a general rule, a focal length of greater than 400 mm is not recommended. Longer focal length lenses are impractical because of their large physical size and weight.

The film for spot film cameras should have a relatively low contrast. An average gradient between 1.0 and 1.6 is recommended by the Inter-Society Commission for Heart Disease Resources.[1] A minimum exposure of 100 μR/film is required to minimize quantum mottle. This is the exposure at the input phosphor of the image tube after the x-ray beam has traversed the patient and grid. Remember that quantum mottle originates in the fluorescent screen so it is not affected by the size of the recorded image. Therefore, the same exposures are recommended for both 70- and 105-mm films.

SUMMARY

The emergence of cinefluorography came about as a byproduct of the development of the x-ray image intensifier. The intensifier is prerequisite for efficient optical coupling and for an image bright enough to expose the film without excessively exposing the patient. Figure 16–25 summarizes the various components of a typical cine system. Beginning on the left side, an 0.6 mm focal spot is recommended. Exposures should be kept in the 3 to 5 ms range with beam energies between 60 to 90 kVp. At least 55 cm should separate the target from the table top or patient support. The beam should be collimated to the framing mode selected. The image intensifier should be chosen for the particular clinical situation and in general should be as small as practical. The collector lens should be as fast as cost and technology permit. The framing mode should be selected and the camera lens designed to produce the appropriate frame size. Lens performance is improved with iris diaphragms. Resolution, contrast, depth of field, and spherical aberrations are all improved with an iris diaphragm. An aperture about two f-numbers less than maximum is recommended.

Cine film should have a wide latitude, low contrast, low base fog and be processed to an average gradient in the 1.0 to 1.6

Figure 16–25 Summary of recommendations for a cinefluorographic system

range. An input phosphor exposure of 20 μR per frame is recommended to minimize quantum mottle. The temperature, replenishment rates and transport times of the cine processors must be precisely controlled and processor performance should be monitored daily. Sensitometric studies should include spot checks of gross fog, speed and contrast. Other components of the cine system should also be monitored on a regular basis.

Spot film cameras are similar to cine cameras in design, but not in function. They are used to produce static images either for GI type radiography in place of conventional spot films or for serial angiography. Film sizes of 70, 90, 100 and 105 mm are in current usage. A per frame exposure of 100 μR is recommended, regardless of film size. The principal advantage of spot film cameras over screen-film radiography is a substantial reduction in patient exposures. The major disadvantages are a relatively small size radiographic field and some loss of resolution in the image intensifier.

REFERENCES

1. Judkins, M. P., Abrams, H. L., Bristow, J. D., et al.: Report of inter-society commission for heart disease resources. Circulation. *53*, No. 2, February 1976.
2. Cameras for image intensifier fluoroscopy. Washington, D. C.: International Commission on Radiation Units and Measurements. Report 15, 1969.
3. Lawrence, D. J.: A simple method of processor control. Med. Radiography and Photography. *49*, 2, 1973.

CHAPTER 17

Television

Before the invention of the x-ray image intensifier, attempts at displaying the fluoroscopic image on television were only partially successful. The large fluoroscopic screen required an elaborate optical system, and suboptimal screen brightness produced a weak video signal. The development of the image intensifier solved both of these problems. Its small output phosphor simplifies optical coupling, and a brightness gain of 3000 to 6000 produces a strong video signal. Two types of television cameras have been used for fluoroscopy, image-orthicon and vidicon cameras. Initially, the image-orthicon camera was the only one sensitive enough to record the limited brightness gains of early image intensifiers. In recent years brightness gains have increased and vidicon cameras have improved, so that now they have completely replaced image-orthicon cameras in fluoroscopy.

CLOSED-CIRCUIT TELEVISION

The components of a television system (Figure 17–1) are a camera, camera control unit, and monitor. To avoid confusion in nomenclature, we will use the terms "television" and "video" interchangeably. Fluoroscopic television systems are always closed-circuit systems; i.e., the video signal is transmitted from one component to the next through cables rather than through the air as it is in broadcast television. A lens system conveys the fluoroscopic image

Television

Figure 17–1   Components of a television system

from the output phosphor of the image intensifier to the video camera, where it is converted into a series of electrical pulses, which are called the **video signal.** This signal is transmitted through a cable to the camera control unit, where it is amplified, and then forwarded through another cable to the television monitor. The monitor converts the video signal back into the original image for direct viewing by the fluoroscopist.

Before discussing the individual components of a television system, we are going to move a little ahead of ourselves and describe the nature of the video picture. An appreciation of its nature will make the design of both the camera and monitor easier to understand. The television image is similar to the screened print shown in Figure 17–2. It is made up of a mosaic of thousands of tiny dots, each contributing a minute bit to the total picture. When viewed from a distance, the individual dots disappear, but at close range, or with magnification, they are clearly visible. The dot

234

Figure 17–2   Dot picture and enlargement of a screened print

distribution is not random or haphazard in a television picture. Instead, they are arranged in a specific pattern along horizontal lines, which are called **horizontal scan lines.** The number of lines varies from one television system to another, but in the United States, most fluoroscopy and all commercial television uses 525 scan lines. To avoid confusion, we must clarify the meaning of television lines. When a radiologist thinks of lines, it is usually in terms of lines per unit length. For example, if a grid has 80 lines, the unit is "lines per inch." Television lines have only the unit of "lines," and no unit of length. The 525 lines in most television systems represent the total number in the entire picture, regardless of its size. The lines are close together in a small picture tube, and spread apart in a large tube, but in both the total number is the same. The television camera converts the features present in the fluoroscopic image into a series of dots because it can only transmit one dot at a time.

The Television Camera

The vidicon camera is the one usually employed for fluoroscopy, and it is the only one that we will discuss in any detail. It is a relatively inexpensive, compact unit (5 inches in diameter, 9 inches long) that weighs approximately 6 lbs. The essential parts of a vidicon camera are shown diagrammatically in Figure 17–3. The most important part is the vidicon tube, a small electronic vacuum tube that measures only 1 inch in diameter and 6 inches in length. The tube is surrounded by two pairs of coils: electromagnetic focusing coils and electrostatic deflecting coils.

The fluoroscopic image from the image intensifier is focused onto the target assembly, which consists of three layers: (1) a glass faceplate, (2) a signal plate, and (3) a target. The only function of the glass faceplate is to maintain the vacuum in the tube. Light merely passes through the faceplate on its way to the target. The signal plate is a thin transparent film of graphite located on the inner surface of the faceplate. It is an electrical conductor with a positive potential of approximately 25 volts. The signal plate is so named because it transmits the video signal.

The vidicon target is functionally the most important element in the tube. It is a thin film of photoconductive material,

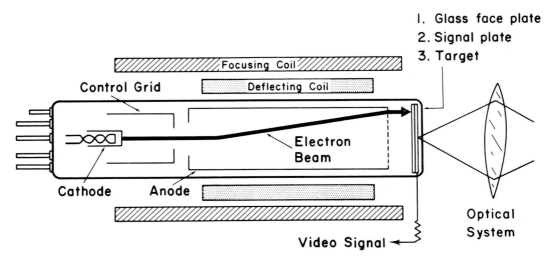

Figure 17-3   Vidicon camera

usually antimony trisulfite suspended as globules in a mica matrix. Each globule measures 1/1000 of an inch in diameter and is insulated from its neighbors and from the signal plate by the mica matrix. The globules form a mosaic of millions of tiny light-sensitive elements, and they form the dot picture that we described earlier. Their function is very complex, but they behave like tiny capacitors. After reviewing the other elements in the camera, we will return to these globules and discuss them in more detail.

The cathode is located at the opposite end of the vidicon tube from the target. It is heated indirectly by an internal electric coil. The cathode-heating coil assembly is called an **electron gun.** The heating coil boils electrons from the cathode (thermionic emission), creating an electron cloud. These electrons are immediately formed into a beam by the control grid, which also initiates their acceleration toward the target. As the electron beam progresses down the tube, it moves beyond the influence of the control grid and into the electrostatic field of the anode. The anode has a positive potential of approximately 250 volts with respect to the cathode, and it accelerates the electron beam to a relatively high velocity. The anode extends across the target end of the tube as a fine wire mesh. The wire mesh and signal plate form a uniform decelerating field adjacent to the target. The signal plate (+25 volts) has a potential of 225 volts less than the wire mesh (+250 volts), so that electrons should flow from the signal plate to the wire mesh. However, the electrons from the cathode are accelerated to relatively high velocities, and they coast through the decelerating field like a roller coaster going uphill. By the time they reach the target, they have been slowed to a near standstill. The decelerating field also performs a second function; it straightens the final path of the electron beam so that it strikes the target perpendicularly.

Since the electron beam scans a dot picture, it must be focused to a point the size of the dots. This is accomplished by two pairs of electromagnetic focusing coils that wrap around the vidicon tube as shown in Figure 17-4A. These coils extend almost the entire length of the tube and create a constant magnetic field that forces the beam of electrons into a narrow

A

SHAPE OF COILS

B

ELECTRON BEAM

FOCUSING COIL

C

ELECTRON BEAM

DEFLECTING COIL

Figure 17–4   Focusing and deflecting coils

over the target in a repetitive scanning motion.

The Video Signal

Now that we have discussed the physical make-up of the camera, we can return to the critical target end of the tube (Figure 17–5A) and the formation of the video signal. When a globule absorbs light, it emits electrons (Figure 17–5B). The electrons are immediately attracted to the anode and removed from the tube. The globule, having lost electrons, becomes positively charged. It is insulated from its

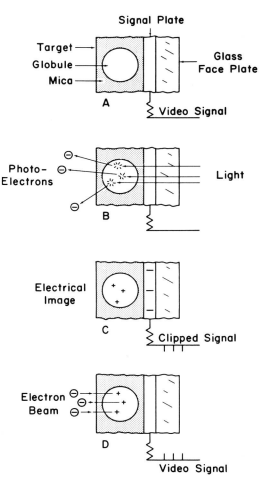

Signal Plate

Target

Globule

Mica

Glass
Face Plate

A

Video Signal

Photo-
Electrons

Light

B

Electrical
Image

C

Clipped Signal

Electron
Beam

D

Video Signal

Figure 17–5   Formation of the video signal

bundle. As the electrons are forced together, they repel each other and diverge, only to be brought back together by the focusing coil. They progress down the tube in a series of oscillating spirals (Figure 17–4B), and strike the target while they are focused at a point.

The electron beam is steered by variable electrostatic fields produced by two pairs of deflecting coils that wrap around the vidicon tube in a manner similar to the focusing coils. Vertical deflecting coils are shown in Figure 17–4C. By alternating the current on the coils, the focused electron beam is moved up and down to scan the target. The other pair of coils moves the beam from side to side along a horizontal line. All four coils, working together, move the electron beam almost instantaneously surroundings so it behaves like one-half of a tiny capacitor, and draws a current into the conductive signal plate. The current that flows into the signal plate is ignored, or clipped, and not recorded (Figure 17–5C). Similar events occur over the entire surface of the target. A brighter area in the light image emits more photoelectrons than a dim area, and produces a stronger charge on the tiny capacitors. The result is a mosaic of charged globules that store an electrical image which is an exact replica of the light image focused onto the target.

The electron beam scans the electrical image stored on the target, and fills in the holes left by the emitted photoelectrons, thus discharging the tiny globule capacitors. Excess electrons from the scanning beam drift back to the anode and are removed from the tube. At the instant of discharge, a current flows through the conductive signal plate and this current forms the video signal (Figure 17–5D). The globules are not all discharged at the same time. Only a small cluster, a dot, is discharged each instant in time. Then, the electron beam moves on to the next dot, and in an orderly sequence, but moving at an enormous speed, it discharges all of the globules on the target. The result is a series of video pulses, all originating from the same signal plate, but separated in time. Each pulse corresponds to an exact location on the target. The task of reassembling these pulses back into a visible image belongs to the camera control unit and the television monitor.

Camera Control Unit

The power supply and all of the controls that regulate the camera are located within the camera control unit. It amplifies the video signal (after preamplification in the camera), regulates the focusing and deflecting coils, and synchronizes the video signal between the camera and monitor.

Television Monitor

The last link in the television chain is the monitor. It contains the picture tube and controls for regulating brightness and contrast.

A picture tube, shown in Figure 17–6, is similar to a vidicon camera tube. Both are vacuum tubes and contain an electron gun, control grid, anode, focusing coils, and deflecting coils. However, a picture tube is much larger. The focusing and deflecting coils are wrapped around the neck of the tube and they control the electron beam in exact synchrony with the camera tube. The brightness of the individual dots in the picture is regulated by the control grid. It receives the video signal from the television camera, and uses this signal to regulate the number of electrons in the electron beam. To produce a bright area in the television picture, it allows a large number of electrons to reach the fluorescent screen. To produce a dark area, it cuts off the electron flow almost completely.

The anode is plated onto the inside surface of the picture tube near the fluorescent screen. It carries a much higher positive potential (10,000 V) than the anode of the camera tube (250 V) so it accelerates the electron beam to a much higher velocity. The electrons strike the fluorescent screen at the flared end of the tube emitting a large number of light photons which form the visible television image. Many secondary electrons are set

Figure 17–6   Television monitor

free by the impact of the electron beam with the screen, and they are attracted to the anode and conducted out of the picture tube.

A large tube, like a television picture tube, can never be completely evacuated. Some residual gas is always present and "outgassing" (release of adsorbed gas) from the components of the monitor adds to the problem. These gas molecules are eventually ionized and then removed from the tube by an ion trap located in the end of the monitor (Figure 17–6).

TELEVISION SCANNING

The television image is stored as an electrical image on the target of the vidicon tube, and it is scanned along 525 lines by a narrow electron beam 30 times a second. Each scan of the entire target is called a frame. The electron beam scans the target in much the same manner that we read a page in a book. Beginning at the top left corner, it drifts across a line sending out a video signal as it moves, and then rapidly returns to the left margin and repeats the process over and over until all 525 lines have been read. When we reach the last line of a page, we move on to the top line of the next page and continue reading. The electron beam does exactly the same thing, only it does not have to turn pages. Instead, as the beam reads, it also erases. As the electron beam discharges the globule capacitors, it erases their image. As soon as a line is read and erased, it is ready to record a new image, and it begins immediately. When the electron beam returns, it sees a different image than it saw the time before. Since the electron beam scans the target 30 times each second, the charge in the image from one scan to the next is slight, and our eyes perceive a continuous motion in exactly the same way that we see motion in a cine film.

In the discussion of cinefluorography, we mentioned that the eye can detect individual flashes of light, or flicker, up to 50 pulses per second (Chapter 16). A television monitor only displays 30 frames per

Figure 17–7   Interlaced horizontal scanning

second, so an electronic trick, called **interlaced horizontal scanning** is employed to avoid flicker. Instead of scanning all 525 lines consecutively each frame, only the even-numbered lines are scanned in the first half of the frame, and only the odd-numbered lines during the second half, as is shown in Figure 17–7. Each pass of the electron beam over the video target is called a field, and consists of 262½ lines. Even though only 30 frames are displayed each second, they are displayed in 60 flashes of light (fields) and flicker disappears.

Frequency of the Video Signal (Bandpass)

Bandpass, which is also called bandwidth, is the frequency range that the electronic components of the video system must be designed to transmit. An analogy with sound will simplify the explanation. Sound is audible at frequencies from about 16 hertz (cycles/sec) to 30,000 hertz. Sound equipment (recorders, amplifiers, speakers, etc.) is designed to transmit this range of frequencies. The range from the lowest to the highest frequency is called the bandpass and it is shown diagrammatically in Figure 17–8. The electronic components are engineered to transmit all of the frequencies in this range as accurately as possible. The cutoffs are not sharply defined at the two frequency extremes and not all frequencies are transmitted with the same quality. Thinking in terms of music, bandpass is the frequency range that the electronic components must "pass" from

Figure 17–8   Frequency range of audible sound and the bandpass required for accurate transmission

the "band" to the listener. A video signal is exactly the same as an audio signal, except that the video signal covers a wider range of frequencies.

As the electronic beam moves along a horizontal scan line, a video signal is transmitted to the camera control unit and then forwarded to the T.V. monitor. The frequency of the video signal will fluctuate from moment-to-moment depending upon the nature of the television image. Figure 17–9 shows one scan line of an image containing four equally spaced black

and white lines, or four line pairs. As the electron beam moves across the image, the video signal increases and decreases in voltage in a cyclic fashion. Like alternating current, one cycle (the shaded area in the illustration) includes one up limb and one down limb and represents two lines, or one line pair. The scanning process is repeated over and over 525 times per frame and 30 frames per second. We can calculate the frequency, or number of cycles/second of the video signal generated by the four line pair image by multiplying the number of cycles/scan line (4 in this case), times the number of scan lines/frame, times the number of frames/sec.

$$\frac{cycles}{scan\ line} \times \frac{scan\ lines}{frame} \times \frac{frames}{seconds} = cycles/sec$$

$$4 \quad \times \quad 525 \quad \times \quad 30 \quad = 63,000$$

When the number of line pairs in the image changes, the frequency of the video signal also changes. The lowest frequency signal occurs with an image of 1 line pair, i.e. a screen that is half black and half white. The highest frequency signal is determined by the amount of money that one is willing to pay for electronic equipment. A reasonable compromise is a system with equal vertical and horizontal resolution.

Figure 17–9   The video signal from one scan line of a line pair phantom

This is accomplished in a 525 line system with 525 vertical lines, or 262½ line pairs. In this case the lowest and highest frequency signals will be as follows:

	cycles / scan line	×	scan lines / frame	×	frames / second	= cycles/second
Minimum	1	×	525	×	30	= 15,750
Maximum	262½	×	525	×	30	≈ 4,130,000

The frequency of the video signal will fluctuate between a minimum of 15,750 hertz and a maximum of 4,130,000 hertz. To accurately transmit the signal, the electronic components should have a bandpass of 4.13 to 0.016 MHz, or approximately 4.1 MHz. Actually, a little higher bandpass is required. About 10% of the scan time is lost in retracing from one line to another. This additional 10% increases the required bandpass to approximately 4.5 MHz for a 525 line system. At this bandpass, vertical and horizontal resolution is equal.

Synchronization

It is necessary to synchronize or coordinate the video signal between the camera and monitor; i.e., keep them in phase with each other. The camera control unit adds synchronization pulses to the video signal at the end of each scan line and scan field. Appropriately, they are called "horizontal" and "vertical synchronization pulses." They are generated during the retrace time of the electron beam, while no video signal is being transmitted. First, the picture screen is blackened by a blanking pulse, and then the synchronization signal is added to the blanking pulse. If the synchronization pulses were added to the video signal while the screen was white, they would generate noise in the form of white streaks, but no visible noise is produced by synchronization on a black screen.

TELEVISION IMAGE QUALITY
Resolution

The number of scan lines and the bandpass of a television system impose an absolute ceiling on resolution. Obviously, a dot picture cannot display an image smaller than the individual dots. The only way that television resolution can be improved is with more and smaller dots, which means more scan lines, and a greater bandpass. A greater dot concentration improves resolution, but it does not remove the ceiling. Regardless of the quality of the x-ray image, the television image has this absolute ceiling on quality.

Television resolution is measured on the face of the TV monitor and expressed in total lines. A resolution of 370 lines means that 370 separate lines, or 185 line pairs (lp), are visible on the entire TV monitor. If the bandpass is properly selected, horizontal and vertical resolution are equal. The ratio between the vertical resolution and the number of horizontal scan lines is called the **Kell factor.** Kell factors are determined experimentally by measuring the maximum number of lines that can be seen with a line pair imaging system. The Kell factor for a 525 line TV system is 0.7. The vertical resolution of this system is as follows:

$$\text{Kell factor} = \frac{\text{Resolution}}{\text{Number of scan lines}}$$

$$0.7 = \frac{\text{Resolution}}{525}$$

$$\text{Resolution} = 525 \times 0.7 \approx 370$$

This is the maximum vertical resolution that can be attained with a 525 line system regardless of the size of the monitor. A resolution of 370 total lines represents 185 black lines separated by 185 equal thickness white lines, or 185 line pairs. Monitor resolution can only be improved by employing more scan lines and a higher bandpass. Such systems are available, but they have numerous disadvantages, including increased cost and incompatibility with the commercial systems currently in use in most hospitals. Also, the higher bandpass is usually associated with more electrical noise, and noise diminishes resolution. At the present time, there is little difference in the quality of the fluoroscopic image between 525 line and 875 line (or any higher number of lines) systems.[1]

The overall resolution of the imaging system, i.e. the image intensifier—lens — TV system depends upon the size of the input image. If the TV monitor resolution of 185 lp is used to show a large picture, resolution will be poor. For example, suppose we use television to display the image from a 9-inch image intensifier. Converting to millimeters, a 9-inch image intensifier is 229 mm in diameter (9 inch × 25.4 mm/inch). The system resolution in lp/mm is as follows:

$$\frac{185 \text{ lp}}{229 \text{ mm}} = 0.8 \text{ lp/mm}$$

Table 17–1 shows system resolution for three different size image intensifiers. The same numbers would apply to a triple mode (4.5, 6 and 9 inches) image intensifier. The television monitor always displays the same 185 lp, but when supplied with the image from a 4.5 inch image intensifier, this 185 lp represents a resolution of 1.6 lp/mm, twice as good as the 0.8 lp/mm of the 9-inch image intensifier. However, even though a resolution of 1.6 lp/mm is a considerable improvement, it

falls far short of displaying the entire resolution of the newer cesium iodide image intensifiers. These tubes have a resolution of up to 4 lp/mm. The only way that this resolution can be adequately displayed at the present time is with a film system such as a 35-mm cine, or 105-mm spot films.

With the appropriate optical system, the 185 lp of television resolution can transmit any desired degree of system resolution, provided the size of the initial image is reduced proportionately. For example, if we start by looking at a radiograph of a whole hand, then gradually zoom in (with the appropriate lens) to look at one phalanx, and finally only a small portion of one cortex, the system resolution increases tremendously. If in the end, we are looking at an area 10 mm in diameter, the system resolution could be as high as 18.5 lp/mm (185 lp ÷ 10 mm). In this case, system resolution would be limited by the input phosphor of the image intensifier and not by the television image.

Figure 17–10 compares the resolution of an older zinc cadmium sulfide image intensifier and television fluoroscopy in terms of dose rate (μR/sec). At low radiation dosages, there are too few x-ray

Table 17–1. Resolution of a TV Imaging System for Various Size Image Intensifiers.

SIZE OF IMAGE INTENSIFIER		TELEVISION RESOLUTION*
inches	mm	(lp/mm)
4.5	114	1.6
6	152	1.2
9	229	0.8

*Based on a 525 line TV system with a total resolution of 185 line pairs (lp).

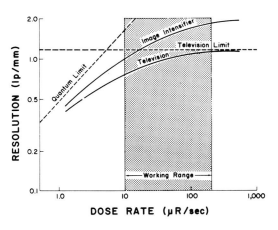

Figure 17–10 Image intensifier and television resolution during fluoroscopy. (Modified from Gebauer, *et al.: Roentgen Television.* New York: Grune & Stratton, 1967)

photons to produce a good image and resolution is quantum limited in both systems. At higher dose rates television resolution continues to be limited, but at a higher level, by the dot composition of the image. A transmitted radiation level of 20 μR/sec produces a good quality image without excessively exposing the patient. A television camera cannot improve image quality beyond that of an image intensifier, since it receives its image from the intensifier.

Contrast

Both the camera and monitor affect the contrast of a television image. A vidicon camera reduces contrast by a factor of approximately 0.8, and the monitor enhances contrast by a factor of 2. The net result is a definite improvement in contrast beyond that of the image intensifier alone. Furthermore, both the brightness and contrast levels can be regulated with the monitor, so the optimum combination can be selected to show a point of interest best.

Lag

An undesirable property of most vidicon tubes is lag, or stickiness, which becomes apparent when the camera is moved rapidly during fluoroscopy; i.e., the image blurs. Lag occurs because it takes a certain amount of time for the image to build up and decay on the vidicon target. In one respect, a certain amount of lag is actually advantageous. It averages out the statistical fluctuations that normally occur with low-dose fluoroscopy and minimizes the annoying effects of quantum mottle.

Brightness

The brightness of the image changes constantly in all fluoroscopic systems as the fluoroscope is moved from one area of the patient to another. Usually, this does not cause any serious problem, and both the chest and abdomen can be examined with preset exposure factors. However, with television fluoroscopy, changes in image brightness seriously affect image quality. As the fluoroscope is moved from the abdomen to the chest, a sudden surge of brightness floods the system, the image becomes chalky, and all detail is lost. Therefore, the brightness level of the television monitor must be controlled within rather narrow limits. This is usually accomplished by varying the x-ray exposure factors. A photocell located between the image intensifier and television camera measures the brightness of the fluoroscopic image, and it transmits a signal back to the x-ray control unit to adjust the exposure factors.

The brightness level of the television monitor can be increased indefinitely, but this does not improve image quality. At low levels of radiation, image quality is limited by quantum mottle and at high levels by the inherent ceiling imposed on resolution by a dot image. Usually, brightness and contrast are adjusted in combination. Contrast is brought to a near-maximum level, and brightness is adjusted to produce a satisfactory level of illumination.

Plumbicon and Image Orthicon Cameras

We have delayed mentioning plumbicon and image-orthicon cameras because we will discuss them only on the basis of their performance, and we will not attempt to describe their mode of operation.

A plumbicon camera is simply a vidicon camera with a lead monoxide photoconductor for its target. Its tube is a little larger than a standard vidicon tube, and it does not fit into a conventional vidicon housing. Plumbicon tubes have two advantages over other vidicon tubes: (1) contrast is not diminished, and (2) lag is considerably less. Motion blurring is almost completely eliminated, but with diminished lag, quantum mottle becomes a problem; in general, plumbicon tubes have considerably more mottle than other vidicon tubes.

Image-orthicon cameras are much larger than vidicon cameras, and they have a completely different electronic design. They are extremely sensitive to light and function well with low levels of illumination. In the early days of television fluoroscopy, image-orthicon tubes were the only ones sensitive enough to transmit a good image with the limited light gain of early image intensifiers. The other advantages are superior resolution, and a complete freedom from lag. However, image-orthicon cameras have serious disadvantages. To begin with, they are too expensive for most radiologists, and their large size makes them cumbersome to operate. Even more important, they are extremely sensitive to temperature changes and require a long warm-up time (up to 20 minutes). In recent years, vidicon cameras have completely replaced image-orthicon cameras for fluoroscopy.

MAGNETIC RECORDERS

The commercial television industry has been storing programs on tape recorders for many years. When magnetic recorders were first developed, their prohibitive cost severely limited their availability for clinical radiology. However, in recent years, less expensive models have been developed and now video tape is commonly used to store fluoroscopic images. A second type of magnetic recorder, a video disc, is also being used in fluoroscopy. The physical principles are exactly the same for tape and disc recorders. We will start by describing tape recorders as a prototype and then briefly point out a few of the characteristics of disc recorders at the end of this section.

Video-tape Recorders

The same unit is used for both recording and playback. As a recorder, it receives a video signal from the camera control unit, and for playback, transmits the signal to one, or several, television monitors. Both of these transmissions are conducted through cables, so it is a closed-circuit television system. The image is stored on either 1- or 2-inch wide mylar tape, coated on one side with a magnetic film. Two-inch video tape records a better-quality image, but costs considerably more, so most fluoroscopy is recorded on 1-inch tape.

A schematic presentation of a tape recorder is shown in Figure 17–11. The three essential components, besides the electronic circuitry, are a magnetic tape, a recording and/or reading head, and a tape transport system. Exactly the same type head is used for both recording and playback, and we will call it a writing head. The writing head converts an electrical signal into a fluctuating magnetic field for recording, and converts a magnetic signal into an electrical signal for replay. Some

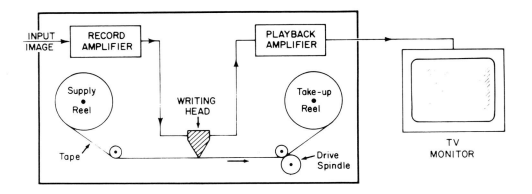

Figure 17–11   Components of a video-tape recorder

Figure 17–12   Video writing head

recorders have separate recording and playback heads, while in others, one head performs both functions. The drive spindle moves the tape past the writing head at a constant velocity. The tape is kept in physical contact with the writing head at all times during both record and playback.

The writing head of a video-tape recorder is shown in Figure 17–12. The head is similar to a transformer (Chapter 3) in that it consists of a magnetic core, such as an iron-nickel alloy, wrapped with two coils of wire. However, the writing head is different in two ways. First, a narrow segment, or gap, is cut from the core as shown in the illustration; second, the two coils are wired together so that their magnetic fields reinforce each other. As a changing electric field moves through the coils, a changing magnetic field is produced in the gap. When the current in the illustration moves from left to right, the magnetic field is in the direction of the arrows. The field reverses when the current changes directions. The magnetic field extends out beyond the gap in the writing head, as shown in Figure 17–13. This extended magnetic field is the critical portion that interacts with the magnetic tape.

The magnetic layer of video tape is composed of oxides of magnetic materials. The molecules of this material behave like tiny bar magnets, called **dipoles.** Each dipole aligns itself in a magnetic field like the needle of a compass. They are randomly arranged on unrecorded tape as shown in Figure 17–13A. As the tape moves past the writing head gap, the alignment of the

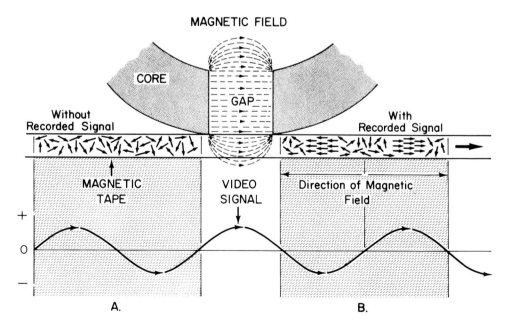

Figure 17–13   The magnetic signal on video tape

dipoles is changed to coincide with the magnetic field impressed upon them while they are passing the gap (B). When the video signal (sine curve in the illustration) is negative, the dipoles are aligned toward the left; when the signal is positive, alignment is in the opposite direction. At the zero points in the video signal, no magnetic field exists in the gap, and dipole alignment is random. The degree of alignment is exaggerated in the illustration to demonstrate the point. The actual alignment is proportional to the strength of the magnetic field. Complete alignment is prevented by the neighboring molecules, which offer some resistance to dipole movement, and by the inertia of the dipoles themselves. Once the tiny magnetic particles leave the magnetic field in the gap, they retain their orientation until some other magnetic force causes them to change.

Playback is exactly the reverse of the recording process, except that the magnetic dipoles are not unaligned in playback. The partially aligned magnetic dipoles have a magnetic field of their own. As this field moves past the gap in the writing head, it induces a magnetic field in the core, which in turn induces an electrical signal in the wire coils. This is the video signal that is forwarded to the display monitor.

Every component of the video signal must be recorded on a different portion of the magnetic tape. The transport system must move fast enough to keep a fresh supply of tape at the writing heads. If the tape moves too slowly, the dipole alignment of one cycle is unaligned by the magnetic field of the next cycle. To record a frequency of several million cycles per second, the tape must move at a very high velocity. This is accomplished by moving both the tape and writing heads as shown in Figure 17–14. The tape moves diagonally past paired writing heads mounted on either side of a rapidly revolving drum. The tape moves in one direction at 10

Figure 17–14   Video-tape recorder. (Modified from *Operating Manual for Ampex Model VR-6000 Videotape Recorder.* Elk Grove Village, Ill.: Ampex Corp., 1966)

Figure 17–15   Video tracks on video tape

inch/sec and the writing heads in the opposite direction at 1000 inch/sec for an effective writing speed of 1010 inch/sec. While one head is recording, the other is away from the tape so that only one writing head is recording at any particular time. Each writing head records one video frame as it passes diagonally across the tape. The signal is laid down in separate tracks approximately 6/1000 of an inch wide as shown in Figure 17–15. The tape moves just fast enough to separate the tracks of the two heads. Consecutive lines are always written by different heads. Video tracks are separated by a narrow guard band. Each 10 inches of video tape stores approximately 1000 inches of magnetic tracks. A reel of tape (3000 feet) plays for approximately 1 hour, and if handled carefully, it can be reused more than 100 times.

Image quality is a little better with direct (live) television than it is with video tape, but the difference is not large. The Ampex Model VR-6000 shown in Figure 17–14 has a bandpass of 3.5 MHz and its resolution is reported by the manufacturer as 350 lines (175 lp) which is very nearly the same as the 370 lines (185 lp) of direct television.

Cassette tape recorders are now increasing in popularity. They have only one advantage over other systems—ease of loading and unloading the tape. Otherwise cassette recorders are exactly the same as other tape recorders.

Video-Disc Recorders

Video-disc and video-tape recorders operate on exactly the same physical principle, but they have completely different functions. Tape recorders are designed to show motion, comparable to a movie camera. Disc recorders are designed to show stationary images, more like a spot film camera. A tape recorder can be used to show a single frame by stopping the tape against the revolving drum, but this subjects the tape to considerable physical wear. Video-disc recorders are designed for stop action. The discs themselves look like phonograph records. The video tracks are laid down in preset grooves. Each groove in a video disc is a completely separate track. The tracks are not continuous from groove to groove. One picture frame is recorded in each track. When a particular frame is selected for replay, exactly the same picture is shown over and over 30 times a second for as long as the operator desires. Most disc recorders can only store a few hundred frames.

Video discs have several advantages over tape. The most important one is **random access.** The video grooves are numbered and the recorder can go directly to any desired number without playing the intervening numbers. This instantaneous access is considerably different than a tape recorder where it may take several minutes to reach a specific frame, even with a rapid wind mode. Another advantage of discs is

that they are not subjected to physical wear in the stop action mode. Actually, they are designed to operate in this mode. Only the disc moves during both recording and playback, so it is not subjected to the physical wear of a rotating drum. In a clinical setting, video-disc recorders are used as a substitute for spot films, and the x-ray exposure factors are frequently increased, just as they would be for spot films. This exposure increase improves the quality of the disc image by decreasing quantum mottle. Primarily because of this exposure increase, image quality is generally better with video discs than with video tape. Resolution is best with the smallest image intensifier mode consistent with the clinical situation.

Comparison of Video Tape and Cine Film

Video-tape recorders have two advantages over cinefluorography: (1) the image is available for instant replay without any intermediate processing system, and (2) the patient's exposure to radiation is not increased. Both of these advantages are important. Instant replay allows the radiologist to examine the record before the patient leaves the room, so that inadequacies in a study can be corrected immediately. Since exposure factors are not increased, the whole fluoroscopic examination can be recorded if so desired. If nothing of permanent value is found, the tape is erased and used again for another patient.

Video tape also has disadvantages, the most important being poor image quality. Cine film (either 16 or 35 mm) produces an image of superior quality. Whether or not this difference is significant depends upon the importance of image quality for the particular examination. For a study like coronary angiography, which requires a high-quality image, cine film is preferable; while for most gastrointestinal examinations, video tape is entirely adequate. Another disadvantage of video tape is its fixed frame speed; i.e., 30 frame/sec in the

United States. Cine cameras can be operated at several different speeds. However, a frequency of 30 f/s is adequate for most fluoroscopic needs.

In summary, video-tape recording offers more convenience with instant playback and decreased patient exposures.

Cine film produces a better-quality image and a greater variety of shutter speeds. Medical needs dictate which is preferable.

REFERENCE

1. Templeton, A. W., Dwyer, S. J., et al.: Standard and high-scan-line television systems. Radiol. *91*, 725, 1968.

CHAPTER 18

Body-section Radiography

Body-section radiography is a special x-ray technique which blurs out the shadows of superimposed structures in order to show more clearly the principal structures being examined. We must point out immediately that it is not a method of improving the sharpness of any part of a radiographic image. On the contrary, it is a process of controlled blurring that merely leaves some parts of the image less blurred than others. Various names have been used to describe body-section radiography. Most of them were initially applied to a specifically designed unit. Over the years considerable confusion has developed over nomenclature. In 1962 the International Commission on Radiologic Units and Measurements[1] adopted the term **tomography** to describe all types of body-section techniques, and we will use this term synonymously with body-section radiography. Some commonly used names are:

1. Tomography (tomogram)—preferred
2. Planigraphy (planigram)
3. Stratigraphy (stratigram)
4. Laminography (laminogram)

A revolutionary new technique, called computerized tomography (CT), was developed in England in 1972. Computerized tomography differs from conventional tomography in almost every way. In fact, about the only point the two have in common is that they both display a thin

layer, or slice of tissue. Since the two tomographic systems are completely different, we will discuss them separately. This chapter will be devoted entirely to conventional tomography, and CT will be discussed in Chapter 24.

THE BASIC TOMOGRAPHIC PRINCIPLE

Many ingenious tomographic methods have been devised. We will begin by describing the simplest, which is shown in Figure 18–1A. The essential ingredients are an x-ray tube, an x-ray film, and a rigid connecting rod that rotates about a fixed fulcrum. When the tube moves in one direction, the film moves in the opposite direction. The film is placed in a tray under the x-ray table so that it is free to move without disturbing the patient. The fulcrum is the only point in the system that

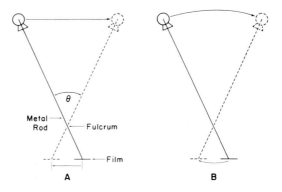

Figure 18–1 Tomographic principle

remains stationary. The amplitude of tube travel is measured in degrees and is called the "tomographic angle" (arc). The plane of interest within the patient is positioned at the level of the fulcrum, and it is the only plane that remains in sharp focus. All points above and below this plane are blurred.

A second type of tube motion is illustrated in Figure 18–1B. Both the x-ray tube and film move along an arc, instead of in a straight line as they did in our previous illustration. Both methods give similar results. The primary advantage of a straight-line motion is that it can be easily adapted to a standard x-ray table and requires no expensive equipment. However, it has more moving parts, including slip joints at both ends of the connecting rod, which eventually wear and get out of adjustment. A tomographic system that moves the tube and film in an arc has fewer moving parts and is less likely to get out of adjustment, but it requires a special table

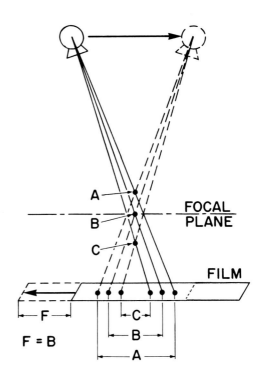

Figure 18–3   Blurring of points outside the focal plane

and tube stand built specifically for tomography, so it is more expensive.

All points that are parallel to the x-ray film and on the same plane as the fulcrum are displayed in sharp focus on the tomogram. A whole plane is in focus, not just a point. In Figure 18–2, points A, B, and C are several centimeters apart on the same plane and their images all move exactly the same distance as the x-ray film. Therefore, they are not blurred. When the tube moves to the left, the distance from point C to its image on the film is greater than the comparable distance of points B and A. However, the ratio of the object-tube and object-film distance for all three points is the same, and there is no difference in magnification of objects on the same plane.

Tomographic techniques blur all points that are outside (above or below) the focal plane. In Figure 18–3, point A is above and point C below the focal plane. As the

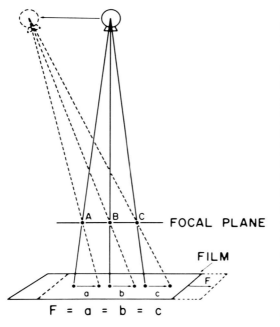

Figure 18–2   Focal plane

x-ray tube moves, only the image of point B, which is on the focal plane, remains in sharp focus, because it is the only image that moves exactly the same distance as the film. The image of point A moves more than the film, and the image of point C less than the film, so both are blurred. The further an object is from the plane of the fulcrum, the more its image is blurred.

Types of Tube Motion

If we look down from the ceiling at the system we have just described, the x-ray tube and film move in a straight line. Appropriately, this is referred to as "linear tomography." Many other types of tube motion have been devised. Most of them circumscribe some sort of arc. (Not to be confused with the arc shown in Figure 18–1B, which is a side view.) The six basic types of tube motion in common usage are shown in Figure 18–4. Remember that these are patterns of tube and film motion as seen from above.

Definition

Before going further with our discussion of tomography, it will be helpful to define a few of the terms we have used. **Blurring** is the distortion of definition of objects outside the focal plane. The **fulcrum** is the pivot point about which the lever arm rotates. It determines the plane that will be in focus. Two mechanically different types of fulcrums are in common usage. In the

first, the relationship between the x-ray tube, fulcrum, and film is fixed. The patient is moved up and down on an adjustable table to bring the level of interest to the plane of the fulcrum. The second type has an adjustable fulcrum that is moved to the height of the desired plane, while the patient remains stationary on the table. The **focal plane** is the plane of maximal focus, and represents the axis (fulcrum) about which the x-ray tube and film rotate. The **focal plane level** is the height of the focal plane above the tabletop. The **tomographic angle** (arc) is the amplitude of tube travel expressed in degrees (Figure 18–1A). The **exposure angle** is the angle through which the x-ray beam (or central ray) moves during the exposure. The tomographic angle and exposure angle are not always equal. Occasionally, x rays are not emitted during part of the tube travel, in which case the tomographic angle is greater than the exposure angle. Sometimes this is intentional, but usually it is the result of an equipment malfunction.

BLURRING

The whole purpose of tomography is to distort, or blur, the objects that might interfere with our perception of a particular radiographic image. In order to use our equipment to best advantage, we must understand the factors that control blurring. In tomography, the term "blurring" is used only with reference to objects outside the focal plane, and the same term should not be used to describe the image unsharpness that is inherent in all tomographic systems.

Width of the Blur

The width of the blur refers to the distance over which the image of an object is spread out on the film. It is determined by the following four factors:

1. Amplitude of tube travel
2. Distance from the focal plane
3. Distance from the film
4. Orientation of tube travel

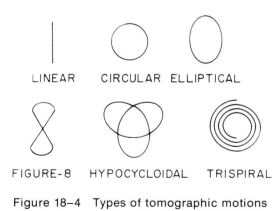

LINEAR   CIRCULAR   ELLIPTICAL

FIGURE-8   HYPOCYCLOIDAL   TRISPIRAL

Figure 18–4   Types of tomographic motions

Each of these four factors will be discussed separately.

Amplitude of tube travel. The width of the blur is a direct linear function of the number of degrees of tube travel. As the amplitude of tube travel increases, the width of the blur increases. When the number of degrees of tube motion is doubled, the amount of blurring doubles.

Distance from the focal plane. The farther an object is from the focal plane, the more it is blurred. Unfortunately, we have no control over this distance in diagnostic radiology. The relationships between anatomic parts and pathological lesions are fixed in the patient, and we cannot change them.

Distance from the film. Objects far away from the film are blurred more than objects close to the film (assuming they are both the same distance from the focal plane). The patient should be positioned so that the objects we want to blur are as far from the film as possible.

Orientation of tube travel. Many body parts are long and narrow and have a longitudinal axis. When the longitudinal axis of an object is oriented in the same direction that the x-ray tube travels, the image of the

object is not blurred, even though it lies outside of the focal plane. Figure 18–5 shows a conventional radiograph (A) and a linear tomographic film (B) taken on a phantom consisting of multiple crossed and curved wires. The wires are located 1 cm below the focal plane on the tomogram. As you can see, the image of one of the wires is not blurred, and the unblurred wire is the one oriented in the direction of x-ray tube motion. Increasing the tomographic arc will not blur this wire, it will merely elongate its image. Maximum blurring occurs when the long axis of the part to be blurred is perpendicular to the direction of tube travel.

Blur Margin

The edge of a blurred image is called the blur margin. Figure 18–6 shows linear (A) and circular (B) tomograms of the same test phantom that was shown in Figure 18–5. As you can see, the blur margins are different with these two types of tube motions. With linear tomography the entire image is uniformly blurred and fades off gradually at its edge. However, with a

Figure 18–5 Blur patterns with linear tomography. (Courtesy of Dr. J.T. Littleton)

Figure 18–6 Character of blur margins for linear and circular tomography. (Courtesy of Dr. J.T. Littleton)

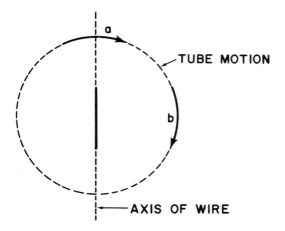

Figure 18-7 Circular tomographic motion superimposed on test wire

circular tube motion the blurred image is not uniform. The margin appears whiter and more sharply defined on the film than the rest of the blur pattern. The reason for the sharply defined border is shown in Figure 18-7, a top view of a circular tube motion superimposed on a test wire. The tube moves both across and parallel to the axis of the wire during different portions of its travel. Maximum blurring occurs as the tube moves across the axis of the wire (a), and this portion of the exposure produces the center of the blur pattern. Little blurring occurs while the tube is moving parallel to the wire's axis (b), and it is during this portion of the exposure that the incompletely blurred image is projected to the edge of the blur pattern. This sharply defined blur margin is important in phantom-image formation which we will discuss later in the chapter.

SECTION THICKNESS

There is no accurate way of defining section thickness. It means the thickness of the section that is in sharp focus on a tomogram. In theory, the focal plane is indeed a "plane" and has no thickness. The image that we see is actually made up of many thin planes superimposed on one

another. The closer these planes are to the true focal plane, the sharper they are in focus. There is no abrupt cut-off in sharpness, just a gradual progressive deterioration of image quality as we move away from the focal plane. The point at which the image is no longer considered in focus is subjective. It varies from one observer to another.

Section thickness is inversely proportional to the amplitude of x-ray tube travel (in degrees) as shown in Figure 18-8. The larger the tomographic angle, the thinner the section. In Figure 18-8C, you can see the length of tube travel does not determine the number of degrees in the tomographic arc. The tube moves the same number of degrees going from point **m** to **n** as it does from point **o** to **p**, although it travels a greater distance between **m** and **n**. With greater target-film distances, the tube must move a greater distance to subscribe the same angle.

While it is always desirable to have objects outside the focal plane maximally blurred, it is not always desirable to have the section as thin as possible. In fact, if we could cut an infinitely thin section, we would not be able to see it. Picture in your mind a coronal section through the human body only one micron thick. If we could take this section out of the body and x ray

Figure 18-8 Section thickness

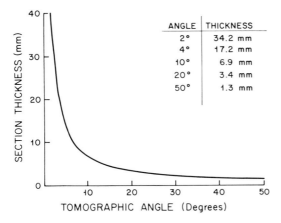

ANGLE	THICKNESS
2°	34.2 mm
4°	17.2 mm
10°	6.9 mm
20°	3.4 mm
50°	1.3 mm

Figure 18–9 Section thickness for various tomographic angles

it, we could not produce an x-ray image. There would be no contrast. Contrast depends on both the density and thickness of adjacent parts. Without some thickness, there is no contrast, and without contrast, there is no image..

Figure 18–9 shows section thicknesses for various tomographic angles, and as you can see, there is little change with angles larger than 10°. However, even though the section thickness does not change with large tomographic arcs, the blurring of objects outside the focal plane does change. Blurring continues to increase as the amplitude of tube travel increases, which is why a film taken with a 10° angle looks a great deal different than one taken with a 50° angle.

NARROW- VERSUS WIDE-ANGLE TOMOGRAPHY

We can use tomography to approach a diagnostic problem in two different ways. One system uses a wide tomographic arc and strives for maximal blurring of obscuring shadows. The other system, usually called "zonography," uses a narrow tomographic arc, and strives to see the whole of an object, undistorted and sharply defined. Which is preferable depends primarily on the type of tissue we are examining and the

nature of the problem. At times the two systems are in conflict, but basically each is designed to do its own particular job.

Wide-angle Tomography

The purpose of wide-angle tomography is to extend the limits of roentgen visibility to enable us to see objects that are completely obscured by overlying shadows on conventional roentgenograms. Figure

Figure 18–10 Extended visibility with wide-angle tomography. (From *The Fundamentals of Radiology.* Rochester, N.Y.: Radiography Markets Division, Eastman Kodak Company)

18–10 illustrates this principle. A series of lead letters are stacked on plastic shelves (top). On a standard roentgenogram all of the letters are superimposed and obscure each other (center), but on the wide-angle tomogram (bottom) the letter "C" becomes clearly visible.

One of the disadvantages of wide-angle tomography is that it decreases contrast. Adjacent thick parts produce greater image contrast than thin parts of the same radiographic density, and since wide-angle tomography produces thin sections, it reduces image contrast. It is most effective in studying tissues that have a great deal of natural contrast, such as bone. It has been used extensively to examine the inner ear, where there is still enough contrast to produce good images, even though the section thickness is very thin.

The sharpness of all images is decreased by wide-angle techniques, including those originating from the focal plane; the wider the tomographic arc, the more unsharp the images become. Theoretically, images from the focal plane should be in sharp focus, but in actual practice, it is impossible to coordinate the motions of the x-ray tube and film perfectly. Minor vibrations cause unsharpness of the focal-plane image, but the newer tomographic units are superbly engineered and unsharpness is minimal.

Narrow-angle Tomography (Zonography)

Narrow-angle tomography refers to body-section roentgenography employing an arc of less than 10°. Zonography is not efficient with linear tomography, and requires a multidirectional tube motion, which in practice is usually circular. Narrow-angle tomography produces undistorted, sharply defined images of the objects on the focal plane. An entire structure is displayed in sharp focus against a background of slight blurring. Our eyes tend to ignore the blurred images. The quality of the primary image is almost as good as it is with conventional roentgenograms, and interference from overlying shadows is diminished.

Zonography is especially useful when the tissues being examined have little natural contrast. Wide-angle techniques diminish contrast, while narrow-angle techniques retain all of the natural contrast that is present. Contrast is usually minimal in soft-tissue radiography, and zonography is the preferred tomographic

Table 18–1. A Comparison of Wide- and Narrow-Angle Tomography

WIDE-ANGLE TOMOGRAPHY	NARROW-ANGLE TOMOGRAPHY
1. Tomographic arc of more than 10° (usually 30° to 50°)	1. Tomographic arc of less than 10°
2. Less "section thickness"	2. Greater "section thickness"
3. Considerable unsharpness of focal-plane images	3. Very little unsharpness of focal-plane images
4. Maximum blurring of objects outside focal plane	4. Minimum blurring of objects outside focal plane
5. Best for tissues with high contrast (bone)	5. Best for tissues with low contrast (lung)
6. Can be done with either linear or circular motion	6. Usually done with circular tomographic motion
7. Unlikely to cause phantom images	7. Frequently causes phantom images
8. Long exposure times	8. Short exposure times (with properly designed equipment)

method. The lung offers an ideal medium for this technique. Contrast is low, and the interfering ribs are usually several centimeters from our plane of interest. Rib blurring is sufficient to prevent them from interfering with visualization of the primary image.

One of the main objections to small-angle tomography is its tendency to produce phantom images. Both the narrow angle and circular motion contribute to phantom-image formation. These images will be discussed in more detail later.

Table 18–1 summarizes the differences between wide- and narrow-angle tomography.

CIRCULAR TOMOGRAPHY

The more a tomographic motion differs from the shape of the object being examined, the less likely it is to produce phantom images, so tomographic units have been designed to operate with a wide variety of curvilinear tube motions, including circles, ellipses, hypocycloidals, sinusoids, spirals and even a random motion. We will limit our discussion to circular tomography, although the same principles apply to all pluridirectional motions.

The movement of the x-ray tube, film, and grid for circular tomography is shown in Figure 18–11A. The x-ray tube and film are located at opposite ends of a rigid connecting rod. The tube moves in a circular motion, and the film follows at the opposite end of the rod. The film does not revolve as it moves. Point (a) in Figure 18–11A identifies one side of the film and as you can see, it remains in the same relative position as the film moves through

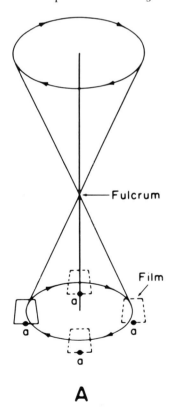

A

Figure 18–11A   Position of film with circular tomography

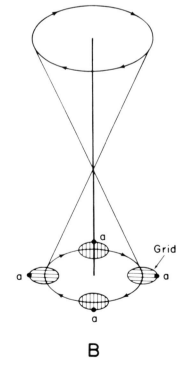

B

Figure 18–11B   Position of grid with circular tomography

a 360° circle. However, the grid must revolve to avoid cutoff, since the entire exposure is made with the x-ray tube angled toward the grid. The only way cutoff can be avoided is to revolve the grid to keep the grid lines pointed toward the tube, as shown in Figure 18–11B. Point (a) on the grid changes its position as the grid revolves so that the lead strips of the grid maintain a constant orientation with the target of the x-ray tube. By examining Figures 18–11A and 18–11B together, you can see that the grid gradually rotates over the film throughout the 360° cycle. Grid lines are obscured by the relative motion of the x-ray tube and film, and no Bucky mechanism is necessary.

Advantages of Circular Tomography

The primary advantage of circular tomography is that it produces a uniform section thickness. Figure 18–6 shows the blur pattern of a test phantom obtained with both linear and circular tomographic motions. With a circular motion all portions of the phantom are uniformly blurred, no matter how they are oriented in space. Linear tomography does not produce a true section thickness. The amount of blurring is completely dependent upon the orientation of the part with reference to tube motion. The only wire in the illustration that is maximally blurred is the one perpendicular to the direction of tube travel. Because linear tomography does not uniformly blur all parts, it frequently produces streaking, or "parasite" lines that remain in sharp focus even though they are several centimeters from the focal plane. These lines represent the edges of linear objects oriented along the line of tube motion. They do not occur with circular tomography.

Disadvantages of Circular Tomography

To most radiologists the principal disadvantage of circular tomography is the high cost of the equipment. Circular tomographic units are much more expensive

than linear units, which can usually be adapted to existing equipment. Another disadvantage is the length of time it takes to obtain an exposure. For a standard radiograph, the exposure time is determined primarily by the thickness and density of the part being examined. However, tomographic exposure times are determined by the length of time that it takes the tube to complete its arc, which is almost always considerably longer than the time that is needed to expose the film. One of the more popular tomographic units* takes 3 seconds to complete a circular motion and 6 seconds for a hypocycloidal motion. These long exposure times are a great disadvantage, especially for chest radiography, where there is considerable involuntary motion.

Another disadvantage of circular tomography is the sharp cutoff of the blur patterns, which is conducive to phantom-image formation.

Table 18–2 summarizes the differences between linear and circular tomography.

COMPLEX TOMOGRAPHIC MOTIONS

The tomographic objective is to blur objects outside of the focal plane as much as possible and as uniformly as possible. This objective can only be fully accomplished with a linear tube motion oriented at right angles to a linear structure. Figure 18–12B shows such an arrangement with three wires displaced 1 cm from the focal plane. The blur pattern of the wire oriented perpendicular to the tomographic motion is perfectly uniform. The blur pattern of the diagonal wire is also uniform, but not maximum. With a circular motion (D), all of the wires are blurred to the same degree, and all are maximally blurred, but the blurring is not uniform, i.e. the blur margin is more sharply defined than the rest of the blur pattern. Since no anatomic part is shaped like a wire, the ideal can never be fully

* Polytome, manufactured by Phillips.

Table 18–2. A Comparison of Linear and Circular Tomography

LINEAR TOMOGRAPHY	CIRCULAR TOMOGRAPHY
1. Equipment is inexpensive	1. Equipment is very expensive
2. Section thickness is dependent upon orientation of body parts (no true section thickness)	2. Section thickness is independent of orientation of parts (produces a uniform section thickness)
3. Blur margins are tapered and indistinct	3. Blur margins are abrupt and sharply defined
4. Objects outside the focal plane may be incompletely blurred, producing "parasite" streaks	4. Objects outside the focal plane are uniformly blurred (no "parasite" streaks)
5. Does not produce phantom images	5. Likely to produce phantom images (with narrow-angle tomography)

Figure 18–12   Three wire phantoms (A), blur patterns for linear (B), elliptical (C), circular (D), hypocycloidal (E) and figure-8 tomographic motions (F)

accomplished in a clinical setting. The more complex tomographic motions, i.e. the ellipses, circles, trispirals, figure-8's and hypocycloidals are all designed to improve the uniformity of blurring.

Figure 18–13 demonstrates how the size of the tomographic arc is determined for complex motions. The number of degrees is measured from the extremes of tube motion. In the illustration, the arc is 35° from all four types of tube motion.

Table 18–3 compares the relative length of tube travel for four different tomographic motions. The numbers are only theoretical since no manufacturer produces a unit that can perform all of these motions with a 48° arc. As the type of motion becomes more complex, the length of tube travel increases. Using the 92 cm

linear motion as the norm, the relative length of tube travel increases about 5 times for the hypocycloidal motion. The result is a considerable improvement in the uniformity of blurring. Figure 18–12 shows the blur patterns for several different tomographic motions. As you can see, blurring is more uniform for the more complex motions. However, increasing the length of tube travel does not necessarily improve blurring. The tomographic motion must be efficiently designed to be effective. For example, running the tube back-and-forth in a linear motion lengthens tube travel, but it does not improve the blur pattern. Section thickness is determined solely by the number of degrees in the tomographic arc, and it is not affected by the complexity of the tube

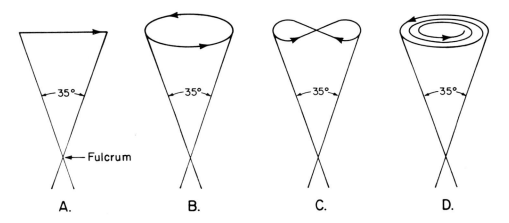

Figure 18–13   Method of determining the tomographic arc for complex motions

Table 18–3.   Approximate Length of Tube Travel for Various Tomographic Motions

TYPE OF MOTION	TOMOGRAPHIC ARC (degrees)	LENGTH OF TUBE TRAVEL (cm)	SECTION THICKNESS (mm)	RELATIVE LENGTH OF TUBE TRAVEL
Linear	48°	92	1.3	1.0
Elliptical	48°	222	1.3	2.4
Circular	48°	292	1.3	3.9
Hypocycloidal*	48°	450	1.3	4.9

*Polytome, Medical Systems Division, North American Phillips Corporation, Shelton, Connecticut. 45″ FFD.

motion. Note in Table 18–3 that the section thickness is 1.3 mm for all four tomographic movements.

PHANTOM IMAGES

Phantom is defined by Webster as "something that appears to the sight but has no physical existence." Phantom images appear on tomograms, but they do not actually exist. These unreal images are always a little less dense, and a little less sharp than real images, but they can still cause considerable difficulty in film interpretation.

Phantom images are produced by the blurred margins of structures outside of the focal plane, and they are most likely to occur with circular tomography and narrow-angle techniques. With a narrow-angle tube motion, objects outside the focal plane are only minimally blurred. The margins are still fairly distinct, and they tend to produce phantom images. Blurring is so complete with wide-angle tomography that phantom images are unlikely.

Phantom images are formed by two different mechanisms which we will discuss separately. However, we should emphasize that the parasite lines that occur in linear tomography are not phantom images. These lines represent the unblurred margins of structures oriented in the same direction as the x-ray tube motion. The images are real and represent structures that do exist.

The first type of phantom image is produced by narrow-angle tomograms of regularly recurring objects, such as the wires shown in Figure 18–14. Three wires are equally spaced a short distance above the focal plane. A represents a standard radiograph, and B and C represent tomograms taken with two different arcs. In A, the images of the wires appear as dots. In B, the images are blurred, but still separate. In C, the blur margins overlap slightly, and the overlapping edges produce the phantom images. These images are not real, and as you can see, it takes

Figure 18–14   Phantom-image formation

Figure 18–15   Phantom-image formation. (Courtesy of Dr. J.T. Littleton)

three wires to produce two phantom wires. Bony trabeculae, teeth, ribs, and dye-filled vessels are several of the anatomic parts that are apt to cause phantom-image formation.

The second type of phantom image is formed by the displacement of the blurred image from an object outside the focal plane to simulate a less dense structure within the focal plane. Frequently, the blurred image of a bone will simulate a soft-tissue structure. Figure 18–15 shows a narrow-angle tomogram of a dried skull. The apparent mucosal thickening along the floor of the nasal cavities represents the blurred images of the bone in front of the focal plane. The films were taken with a circular tomographic motion, so the blur margins are fairly sharp. Since the images are from a dried skull, the apparent mucosal thickening must represent a phantom image. Bone is quite dense and when it is minimally blurred by narrow-angle tomography, it retains enough density to simulate soft tissue. This type of phantom-image formation is most likely to occur when the shape of the part being examined is similar to the x-ray tube motion, so it is common with circular tomography about the skull. However, the same mechanism may produce phantom images in other anatomical areas. For example, a densely calcified granuloma in the chest, when incompletely blurred, may appear on a tomogram as a somewhat larger soft-tissue nodule. The density of the calcification is spread out over a larger area, so it becomes that of soft tissue, and the margins are sharply defined because of the circular tube motion.

Figure 18–16 shows a conventional radiograph of a nickel (A) and three circular tomograms taken with the same coin at slightly different distances from the image plane. One side of the coin is marked with a line that identifies the position of the same edge on all four films. The coin's image is blurred to exactly twice its original diameter in C, a little less than twice its diameter in B and a little more in D. If the original coin had represented a densely calcified pulmonary granuloma, then the exactly doubled image (C) would look like a larger, less dense soft tissue nodule; the less than doubled image (B) would look like a nodule with a calcific center; and the more than doubled image (D) would exactly mimic a thick-walled cavitary lesion. Interpretive errors of this type can be avoided by carefully correlating the tomograms with the plain films.

In summary, phantom images are produced in two ways: (1) by the superimposition of the blur margins of regularly recurring structures, and (2) by displacement of the blur margins of dense objects to simulate less dense objects. They are most likely to occur with narrow-angle circular tomography, and they are never as dense or as sharply defined as real images.

SIMULTANEOUS MULTIFILM TOMOGRAPHY

The basic principle of simultaneous multifilm tomography is very simple. Several layers of x-ray films are placed in a special "book cassette," and all of the films are

A   B   C   D

Figure 18–16 Plain film of a coin and three circular tomograms taken with the coin at different distances from the focal plane

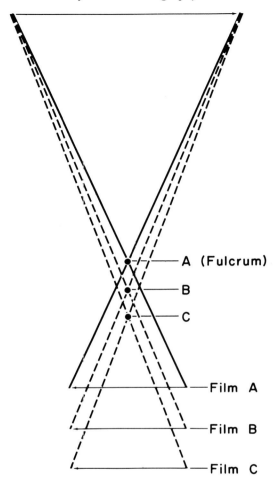

Figure 18–17 Simultaneous multifilm tomography

has its own separate fulcrum level. As you can see in Figure 18–17, the top and bottom layers are equally magnified. Even though the lower films are farther from the mechanical fulcrum, the ratio of the tube-fulcrum (real or virtual) distance to the fulcrum-film distance is the same for all levels.

The Book Cassette

Simultaneous multifilm tomography is done with a specially designed film holder called a "book cassette." Books are usually made up of from three to five sets of x-ray screens separated by x-ray transparent spacers. The spacers are composed of polyurethane sponge, the thickness of which can be varied from ½ to 2 cm. Figure 18–18 shows a five-film cassette with 1 cm spacers. The total thickness of the cassette is 4 cm. The resiliency of the sponge helps maintain good screen-film contact.

As x rays pass through the book cassette, their intensity decreases because of absorption by the screens and films, and to a lesser extent because of the inverse square law. If all of the screens in a book were of the same speed, the first film would be properly exposed, and the succeeding films would become progressively lighter. In order to produce a series of equally exposed films, we must "balance the book."

exposed simultaneously during a single tomographic sweep. The only difference between multifilm and single-film tomography is in the cassette. Figure 18–17 illustrates the principle diagrammatically. There is one mechanical fulcrum (point A) for the top film in the book cassette, and a virtual axis (points B and C) for every other film. The virtual axis is a point in space about which the x-ray film and tube rotate. Its position is determined by the spacing of the films in the cassette. When the films are spaced 1 cm apart, the virtual axes are 1 cm apart, and each object layer

Figure 18–18   Book cassette

This is accomplished by increasing the speed of the screens in each successive layer. The first layer of screens is very slow, the next layer is a little faster, and the last layer is very fast. In this way, all of the films are exposed to the same degree of blackness, even though they receive different quantities of radiation. No serious loss in film quality results from the use of the faster screens, since tomographic image quality is not good to begin with.

Plesio-sectional tomography refers to a somewhat different multifilm system. It is used to obtain tomograms at 1-mm intervals. No spacers are used in the book cassette. A pair of screens is about 1 mm thick, so they serve as their own spacers.

A properly balanced book only functions effectively in a limited kVp range. Most books are balanced to produce films of uniform density at about 80 kVp, and if you use them at much lower or higher energies, they are likely to be out of balance. At lower energies, the lower films in the cassette become progressively lighter.

Advantages of Simultaneous Multifilm Tomography

One obvious advantage of simultaneous multifilm tomography is a saving in technician time and equipment load, but this should only be a secondary consideration. Patients receive smaller doses of radiation with multifilm tomography, and this is its greatest advantage. When five films are produced with a single exposure, there is a definite decrease in the patient's radiation dose. However, the saving is not as great as the five-to-one film-production ratio suggests. Remember, the first pair of screens in a book cassette is slow, so the exposure factors must be increased over those required for a single-film technique. The patient's exposure dose per film is approximately one-half as much with simultaneous multifilm tomography. This means that two films can be exposed with the same amount of radiation that would be required to expose a single film with conventional tomography. The exact figure will vary somewhat depending on the thickness of the book cassette. Another advantage of the book cassette is that it allows us to obtain tomograms at various levels during one physiological cycle. We can be sure that the difference between films represents a real change in the structure that we are examining, and not merely a change in position that took place in the interval between exposures.

Disadvantage of Multifilm Tomography

The one serious problem that plagues simultaneous multifilm tomography is uncontrolled scatter radiation. Film quality is never as good as it is with a single-film technique. The lower films in the book cassette are fogged by scattered photons from the upper layers, and the amount of scatter radiation increases as the thickness of the book cassette and energy of the radiation increase. Because of the poor image quality associated with multifilm techniques, most radiologists prefer single-film tomography.

DETERMINATION OF THE TOMOGRAPHIC ANGLE

Hundreds of different phantoms and multiple ingenious methods have been devised to study the characteristics of tomographic units. We will only discuss one, the pinhole camera technique described by Hodes and his co-workers.[2] Figure 18–19 illustrates the principle. The only special equipment you need, besides the tomographic unit, is a sheet of lead with a small hole in its center. The lead is positioned at the level of the focal plane and a film is placed on the x-ray table directly under the center of the pinhole. The film remains stationary throughout the test. It is exposed twice: the first time with the x-ray tube perpendicular to the center of the film to mark the center of the tomographic arc; the second time while the tube swings through its arc to record a series of superimposed dots which are a record of

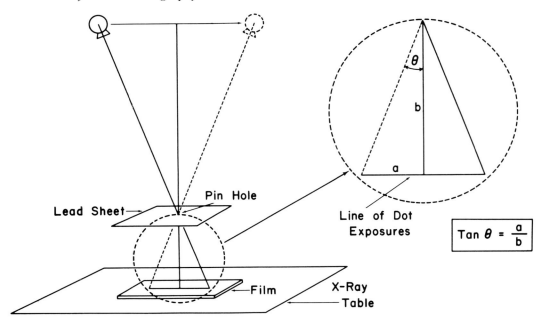

Figure 18–19 Determination of the tomographic angle by the pinhole camera technique

the tomographic motion. The line of dots produced on the film by the pinhole technique gives us the following information:

(1) It is a geometric presentation of the type of tube motion; i.e., linear, circular, hypocycloidal, etc.

(2) It makes it possible for us to calculate the length of the exposure angle, which is the number of degrees of tube motion during which x rays are emitted. We only need to know two sides of a triangle for the calculation. The first side is the distance between the pinhole and the film, and the second side is recorded on the film as shown in Figure 18–19 (insert). We can calculate the tomographic angle from the formula given in the illustration.

(3) It shows us the symmetry of the exposure angle. With a properly functioning unit, the exposed dot-line will be equal in length on either side of the center of the tomographic arc. If the line is asymmetrical, each side must be calculated separately, and then the two sides added to find the true exposure angle.

J.T. Littleton described "a phantom method to evaluate the clinical effectiveness of tomographic devices" in Amer. J. Roentgen. *108*,847, 1970; you are encouraged to read this article, especially if you anticipate purchasing new equipment.

SPECIAL TOMOGRAPHIC TECHNIQUES

Axial Transverse Tomography

In all of the tomographic techniques that we have described, tomographic sections are cut through the coronal plane of the patient. In axial transverse tomography, the plane of the section runs through the patient transversely as shown in Figure 18–20. The patient sits in a special rotating chair in an upright position. The x-ray film lies flat on a rotating horizontal table beside the patient as shown in Figure 18–21. The table is positioned a little below the desired focal plane. X rays are directed

CONVENTIONAL   AXIAL TRANSVERSE
TOMOGRAPHY   TOMOGRAPHY

Figure 18–20 Orientation of the focal plane with conventional and axial transverse tomography

Figure 18–21 Axial transverse tomography

toward the film the thinner the tomographic section. Since the x-ray beam passes through a considerable thickness of tissue, it is usually necessary to use an x-ray grid. The grid is placed as close to the x-ray film as possible, and it remains stationary while the film rotates. Grid lines are blurred by the relative motion between the film and grid.

Axial transverse tomography does not distort the radiographic image. Distortion is produced by unequal magnification. When one portion of an object is more magnified than another portion, its image is distorted. But in axial transverse tomography, points close to the film are also close to the x-ray target, and points far from the film are far from the target, so the object-film to object-target ratios are all the same. Since all points are equally magnified, the image is not distorted.

"Skip" Techniques

Skip tomography is a tomographic method that stops the exposure through a portion of the tube's motion. Occasionally,

obliquely through the patient and onto the film. The x-ray tube remains stationary throughout the exposure. The patient and film both rotate in the same direction and at the same velocity. Only those points actually on the focal plane remain in sharp focus throughout a rotation. Points above and below the focal plane are blurred. The section thickness is determined by the angle between the x-ray tube and film. The more obliquely the central ray is directed

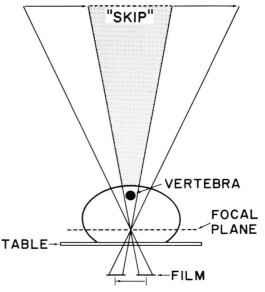

Figure 18–22 "Skip" exposure tomography

our point of interest is completely obscured during the central portion of the tomographic arc by dense superimposed structures. Since no useful image is produced on the film during this portion of the exposure, if it is omitted, the overall tomographic effect is improved. Figure 18–22 illustrates the principle. The exposure is skipped during the central portion of the tomographic arc, when the dense vertebral structures are superimposed over our point of interest. The method is only applicable to wide-angle techniques where our goal is to broaden our limits of visualization. Usually, about 20° of the tomographic angle is skipped. The technique only works well when there is a fairly large distance between the object of interest and the object to be blurred.

Autotomography

Autotomography is a technique that is designed to show the midline structures of the brain stem (aqueduct and 4th ventricle) during pneumoencephalography. It is illustrated in Figure 18–23. The x-ray tube and film both remain stationary while the head is rotated back and forth through an angle of approximately 10°. The only structures that remain in focus are those located along the axis of rotation. Other structures are blurred, including the dense petrous portion of the temporal bone which tends to obscure the delicate architecture of the brain stem.

Figure 18–23   Autotomography

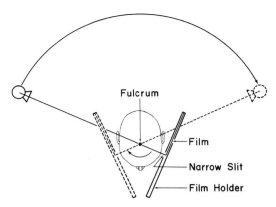

Figure 18–24   Pantomography

Pantomography

Pantomography is a special radiographic technique which produces a panoramic roentgenogram of a curved surface. The patient sits in a chair and remains stationary throughout the examination as shown in Figure 18–24. The x-ray tube and film holder both rotate during the exposure. The film holder has a protective lead front, and is considerably longer than the film. The film is exposed through a narrow slit in its holder. The film moves across this slit as the x-ray tube rotates, and the radiographic image is "laid out" as the film passes by the slit, in much the same way that paint is applied to a wall with a roller. The resultant roentgenogram is a flattened out image of a curved surface. The rounded configuration of the mandible and teeth are especially well suited to pantomography, and it is widely used in dentistry. Pantomograms of the jaw show the temporomandibular joints on either side of the film with the teeth laid out between them as shown in Figure 18–25.

SUMMARY

Body-section radiography is a special x-ray technique which blurs out the shadow of superimposed structures in order to show more clearly the principal structures being examined. The x-ray tube

Figure 18–25 Pantomogram of the mandible

and film are connected by a rigid rod which rotates about a fulcrum. When the tube moves in one direction, the film moves in the opposite direction. The level of the fulcrum is called the focal plane. Images originating at the focal-plane level are in sharp focus on the film. The thickness of the section that is in focus depends upon the amplitude of tube travel (in degrees). The larger the amplitude, the thinner the section.

If an object is located above or below the level of the focal plane, its image is blurred. The amount of blurring depends upon the amplitude of tube travel, distance of the object from the focal plane and film, and, in linear tomography, the orientation of the long axis of the part in relation to the direction of tube travel.

Pluridirectional tube motions (circles, ellipses, hypocycloidals, and spirals) are superior to linear motion because they produce a uniform section thickness; i.e., one that is independent of the orientation of the long axis of the part to be blurred. However, pluridirectional motions produce a sharply defined blur margin, and they are more likely to produce phantom images, especially with small tomographic angles.

Simultaneous multifilm tomography, employing a book cassette, exposes more than one film with a single tomographic exposure. These techniques diminish the patient's radiation exposure, but they produce poorer-quality tomograms. In recent years, most radiologists have abandoned simultaneous multifilm techniques.

Axial transverse tomography is a special technique that produces a cross-sectional tomogram. Autotomography, in which the patient is rotated along his central axis, produces a linear image plane in which all points are blurred except those along the axis of rotation. Pantomography is a special x-ray technique which produces a panoramic roentgenogram of a curved surface.

REFERENCES

1. *Methods of Evaluating Radiological Equipment and Materials.* National Bureau of Standards, Handbook 89, August 1963.
2. Hodes, P.J., De Moor, J., and Ernst, R.: Body section radiography: Fundamentals. Radiol. Clin. N. Amer., *6,* 229, 1963.

CHAPTER 19

Stereoscopy

J. MacKenzie Davidson introduced stereoscopy to radiology in 1898, and it won immediate and widespread acceptance. Stereoscopy grew in popularity, and by 1930 most radiographs were taken stereoscopically. You can gain some insight into its popularity from a statement made by Jarre and Teschendorf[1] in 1933: "A discussion of roentgen stereoscopy and some of its phases may seem rather unnecessary; no American roentgenologist doubts the advantages to be derived from the study of stereo-roentgenograms. To the well-informed observer it is even apparent that frequently overemphasis is placed upon the esthetic satisfaction of the tridimensional image, especially by many a young clinician using roentgenograms rather casually to the point of refusal of any non-stereo projection no matter how instructive it may be." Stereoscopy had reached the height of its popularity. Then, gradually, the pendulum began to swing.

The first step in the decline of stereoscopy was probably the result of its earlier overemphasis. When we expect too much, we are frequently disappointed, and stereoscopy was no exception to this dictum. In addition, routine stereoscopy is expensive and time consuming. The death blow came with the discovery that radiation causes mutations. The popularity of stereoscopy dropped precipitously, and the pendulum made its full swing. Unfortunately, in recent years stereoscopy is no longer used by many radiologists. Throughout the country stereoscopes are collecting dust, being placed in x-ray museums along with gas x-ray tubes as a remembrance of the past, or even more humiliating, serving as stands for coffee pots.

While we agree that stereoscopy was overemphasized in the past, this does not justify its present abandonment. Stereoscopic roentgenograms can give information that cannot be obtained in any other way, or at least not as easily in any other way. When properly used, it is still a valuable tool, and worthy of the attention of all radiologists.

PHYSIOLOGY OF DEPTH PERCEPTION

A basic knowledge of the physiology of depth perception is essential to an understanding of the principles behind stereoscopic filming and viewing systems. Depth perception is extremely complex and has some serious limitations. It depends upon two completely independent mechanisms: the first, monocular or photographic depth perception, requires only one eye; the second, stereopsis, requires binocular vision. We will discuss each mechanism separately.

Monocular Depth Perception

Monocular depth perception is familiar to all accomplished artists. The artist depicts depth the same way we see depth with one eye. The mechanisms are as follows:

1. **Size.** Near objects are larger than distant objects.
2. **Overlapping contours.** Near objects overlap distant objects.
3. **Perspective.** We see objects from a particular vantage point, or perspective. By following lines and contours we gain a sense of depth.
4. **Shading.** A sphere has the contour of a circle, but with proper shading we perceive its true shape.
5. **Air haze.** Water vapor, dust and smoke in the atmosphere absorb and reflect light casting a veil over distant objects causing them to appear farther away and less sharp.

These monocular mechanisms of depth perception are of little value in interpreting radiographs. Object size may occasionally give us some concept of depth, provided that two objects known to be the same size are both visible on one film. Perspective is of some value in determining depth, but only after we have become thoroughly familiar with anatomy. In a crude sort of way, unsharpness from penumbra is comparable to air haze; i.e., objects close to the film are sharper than objects far from the film. Overlapping contours and shading contribute nothing to depth perception in radiography. In general, there is little that allows us to see depth on a single radiograph.

Stereopsis

Binocular depth perception, which is called "stereopsis," is a unique characteristic of man and other primates. It is dependent upon the brain's ability to receive slightly different images from each eye, **discrepant images,** and then fuse them into a single image that has depth. Discrepant images are the heart of stereopsis, and fusion occurs in the brain. The degree of discrepancy is of vital importance. If the images are too different, the brain cannot fuse them, and the stereoscopic effect is lost. If the difference is too small, the fused images appear flat.

Accommodation and Convergence

In the past, physiologists thought that accommodation and convergence were responsible for stereoscopic depth perception, but now it is known that they play only a passive role. Accommodation is the ability to change the curvature of the lens with a change in visual distance. Convergence is a turning in of the optical axes so that both eyes can see the same object. The ciliary muscles, which regulate the curvature of the lens, and the internal rectus muscles, which converge the eyes, do not send the impulses that allow us to perceive depth. However, they are responsible for the mechanical changes which produce discrepant images from the two eyes, so they play a major role in stereopsis, but only in a subservient manner. They are involved in the mechanism of image formation, but not in the actual perception of depth.

Relative and Absolute Depth Perception

There are two types of depth perception: one relative, the other absolute. Relative depth perception is the ability to distinguish which of two objects is closer to the observer. Absolute depth perception is the ability to judge how far away an object is, or the distance between two objects. One is qualitative, the other quantitative. Stereopsis is relative. It only allows us to distinguish which of two objects is closer to us. To judge the distance between them accurately, we rely exclusively on monocular depth perception. Since monocular depth perception is of no value in interpreting radiographs, x-ray stereoscopy is only relative. It is a rank-order type of depth perception. We can accurately rank objects in their order of closeness, but we cannot accurately judge the distance between them. A failure to appreciate this fact is one of the reasons why some

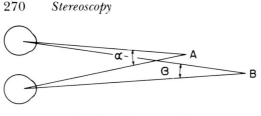

PARALLAX = α - β

Figure 19-1   Parallax

radiologists have been disappointed in stereoscopy.

Parallax

Parallax is the apparent displacement of an object when viewed from two different vantage points. In Figure 19–1, point A moves with respect to point B as the view shifts from one eye to the other eye. The convergent angle is larger from A than from B, and the difference is called the angle of instantaneous parallax. As points A and B are moved closer together, eventually the angle of instantaneous parallax becomes so small that the brain can no longer recognize a difference between the images from the two eyes. The smallest recognizable angle has been found experimentally to be between 1.6 and 24 seconds of arc, depending upon the investigator.[2] We can use this information to calculate the in-depth resolution of a stereoscopic filming system. If we use the largest reported angle of instantaneous parallax (24 sec), a 40-inch filming distance, and a 4-inch stereo tube shift, we should be able to recognize a difference in depth between two adjacent objects of slightly less than $\frac{1}{16}$ inch, which is sufficiently accurate to meet most of our radiological needs.

STEREOSCOPIC FILMING

Stereoscopic filming techniques are simple and usually require no special equipment. Two films are exposed, one for each eye. Figure 19–2 shows the relationship between the x-ray tube, patient, and film.

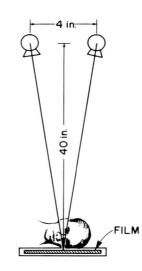

Figure 19-2   Stereoscopic filming

The film is changed between exposures. The second film should be placed in exactly the same position as the first film. The tube is shifted from the left to the right eye position between exposures, and it is the only part that moves. The patient must remain absolutely still. Usually, the film is placed in a Bucky tray under the grid, so that it can be changed without disturbing the patient. If the examination does not require a grid, the film is placed in a flat box with an open end (stereo tunnel), as shown in Figure 19–2.

Magnitude of Tube Shift

In the past, radiologists thought that the stereoscopic tube shift had to be equal to the interpupillary distance (2.6 inches), but now we know that this is neither necessary nor desirable. The optimal quantity of tube shift is empirical. We have learned by trial-and-error that a tube shift equal to 10% of the target-film distance produces satisfactory results. A 10% shift is simple to apply, and it produces discrepant images, which is the only prerequisite to stereoscopic image formation. For example, if the filming distance is 40 inches, the tube shift will be 4 inches.

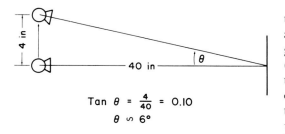

$$\text{Tan } \theta = \frac{4}{40} = 0.10$$
$$\theta \backsim 6°$$

Figure 19–3   Stereoscopic tube shift

In some radiographic units, especially head units, the x-ray tube and film are mounted on rigid connecting rods, so that the tube moves in an arc. With these units, it is easier to shift the tube a certain number of degrees rather than a specific distance. Referring to Figure 19–3, and applying the 10% rule, you can see that a 10% tube shift is equal to an angle of approximately 6°. This angle will always be the same, regardless of the filming distance. The entire 4-inches (or 6°) tube shift in Figure 19–3 is in one direction, which is perfectly acceptable, although it is more customary to shift 2 inches on either side of center.

Direction of Tube Shift

The direction of tube shift is important for two reasons. First, many stereoscopic examinations are done with grid techniques, and it is undesirable to shift across the long axis of a grid because of grid cutoff from lateral decentering (Chapter 8). In general, all grid-type techniques should be done with a longitudinal tube shift; i.e., along the long axis of the grid. If there is a compelling reason for using a cross-shift, then you should use a low-ratio grid. Usually, you can expect satisfactory films with a 10% cross-shift on an 8:1 or lower-ratio grid, but at the expense of increased patient exposure. Both exposures should be made with exactly the same tube shift to either side of grid center. If the shift is greater to one side, the films will not be equally exposed. Under no circumstances should you attempt a cross-shift with a 12:1 or higher-ratio grid. The chances of obtaining a satisfactory study are slight, and patient exposures are excessive because of grid cutoff from lateral decentering.

The direction of tube shift is important for a second reason. The objective in stereoscopic filming is to produce discrepant images. The tube shift should be in the direction that produces maximum discrepancy. In Figure 19–4, the tube was shifted across the axes of the lines to produce maximum image discrepancy. If the tube had been shifted along the longitudinal axes of the lines, the difference between the two images would be less, and

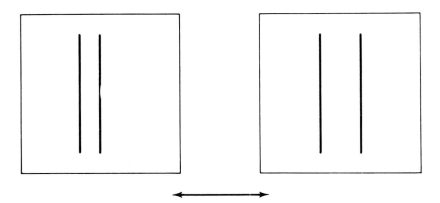

Figure 19–4   Stereoscopic images

the stereoscopic effect would be correspondingly less. In this respect, stereoscopy is a close cousin to tomography. Both use a tube shift, and both yield best results when the tube is shifted across the long axis of the part being examined. You can think of the lines in Figure 19–4 as the tibia and fibula, the anterior and posterior ribs, or the front and back cortices of a joint. In each case the stereoscopic effect is greatest when the tube is shifted across the lines of interest.

STEREOSCOPIC VIEWING

The stereoscope is an optical instrument used to superimpose two pictures taken from slightly different vantage points. It was invented by Wheatstone in 1838, long before Roentgen discovered x rays. Since that time many different designs have been described.

Preliminary Steps

Before we can view films stereoscopically, there are three preliminary steps we must follow to determine how the films should be oriented for stereoscopic viewing.

1. The first step is to **identify the tube side of the film,** i.e., the side that was closer to the patient and thus facing the x-ray tube during the exposure. Usually, we read x-ray films as if the patient is facing us. For example, frontal films of the skull are usually taken PA; i.e., with the patient facing the film. However, most radiologists read the films as if the patient is facing him. For stereoscopic viewing, we should think of our eyes as the tube, and view the patient as if he is standing between us and the film. If we do not do this, the left and right sides are likely to be reversed.

2. The next step is to **determine the direction of the x-ray tube shift.** In Figure 19–5, the films in the upper illustration were obtained with a cross-shift, and those in the lower illustration with a longitudinal shift. The films must be viewed as shown in order to present the eyes with discrepant

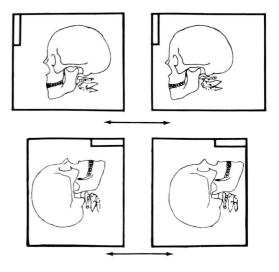

Figure 19–5   Direction of tube shift and position of films for viewing

Figure 19–6   Right and left eye films

images. If the films are viewed in any other way, there will be no stereoscopic effect. Usually, the direction of tube shift is determined by superimposing the images on the films, as shown in Figure 19–6. The two edges of the film that superimpose (upper and lower in the illustration) represent the axis along which the x-ray tube shifted.

3. The last preliminary step is to **determine which film is to be viewed by the left eye, and which by the right eye.** Each eye must view its appropriate film. The whole concept of film placement is simplified if we merely think of ourselves as the x-ray tube. Our right eye represents the tube when it is on the right side, and our left eye represents the tube from the left side. Now if we place the patient between us and the film, we are duplicating the manner in which the films were taken, and this is exactly the manner in which they must be viewed. Referring again to Figure 19–6, when the two films are superimposed, the right eye film will project out on the right side. If you just think of how they are taken, you can usually tell by inspection which is the right eye film. When the exposure is made from the right eye side, the image is projected over toward the left side of the film and vice versa for the left eye exposure.

If you superimpose the images on a pair of stereo films, and two edges of the films do not superimpose, then one (or more) of three things went wrong: (1) the patient moved and the stereoscopic effect was lost; (2) the second film was put in a different position than the first film, in which case the study is still perfectly satisfactory, but

Figure 19–7 Stereoscopic viewing of films taken improperly

the films must be viewed a little askew, with one film higher in the view box than the other (Figure 19–7A); or (3) the tube moved in two directions during the stereo shift. Again, the study is usually salvageable, but the films must be viewed diagonally so that our eyes converge along the true direction of tube shift (Figure 19–7B). The only way of determining which of the three errors actually occurred is to put the films up in various positions and attempt to view them stereoscopically.

In summary, in order to keep the image of the patient properly oriented with regard to left and right, we must view stereoscopic films from the tube side, with our eyes converging along the direction of tube shift, and with each eye viewing its appropriate film.

Viewing Systems

In the past, it was felt that the filming and viewing distances had to be the same or the distance between objects would be distorted. Before discussing individual viewing systems, we must clarify this point. Stereopsis, or binocular depth perception, is only qualitative. **With stereoscopic radiographs we are incapable of judging the absolute distance between objects.** All we can appreciate is which of two objects is closer to us; i.e., a rank-order type of depth perception. All we need for stereopsis are discrepant images, and the degree of discrepancy must be sufficiently great to permit an appreciation of depth, and yet not so great that the brain cannot fuse the images. With this fact in mind, we can understand why the film reading distance is not important. Whatever distance is convenient and comfortable is perfectly adequate. The same stereoscope can be used to interpret all stereoscopic films, no matter what distance was used for the exposure.

Cross-eyed Stereoscopy

In the routine interpretation of roentgenograms, both eyes are focused at

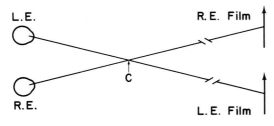

Figure 19–8   Cross-eyed stereoscopy

a single area of interest, accommodation and convergence are coordinated, and both eyes see identical structures in sharp focus. With cross-eyed stereoscopy two films are interpreted at the same time (Figure 19–8). Accommodation and convergence must be dissociated. Our eyes cross so the right eye sees the film on the left side and both eyes converge to point C in the illustration. If our eyes also accommodated for point C, the films would be out of focus, since they are much farther away. So we must converge on a point considerably in front of the films and still accommodate to the plane of the films. This dissociation requires a lot of practice, causes eye strain, and for many people, produces an image that is reduced in size or out of focus. However, in spite of all these difficulties, many radiologists have become quite proficient at cross-eyed stereoscopy. You can test your own ability on Figure 19–4. Hold a finger between your eyes and the illustration, and focus both eyes on your finger. In the background you will see three images. The image in the center is formed by the fusion of the left and right eye images and it has depth. Concentrate on it. If you are seeing stereoscopically, the right line will be suspended in space above the page. It takes a lot of practice to become proficient, but with enough effort you can master it.

Since no special equipment is needed, cross-eyed stereoscopy has two advantages over any other system. It costs nothing and is always available. It is certainly the most convenient system to use.

Wheatstone Stereoscope

The principal disadvantage of cross-eyed stereoscopy is that it requires a dissociation of accommodation and convergence. All other stereoscopic systems are designed to overcome this disadvantage. The Wheatstone stereoscope will be used to illustrate how they function. With a Wheatstone unit, convergence is assisted by a pair of mirrors that are located halfway between the films as shown in Figure 19–9. We accommodate to the plane of the films and view reflected mirror images. The mirrors are adjusted to superimpose the right and left eye films without changing our convergent effort from what it would normally be for the viewing distance. We see a stereoscopic image hanging in space behind the mirrors, and since accommodation and convergence are coordinated to the same distance, our eyes feel no strain. All other stereoscopes operate on the same principle using either mirrors or prisms to assist the eyes in convergence. In stereoscopes containing mirrors, the mirrors reverse the left and right sides of the patient's image; i.e., they produce mirror images. To compensate for the reversal, the films must be turned over, so that they are viewed from the side away from the x-ray tube. This reverses

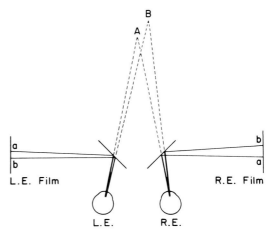

Figure 19–9   Wheatstone stereoscope

the image again and brings it back into proper orientation.

Many other stereoscopes have been designed, but we will mention only a few of them. Figure 19–10 shows a stereoscope that was designed by Caldwell in 1906.[3] It consists of a pair of prisms mounted into binoculars. The unit is compact and convenient to use. Gass and Hatchett[4] have described a similar system in which they mounted a pair of thin prisms into eyeglasses. The simplest stereoscope, described by Kerekes,[5] requires only a small pocket mirror and a steady hand. The mirror is held against the side of the nose and both eyes focus on the left eye film, as shown in Figure 19–11. The mirror is adjusted to interrupt the view of the right eye, which then sees a mirror image of the right eye film. The mirror is carefully adjusted until the left and right eye images superimpose and are fused into a combined image having depth. Since the right eye sees a mirror image, the film must be reversed so that both images are seen in the same orientation. The mirror should be silvered on its front surface because of the high angle of reflection. The primary disadvantage of this system is that it is difficult to hold the mirror steady.

Many other stereoscopes have been designed, most of them using two or more mirrors to assist the eyes in convergence. They all work well, but they have one disadvantage in common. They greatly limit the number of viewers. In fact, most of them allow only one person to see the films. Two other systems have been devised which at least partially overcome this difficulty. One system uses polarized light,[6] and the other colored filters.[7] They will be discussed under stereofluoroscopy.

ADVANTAGES AND DISADVANTAGES OF STEREOSCOPY

Advantages

The advantages (or perhaps **uses** is a better term) of stereoscopy depend upon the skill of the stereoscopist. We will discuss only a few of the situations in which we have found stereoscopy helpful. The list could be extended considerably.

1. Education. The teaching of normal anatomy is simplified with stereoscopic images. Lines that are superimposed into a confusing array for the novice migrate to their true position in depth, and they create a perspective that is not possible on a single film.

2. Foreign-body localization. Stereoscopy cannot compete with a pair of right-angle radiographs for localization of a single foreign body. However, stereoscopy is superior for the localization of many foreign bodies, such as multiple pellets from a shotgun wound. It allows us to localize each object from a single vantage point. With two right-angle films, it is not always possible to identify one particular foreign body on both films, since they all look alike.

3. Localization of intracranial calcifications. Some intracranial calcifications are so small that they can only be seen on the lateral view, and the only way they can be

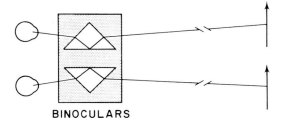

BINOCULARS

Figure 19–10   Binocular prism stereoscope

Figure 19–11   Single-mirror stereoscope

localized is with stereoscopic films. In fact, some calcifications can only be recognized stereoscopically.

4. Unimposing confusing shadows. The more confusing a radiograph is, the more likely stereoscopy is to be helpful. For example, a collection of gas in the colon may be impossible to differentiate from a destructive lesion in the pelvis on a single film. A good stereoscopist can recognize the true situation with ease. You can argue that a repeat film the next day would solve the problem, and you are correct. Almost all problems can be solved without resorting to stereoscopic films, but frequently stereoscopy offers the simplest solution.

Disadvantages

The disadvantages of stereoscopy are much better defined than the advantages.

1. Expense. Stereoscopy requires two films which adds to the cost of an examination. It requires more technician time, is wearing on the equipment, and doubles the cost of films and processing.

2. Patient exposure. The principal disadvantage of stereoscopy, the reason it should not be used routinely, is the increased patient exposure which is required to produce two films.

3. Need for patient cooperation. Since the patient must remain perfectly still between exposures, stereoscopy cannot be used on patients who are unable to cooperate.

4. Need for practice. In order to become, and remain, a good stereoscopist, you must practice. The more stereoscopy you do, the better you will become. Most of us only dust off our stereoscopes when we have a problem, and in the long interval between examinations, we become rusty and lose our confidence. Stereoscopy should be practiced daily; routine lateral skull films are probably the most satisfactory study to use, for they frequently give information that cannot be obtained in any other way.

STEREOFLUOROSCOPY

Researchers have been working on stereofluoroscopy for almost 70 years, but have not developed a system that has gained widespread clinical acceptance. Stauffer and his co-workers[8] have reported on two different methods. The first, which is shown in Figure 19–12, employs two x-ray tubes and two image-orthicon television cameras. The x-ray tubes fire alternately, and the cameras are synchronized with the tubes. One camera records a right, and the other a left eye image. The images are displayed on two television monitors that are mounted at right angles to each

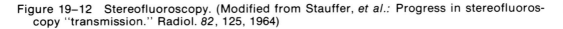

Figure 19–12 Stereofluoroscopy. (Modified from Stauffer, *et al.:* Progress in stereofluoroscopy "transmission." Radiol. *82,* 125, 1964)

Figure 19–13   Polarized light

other. A semitransparent beam-splitting mirror permits observation of both monitors at the same time. The light from the monitors is polarized and viewed through polarized eyeglasses. One image is polarized vertically, the other horizontally, and the glasses are similarly oriented. If you follow the light waves in Figure 19–13, you can see that after light is polarized vertically, it can only be seen with a vertically oriented polarized lens. Similarly, the other eye sees the light that is polarized horizontally. The beam-splitting mirror reflects and transmits equal quantities of light, which permits superimposition of the slightly different, or discrepant, images.

A second, more compact system has been described by Stauffer *et al.*[7] This system employs a twin-target stereoscopic x-ray tube, one image intensifier, and one image-orthicon color camera. The x-ray tube and color television camera are synchronized so that the camera records both a right and a left eye image alternately 30 times per second. Both images are displayed on a single television monitor; one image in red, and the other in green. Each second the monitor alternately flashes 30 red and 30 green images, which are viewed by an observer wearing red and green glasses. Each eye sees a slightly different image from a single monitor; the fusion of these two images produces a stereoscopic picture.

Polarized light and colored filters can also be used to view standard stereoscopic radiographs. The polarized system is set up exactly as shown in the right hand side of Figure 19–12. Conventional view boxes are used in place of the television monitors, one holding the left, and the other the right eye film. With a color system the view boxes are arranged in the same manner, but the polarizing material is replaced with colored filters. Each eye sees its appropriate film through colored glasses with the aid of a semitransparent beam-splitting mirror.

SUMMARY

Stereoscopic filming techniques are simple and require no special equipment. Two films are exposed, one for each eye. Between exposures, the x-ray tube is shifted 10% of the target-film distance (6°); the films are changed, taking care to position the second film in exactly the same position as the first film. The films of the stereoscopic pair present the eye with slightly different, or discrepant, images. Many viewing systems are available, but they all accomplish the same purpose. They assist the eyes in coordinating accommodation and convergence. Stereosopic depth perception is only relative, a rank-order type of depth perception, which ranks objects in their order of closeness, but does not disclose the distance between them. A failure to appreciate this fact is one of the reasons why some radiologists have been disappointed in stereoscopy.

Stereoscopy has several serious disadvantages. The examination requires two films, so that it is costly and doubles the patient's radiation exposure. Since the patient must remain perfectly still between exposures, it cannot be used on patients who are unable to cooperate. In spite of these disadvantages, stereoscopy is still a valuable tool and frequently offers the simplest solution to a difficult radiological problem.

REFERENCES

1. Jarre, H. A., and Teschendorf, O. E. W.: Roentgen stereoscopy: A review of its present status. Radiol. *21*, 139, 1933.
2. Davson, H.: *The Physiology of the Eye.* 2nd ed. Boston: Little, Brown and Co., 1963.

3. Caldwell, E. W.: The stereoscope in roentgenology. Amer. J. Roentgen. *5*, 554, 1918.
4. Gass, C. C., and Hatchett, C. S.: A simple inexpensive set of prisms for viewing stereoscopic roentgenograms. Amer. J. Roentgen. *61*, 715, 1949.
5. Kerekes, E. S.: A simple device for stereoscopic viewing of films. Amer. J. Roentgen. *75*, 140, 1956.
6. Stamm, R. W.: The polaroid stereoscope. Amer. J. Roentgen. *45*, 744, 1941.
7. Stauffer, H. M., Haas, C. and Blackstone, A. W.: Progress in stereofluoroscopy "transmissions." Radiol. *82*, 125, 1964.
8. Stauffer, H. M., Henny, G. C., and Blackstone, A. W.: Stereoscopic television fluoroscopy. Radiol. *79*, 30, 1962.

CHAPTER 20

Magnification Radiography

We have previously discussed the geometric principles of direct x-ray magnification. If the distance between the x-ray tube and the film (focus-film distance) remains constant, magnification of the image of an object will increase as the object is moved away from the film and closer to the tube. The degree of magnification is the ratio of the focus-film distance and focus-object distance:

$$\text{Magnification} = \frac{\text{Focus-film distance}}{\text{Focus-object distance}}$$

The standard focus-film distance is 40 inches. If a magnification of 2 is desired, the object is placed halfway between the x-ray tube and film (focus-object distance = 20 inches):

$$M = \frac{40}{20} = 2$$

Using a focus-film distance of 40 inches, what will the focus-object distance be if magnification of 1.5 is desired?

$$1.5 = \frac{40}{X}$$

$$x = \frac{40}{1.5} = 26.6, \text{ or about 27 inches}$$

Remember, 27 inches is the focus-object distance. The object-film distance will be 40 minus 27, or 13 inches.

TRUE MAGNIFICATION VERSUS GEOMETRIC MAGNIFICATION

If x rays were generated from a point source, the preceding discussion of mag-

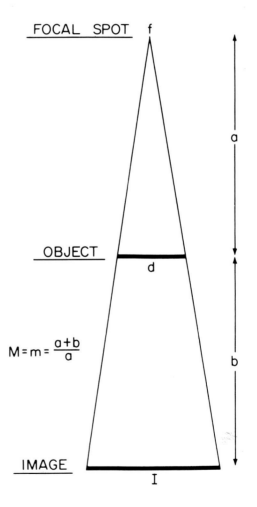

Figure 20–1 Geometry of a magnified image produced by a point source focal spot

nification would be correct, and true magnification (M) and geometric magnification (m) would be the same. Figure 20–1 diagrams this situation. If "a" represents focus-object and "b" represents object-film distance, then the equation for both true (sometimes termed total) magnification and geometric (sometimes termed nominal) magnification is the same (i.e., we are using a point source focal spot).

$$M = m = \frac{a + b}{a}$$

Unfortunately, real focal spots have a finite size. If we assume that x-ray production is of uniform intensity across the focal spot (that this is often untrue will be emphasized subsequently), and that the object is about the same size or smaller than the focal spot, the image of the object will be formed as diagrammed in Figure 20–2. Notice that the total image size now contains a central (U) region and two areas of edge gradient (E). (The term edge gradient, rather than penumbra, is preferred.) Derivation of the equation which must be used to calculate true magnification in this situation is an interesting exercise, but we will be content to record the equation which relates total magnification (M) to geometric magnification (m)

$$M = m + (m-1)\left(\frac{f}{d}\right)$$

M = true magnification
m = geometric magnification

$$\left(\text{calculated from } m = \frac{a + b}{a}\right)$$

d = object size
f = focal spot size

Notice that as objects become smaller than the focal spot, the term $\frac{f}{d}$ becomes large, and true magnification becomes much greater than geometric magnification. Conversely, if an object is large compared to focal spot size (i.e., radiography of the femur with a 1.2-mm focal spot tube), the term $\frac{f}{d}$ becomes small and for practical

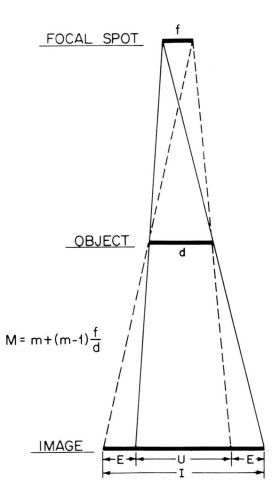

$$M = m + (m-1)\frac{f}{d}$$

Figure 20–2   Geometry of a magnified image produced by focal spot with finite size

purposes we may conclude that M and m are identical.

To summarize: **true magnification (M) is a function of the ratio of focal spot size to object size ($\frac{f}{d}$).**

An example will help in understanding this concept of true versus geometric magnification. Assume you are filming a renal angiogram using a 40-inch target-film distance and an 0.6-mm focal spot. What will be the size of the image of a 200 micron (0.2 mm) renal artery located 4 inches from the film? First we must calculate

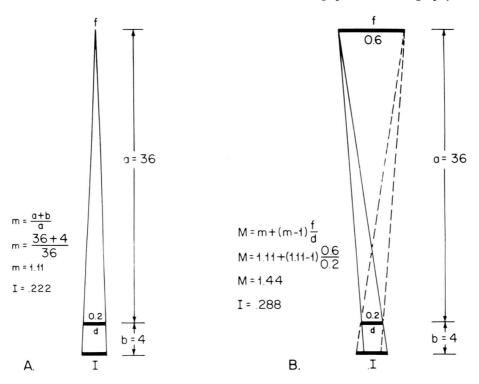

Figure 20–3   Calculation of geometric magnification (m) and true magnification (M)

geometric magnification (m). Refer to Figure 20–3A.

$$m = \frac{a + b}{a} = \frac{36 + 4}{36}$$

$$m = 1.11$$

With a punctiform focal spot, image size would be .222 mm or 222 microns (200 × 1.11 = 222). But, since the object is small compared to the focal spot (.2 mm vs. .6 mm), the term $\frac{f}{d}$ will be large and we must calculate how the term $(m-1)\frac{f}{d}$ will affect true image size (Figure 20–3B).

$$M = m + (m-1)\frac{f}{d}$$

$$M = (1.11) + (1.11-1)\frac{.6}{.2}$$

$$M = 1.11 + (.11)(3) = 1.44$$

Thus, true magnification is 44% vs. geometric magnification of only 11%, and true image size will be .288 mm or 288 microns (200 × 1.44 = 288). Keep in mind that the various causes of unsharpness (i.e., screen, geometric, absorption and motion) will make the precise boundaries of the image of our hypothetical vessel difficult to identify.

X-RAY TUBE FOCAL SPOTS

Magnification radiography demands use of the smallest practical focal spot because geometric unsharpness must be reduced as much as possible. A focal spot size of 0.3 mm or less is required for magnification, but simply purchasing a standard 0.3-mm focal spot tube may not get the job done. We must examine the following:

1. What does focal spot size mean
2. How is focal spot size measured

and how are the measurements useful

3. How does focal spot size vary with change in tube operating conditions (mA and kVp).

Focal Spot Size

In the United States, the National Electrical Manufacturers Association (NEMA) has established a standard method for measuring focal spot size and has specified the amount that a focal spot can vary from its stated size (NEMA Standards Publication No. XR5-1974, Measurement of Dimensions of Focal Spots of Diagnostic X-Ray Tubes, 155 East 44th St., New York, N.Y., 10017). The 1970 NEMA standards for measurement of focal spot size are shown in Table 20–1. These standards allow measurement of focal spot size at signficantly lower mA settings than those usually used in clinical applications. It is important to recognize that focal spot size changes with different kVp and mA settings (focal spot blooming at high mA), so the 1970 NEMA standards allow one to compare focal spot measurements but often do not define the size of the focal spot under normal use. In recognition of this, the NEMA 1974 standard differs from that shown in Table 20–1 as follows: "spots are to be taken at one-half the maximum allowable current for 0.1 second exposure."[3] We will discuss focal spot size

Table 20–1. 1970 NEMA Recommendations for Proper kVp and mA Settings Used to Measure Focal Spot Size

FOCAL SPOT SIZE (mm)	MILLIAMPERES
0.4 and Less	15
0.5 to 0.9	50
1.0 to 1.4	100
1.5 to 1.9	200
2.0 and Greater	300

Measurements are made at 85 kVp with rotating anode tubes and single-phase full-wave rectification.

Table 20–2. NEMA Tolerance Limits for Focal Spot Variation

FOCAL SPOT SIZE (mm)	TOLERANCE MINUS	TOLERANCE PLUS
Less than 0.8	0%	50%
0.8 through 1.5	0%	40%
Greater than 1.5	0%	30%

variation under different operating conditions later.

NEMA standards also define the tolerance limits by which a focal spot can vary from its stated size. These tolerances are shown in Table 20–2. Since tolerance limits for an 0.3 mm focal spot are 50%, such a focal spot may measure 0.45 mm and meet specifications. When purchasing a small focal spot tube for use in magnification radiography one should consider specifying a true 0.3 mm focal spot in the contract (and expect to pay more for this special consideration). For routine radiography the tolerance standards are generally considered acceptable.

Measuring Focal Spot Size

After the tube is installed, it is necessary to measure focal spot size under conditions of clinical use. NEMA specifications call for focal spots of size 0.3 mm or smaller to be measured with a line-pair resolution test pattern (such as a star test pattern), and those greater than 0.3 mm to be measured with a pinhole camera. There are significant differences in interpreting focal spot "size" as determined by these two methods, and we must understand both the measurement techniques and the appropriate application of the data to clinical magnification radiography.

The Pinhole Camera

The pinhole technique measures the physical size of the focal spot and demonstrates the intensity distribution of radiation from the focal spot. The pinhole consists of a small hole in a sheet of lead.

FOCAL SPOT

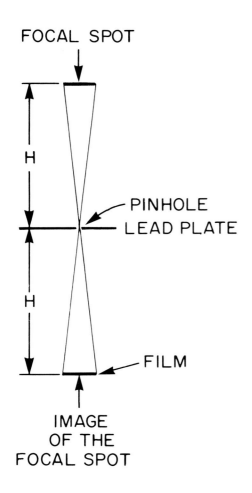

H

PINHOLE
LEAD PLATE

H

FILM

IMAGE
OF THE
FOCAL SPOT

Figure 20–4   Formation of an image of the focal spot by a pinhole camera

The pinhole assembly is placed between the x-ray tube and a sheet (no intensifying screens) of x-ray film (Figure 20–4) and an exposure made that produces a density of 0.6 to 1.0 on the film. If the pinhole is placed exactly halfway between the focal spot and film, as in Figure 20–4, the image of the focal spot will be the same size as the actual physical dimensions of the focal spot. The pinhole technique will also demonstrate the intensity distribution of radiation from the focal spot. Figure 20–5 is a photographically magnified pinhole image of a focal spot showing that x-ray intensity is much greater along the edges of a focal

spot than in its central area. This is termed edge-band distribution, and while it is the most common type of intensity distribution, it is the least desirable, as we will discuss later. There are several problems with the pinhole technique of measuring focal spots:

1. The size of the pinhole must be small with respect to the size of the focal spot. Recommended pinhole diameters are:

   0.03 mm for focal spots below 1 mm
   0.075 mm for focal spots from 1.0 to 2.5 mm

   The 0.03 mm pinhole transmits so little radiation that producing a film image of the focal spot requires multiple exposures at high mA values.
2. The size of the image of an 0.3 mm focal spot is so small that accurate measurement without special equipment is difficult.
3. Accurate measurement of the length of the focal spot is difficult. X-ray intensity along the cathode-anode axis (length) peaks near the center of the focal spot and fades toward each extremity. To compensate for this uneven distribution, it is recommended that the measured length of the focal spot (cathode-anode axis) be reduced by multiplying it by 0.7. The accuracy of this correction factor is questionable.
4. It is important to accurately align the pinhole to the central beam of the x-ray tube. This location is difficult to determine.

The pinhole technique provides a measurement of the size of the focal spot and its intensity distribution. Focal spot size measured by this technique is used to calculate anode heat loading characteristics of the x-ray tube and is the measurement (f) used in the formula to calculate true radiographic magnification (M). We will return later to the importance of intensity distribution.

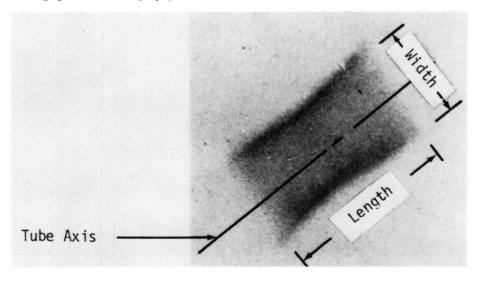

Figure 20–5 Pinhole image of a focal spot with edge-band distribution (from Bull,[4] with permission)

Figure 20–6 Photograph of a star resolution pattern. Notice inability of the camera lens to record the inner spokes

Line-Pair Resolution Test Patterns

Because of the problems associated with use of a small pinhole, line-pair resolution test patterns are now recommended for imaging focal spots of 0.3 mm or less. Commonly, a star test pattern, illustrated in Figure 20–6, is used. This pattern consists of a circular sheet of lead 50 microns thick, with a diameter of 45 mm, divided into 180 spokes of which 90 are lead and 90 are blank. Each spoke subtends an angle of 2°. A star test pattern can be viewed as consisting of many line-pair test patterns, each diameter of the star corre-

sponding to a line-pair of different size. To measure focal spot size, the star test pattern is positioned about midway between the focal spot and film (do not use screens), exactly parallel to the film, and in the central axis of the x-ray beam. Figure 20–7 is a diagram of this technique, and Figure 20–8 is a picture of an actual star test pattern. As one moves toward the center of the image, an area is encountered where the image of the rays of the star gradually disappears (D, Figure 20–7). This is termed the area of failure of resolution, and the diameter (D) of the blurred image is measured both parallel and perpendicular to the cathode-anode axis of the tube. It must be noted that D is measured perpendicular to the desired dimension of the focal spot (in Figure 20–8 one would measure D for the cathode-anode axis of the focal spot in the dimension perpendicular to the cathode-anode alignment of the tube when the exposure was made). One then calculates focal spot size by the formula:

$$f = \frac{\theta D}{57.3 \, (M - 1)}$$

f = focal spot size
θ = the angle of one of the lead spokes
D = diameter of the blurred image of the star phantom parallel or perpendicular to the tube axis (cathode-anode axis)

M = magnification (true).

Since $\theta = 2°$ in the star phantom, the equation used with this phantom reduces to:

$$f = \frac{D}{28.65 \, (M - 1)}$$

M is easily measured. The diameter of the star pattern is always known (the one illustrated has a diameter of 45 mm), and the diameter of the image of the pattern is quickly measured. Magnification is calculated:

$$M = \frac{\text{Image size}}{\text{Object size}}$$

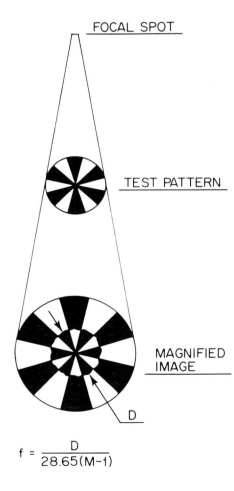

FOCAL SPOT

TEST PATTERN

MAGNIFIED IMAGE

D

$$f = \frac{D}{28.65(M-1)}$$

Figure 20–7 Using a star resolution pattern to determine focal spot size (not drawn with correct perspective)

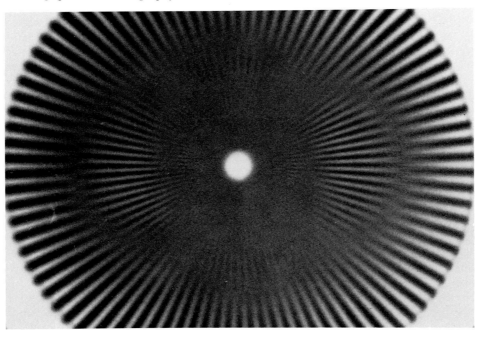

Figure 20–8   Appearance of a star test pattern image used to calculate focal spot size

Notice in Figure 20–7 that continuing inward from the region of failure of resolution the image of the test pattern reappears, but the light and dark lines will have shifted 180° in their alignment (called a phase shift). This is the area of spurious resolution which is seen with focal spots with edge band intensity distribution, and corresponds to spatial frequencies where the modulation transfer function (MTF) of the focal spot is negative. Milne[8] describes this phenomenon in detail, so we will not further consider phase shift and spurious resolution. Focal spot size measured with a star phantom depends on two characteristics of the focal spot:

1. Focal spot size
2. Radiation intensity distribution within the focal spot.

Thus, **this technique does not measure the actual physical size of a focal spot** (size is measured with the pinhole camera), but measures the **resolving capacity of the focal spot** (which is a function of both size and radiation intensity distribution).

The effect of the intensity distribution of a focal spot has been discussed by Milne.[9] There are three types of intensity distribution encountered in focal spots (we will not consider the ring distribution of a field emission x-ray tube):

1. Edge band distribution (illustrated in Figure 20–5)
2. Homogeneous distribution, in which radiation intensity is uniform throughout the focal spot.
3. Centrally peaked distribution, in which radiation intensity is peaked in the central portion of the focal spot and tapers toward the margin (i.e., the "opposite" of edge band distribution), also termed Gaussian distribution.

The type of intensity distribution has an important influence on the resolving capacity of a focal spot. Milne advises that the term **Effective** focal spot size be used to describe the physical size of a focal spot as measured with a pinhole camera. To this is added another measurement: the **Equivalent** focal spot size (this is the size measured with a star pattern). The definition of equivalent size is: "The equivalent size (F_{eq}) of a focal spot F with any type of intensity distribution is equal to that size of homogeneous focal spot which has the same resolving power as F."[9] The focal spot with the best resolving power has a peaked intensity distribution, next best is homogeneous, and worst is edge-band distribution. Table 20–3 illustrates the difference in equivalent (star test pattern) focal spot size which results from differences in radiation intensity distribution in three focal spots which have identical effective (pinhole) focal spot size measurements. Notice that the focal spot with edge band distribution has an equivalent size twice that of the one with homogeneous distribution, while the centrally peaked focal spot has an effective size only half that of the homogeneous one. Many measurements of focal spot resolving power have been made assuming a homogeneous intensity distribution. Obviously, such measurements will not be accurate if applied to focal spots with other types of intensity distribution.

Let us digress a moment to emphasize that the star pattern measurement of focal spot size gives information about resolving power, which is the ability of the focal spot to record separate images of small objects placed close together (i.e., a series of 100μ

interlobular vessels in the renal cortex). The ability of the focal spot to image a single, isolated 100μ vessel is determined by the physical size of the focal spot (pinhole size); although the intensity distribution will influence the shape of the edge gradient (i.e., how sharp the edge of the vessel will appear). If one wishes to calculate true magnification (M) of a small object, the focal spot size (f) used in the equation must be that determined by the pinhole camera. If one wishes to determine the resolving power of a particular focal spot, he may use the size determined from a star pattern, or adjust the size measured with a pinhole for the type of intensity distribution (this usually requires photographic enlargement of the tiny pinhole image or use of a microdensitometer, both of which are not usually available in clinical situations).

Variation of Focal Spot Size with Changes in Tube Operating Conditions (mA and kVp)

Two articles by Chaney and Hendee[5,7] nicely document the fact that focal spot size varies depending on tube operating conditions.

Focal spot size increases in direct proportion to tube current. This is called **blooming** of the focal spot, and is much more marked at low kVp and high mAs techniques. Weaver[14] has reported the effect of the current on focal spot bloom at 40 kVp and 80 kVp to be as shown in Table 20–4. Focal spot bloom is much more marked parallel to the tube axis.

Table 20–3. Comparison of Effective and Equivalent Focal Spot Sizes for Various Radiation Intensity Distribution

EFFECTIVE FOCAL SPOT SIZE (Pinhole Size)	RADIATION INTENSITY DISTRIBUTION	EQUIVALENT FOCAL SPOT SIZE (Star Test Pattern)
1.0 mm	Homogeneous	1.0 mm
1.0 mm	Edge-Band	2.0 mm
1.0 mm	Centrally Peaked	0.5 mm

Table 20–4. Measured Sizes of a Typical Focal Spot at Various Exposure Factors[14]

TUBE kVp	TUBE mA	FOCAL SPOT SIZE
40 kVp	100 mA	2.0 mm
40	300	2.3
80	100	1.7
80	300	1.8

proximately proportional to $\frac{1}{f_0 V^{3/2}}$ where f_0 = focal spot size for a small tube mA, and V = tube kVp. Weaver[14] has illustrated decreasing focal spot size with increasing kVp as shown in Table 20–5. There is no industry standard regarding focal spot blooming. Since blooming will vary significantly between supposedly

Focal spot bloom perpendicular to the cathode-anode tube axis depends on the accuracy of the focusing of the electron beam, and measurements with a star pattern showed wide variation between identical models of tubes.

Focal spot size will decrease slightly with increasing kVp. As measured by Chaney and Hendee this change was ap-

Table 20–5. Measured Size of a Typical Focal Spot at Various kVp Settings, mAs Constant[14]

TUBE kVp	TUBE mA	FOCAL SPOT SIZE
40 kVp	100 mA	2.0 mm
60	100	1.8
80	100	1.7
150	100	1.7

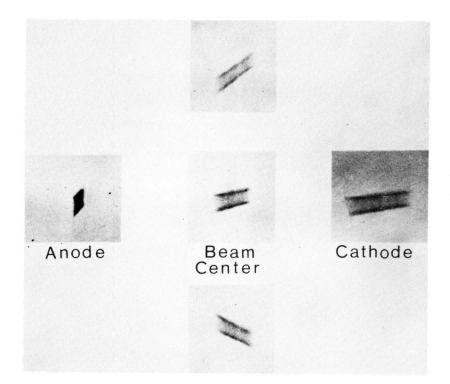

Anode   Beam Center   Cathode

Figure 20–9 Pinhole images showing variation of focal spot size and shape at various positions in the x-ray beam (from Bull,[4] with permission)

identical tubes, one may need to specify the acceptable amount of focal spot blooming when purchasing a tube to be used for magnification radiography. As an alternate approach, one may wish to specify the tube mA and kVp which must be used to produce a star pattern equivalent to an 0.3 mm focal spot in both parallel and perpendicular dimensions relative to the tube axis.

Off-Axis Variation in Focal Spot Size

Focal spot measurements must be made in the central part of the x-ray beam. As one moves away from the central ray, the apparent size of the focal spot will change. **The projected focal spot length is much shorter in the heel (anode side) of the beam than at the cathode side.** Figure 20–9 illustrates the marked variation in focal spot length as one moves from the beam center to 10° toward the anode and 10° toward the cathode on the cathode-anode tube axis. Focal spot changes are less significant in the cross axis direction, where focal spot shape may become more diamond shaped but the width and length remain almost constant. The pinhole camera or resolution test pattern must always be accurately aligned with the x-ray beam center if focal spot measurements are to be reliable.

Let us conclude this short review of focal spots by emphasizing what is now an obvious fact: the radiologist who hopes to make successful use of magnification radiography must use great care in selecting an appropriate x-ray tube.

QUANTITATIVE EVALUATION OF RESOLUTION

With magnification techniques it is necessary to combine the most appropriate film-screen combination with the correct focal spot, then determine which amount of magnification is optimum. The serious problem of object motion must also be considered. In this respect, it is useful to study the resolution properties of the

components of the entire radiographic system with the aid of the modulation transfer function (MTF) of the individual and combined components. To review briefly: an MTF is a curve which describes the ability of an imaging system, or any part of the system, to reproduce (or record) information. An MTF of 1.0 is perfect, indicating that the system can record all the information it has received. An MTF of 0 indicates that none of the information has been reproduced. We shall use the MTF curves to compare various system components. Precise data about how the curves are derived and detailed analyses will not be considered, but are available in the literature.[11,12] For example, Figure 20–10 depicts the MTF curves of 3 imaginary x-ray tube focal spots up to an object frequency of 10 line pairs per mm. Focal spot 1 images perfectly (MTF = 1) at all frequencies. Focal spot 2 is not nearly as good, with its MTF dropping to 0.5 at 5 line pairs per mm., and focal spot 3 is lousy with an MTF of 0 by 6 line pairs per mm. Obviously, one need not know much about MTF curves to be able to glance at Figure 20–10 and determine curve 1 is the best, 2 is next best and 3 is worst. This is the use we will make of the following MTF curves,

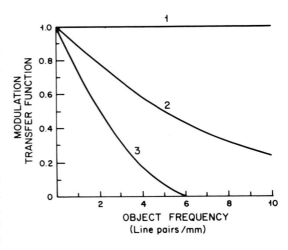

Figure 20–10 Illustrative MTF curves

they allow quick graphic comparisons. There is one additional use we must make of the MTF. If one knows the MTF of each of several components of an imaging system (i.e., film, intensifying screen and focal spot), the MTF of the entire system is calculated by multiplying the MTF of each component. We will now briefly consider the MTF of:

> Film
> Focal spots
> High speed intensifying screens
> Object motion

and show how magnification influences the MTF of film, focal spots and screens.

Film

The ability of x-ray film to image objects with a frequency of 10 to 20 line pairs per mm is so good that we may consider film to have an MTF of 1.0 for all clinical applications of magnification radiography.

Focal Spots

We will assume focal spots of uniform intensity distribution. Figure 20–11A is a set of calculated MTF curves of an 0.3 mm focal spot for magnification factors of 1.0 (contact radiography, not possible clinically), 1.2 and 2.0. **Notice how rapidly the MTF deteriorates as the magnification factor increases,** even in the case of this small focal spot. Figure 20–11 B shows similar data for a 1.0-mm. focal spot, emphasizing that the larger the focal spot the more drastic the deterioration of MTF produced by magnification. **Focal spot MTF is adversely affected by magnification.**

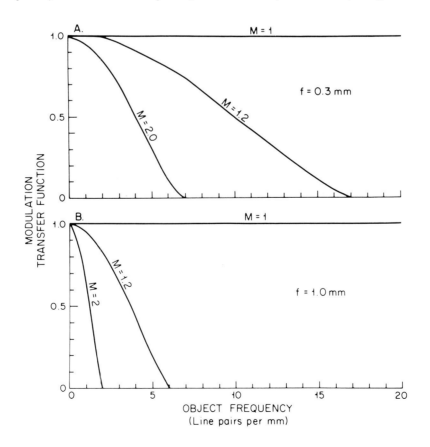

Figure 20–11   Calculated MTF curves for an 0.3 mm (A), and a 1.0 mm (B) focal spot (f) at magnification of 1, 1.2 and 2

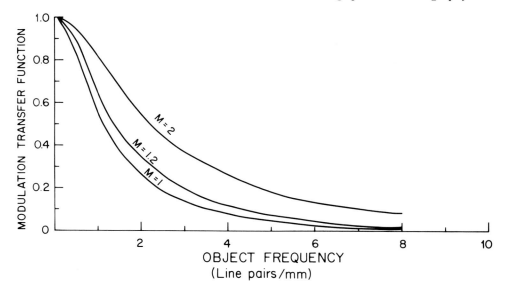

Figure 20–12   Approximate MTF curve of a Quanta II intensifying screen at a magnification of 1.0, 1.2 and 2.0 (courtesy E. I. du Pont de Nemours and Company, Inc.)

Intensifying Screens

We will consider only high speed screens, since they are the ones usually employed for magnification angiography. Figure 20–12 diagrams the approximate MTF curves of the DuPont Quanta II (barium fluorochloride) screens at a magnification of 1.0, 1.2 and 2.0. It is clear from Figure 20–12 that **screen MTF improves with magnification.** In fact, the worse the MTF curve of the screen, the more improvement one sees with magnification, which is fortunate because we are usually using high speed screens in clinical situations in which magnification is attempted. It is quite easy to understand why screen MTF improves with magnification when one considers what magnification does to the frequency (line pairs per mm) of information in the image presented to the intensifying screen. Assume that a test object has a frequency of 4 line pairs per mm (Figure 20–13). When the object is magnified by a factor of 2, the 4 line pairs are presented to the intensifying screens over an area of 2 mm, thus reducing the frequency of the image presented

Figure 20–13   Resolution demanded at the level of the screen decreases as magnification increases

to the screen to 2 line pairs per mm. The frequency of the image is less than the frequency of the object and is calculated by dividing object frequency by the magnification factor. For example, assume a test object has six line pairs per mm. When the object is magnified by a factor of 1.5, the 6 lines will cover 1.5 mm at the level of the intensifying screens, corresponding to an image frequency of $\frac{6}{1.5}$, or 4 line pairs per mm. Similarly, at 2× magnification, the object frequency of 6 line pairs per mm is reduced to an image frequency of 3 line pairs per mm. Since magnification reduces the frequency (i.e., line pairs per mm) of information which the intensifying screen must resolve, the screen is able to do a better job.

Focal Spot and Screens

Since focal spot MTF gets worse with magnification, and screen MTF improves, what degree of magnification is best when only focal spot and screen are considered (assume film MTF of 1.0 in all situations)? Under these conditions (no object motion), the best resolution (MTF) is obtained by using detail screens and as little magnification as possible. In the clinical situation, object motion must be considered, and this changes all the answers.

Object Motion

The amount of unsharpness caused by motion of an object is independent of the amount of magnification. Motion unsharpness depends only on

Velocity of motion
Exposure time.

Velocity (**v**) is expressed in mm per second, and exposure time (**t**) is expressed in seconds. The product **vt** can be used to determine the MTF due to object motion. For example, if an object is moving at a rate of 10 mm per second (such as a pulmonary artery), and an exposure time

of .025 seconds is used, the product **vt** will be 10 × .025 = 0.25. Assume an object frequency of 2 line pairs per mm (i.e., an opacified pulmonary artery 0.250 mm in diameter, giving 2 arteries and 2 spaces of 0.250 mm each per 1 mm), Table 20–6 shows that the MTF due to motion will be 0.64. Table 20–6 lists the MTF due to object motion for an object frequency of 2, 3, 5, 8 and 10 line pairs per mm at **vt** values of 0.1, 0.25, 0.5 and 1.0. The equation used to calculate these MTF values is terrifying, but is available to those able to deal with such things in reference 12. From Table 20–6, it can be appreciated that knowledge of object motion is required if one is to seriously evaluate the optimal exposure factors in the case of moving objects. As a general rule, if it is determined that the product of object motion (v) and exposure time (t) is less than 0.1, motion unsharpness will be minimal. If the value of **vt** is large (1.0 or greater), motion unsharpness becomes the dominant factor in total imaging system MTF and one will sacrifice any other component of the imaging system to make the exposure time shorter (i.e., use the fastest available film and screen regardless of quantum mottle and screen unsharpness). If the product of **vt** is greater than 0.1 but less than 0.5, a compromise is usually best: use a fast (but not the fastest) film-screen system, which will keep quantum mottle and screen unsharpness as favorable as possible and still allow reasonably short exposure times. Since magnification is useful when fast screen film systems are used, the MTF of angiographic studies

Table 20–6. The Calculated MTF Due to Object Motion

OBJECT MOTION (vt) mm	MOTION MTF				
	2 line prs/mm	3 lp/mm	5 lp/mm	8 lp/mm	10 lp/mm
.1	.94	.85	.64	.24	0
.25	.64	.30	0	0	0
.5	0	0	0	0	0
1.0	0	0	0	0	0

Table 20–7. Example Calculations of MTF Values of Various Components of a Magnification Radiographic System

Focal spot size: 0.3 × 0.3 mm
Object motion: 3 mm per sec.
Exposure time: 0.033 sec.
Image frequency: 4 line pairs per mm
Very fast screens (Du Pont Quanta II)

MAGNIFICATION	SCREEN MTF	FOCAL SPOT MTF	MOTION MTF	TOTAL SYSTEM MTF
1.0	0.08	1.0	0.76	0.06
1.2	0.12	0.91	0.76	0.08
1.5	0.16	0.76	0.76	0.09
2.0	0.27	0.51	0.76	0.10
3.0	0.44	0.24	0.76	0.08

of moving vessels can usually be improved with magnification if the focal spot is of the correct size and shape. For example, consider an abdominal angiogram in which vessel motion is about 3 mm per second. Assume one uses Quanta II screens (Figure 20–12), an 0.3-mm focal spot with uniform intensity distribution (Figure 20–11A) and an exposure time of 0.033 seconds (vt = 3 × 0.033 = 0.1). At an information content of 4 line pairs per mm (i.e., blood vessels 0.125 mm in diameter), will system MTF be better at a magnification factor of 1.0, 1.2, 1.5, 2.0 or 3.0? The appropriate calculations are shown in Table 20–7, which shows system MTF to be best at a magnification of 2×. While calculation of MTF values does not tell the entire story of useful information content of the radiographic image, it does provide us a means of beginning an objective analysis of a complex subjective problem (for example, this treatment neglects system noise, or quantum mottle).

HOW MUCH MAGNIFICATION IS BEST?

With an 0.3-mm focal spot there is a rather narrow range of magnification which will result in improvement in resolution. No significant improvement greater than a magnification of about 2 is possible, so 2× magnification is the upper limit with an 0.3-mm focal spot. This amount of magnification is calculated for structures inside the body, so magnification as calculated from the skin surface of the body nearest the tube will be about 1.6 to 1.8. Since the correct magnification factor will vary between tubes (i.e., focal spots are not the same), Milne[10] suggests that one should perform some experiments before clinical work is done. For example, place a resolving power target in an appropriate phantom, then make a series of exposures at different degrees of magnification using the same mA as will be used with patients. One then determines which degree of magnification gives the best resolution. With small focal spots, information content will increase over much higher ranges of magnification (up to 8.0× with a 0.1-mm focal spot).

QUANTUM MOTTLE

Quantum mottle is statistical fluctuation in the number of x-ray photons used by the imaging system to form the image. With magnification radiography, the number of x-ray photons per mm² required to produce the image is the same (if film density is the same) for any degree of magnification. That is, **quantum mottle does not change with radiographic magnification.** If one photographically enlarges a radiograph there is a change in quantum mottle. If 40,000 photons per mm² were used to form the radiographic image, photographic magnification of 2× will increase the area of 1 to 4 mm² and reduce the number of x-ray photons to 10,000 per mm². Thus, photographic enlargement increases quantum mottle in the magnified image by a factor of $\frac{N}{m^2}$ in which:

> N = the number of photons used
> m = magnification

How does quantum mottle (noise) affect the radiographic image? Quantum mottle influences the perception of low contrast objects with poorly defined borders. By comparison, system MTF largely defines the ability to record small objects with sharp borders and high contrast. Therefore, radiographic magnification (as opposed to photographic or optical magnification) may improve visualization of low contrast images because it does not increase noise.

Patient Exposure

If 2 times magnification radiography requires that the patient's body surface be twice as close to the x-ray tube as in non-magnification radiography, one would conclude that exposure to the skin would be increased by a factor of 2^2 or 4 (inverse square law). This conclusion is not correct for the following reasons.

First, in routine radiography there is always some amount of magnification, usually by about 1.1 to 1.2 at the skin on the tube side of the body. The inverse square law calculated with these values shows skin exposure to increase by:

$$\frac{2^2}{1.1^2} = 3.31 \quad \text{or} \quad \frac{2^2}{1.2^2} = 2.78$$

Second, with magnification radiography a smaller portion of the body is exposed to x rays because a smaller body area now covers the film. With magnification only relatively small anatomical areas can be recorded. Because of the limited area which can be encompassed, careful collimation of the x-ray beam and accurate alignment of the part being examined with the central beam are mandatory. This improves image quality and decreases patient exposure.

Third, with magnification one is always using high speed or ultra-high speed screens, and does not need a grid.

Because of these considerations, the increase in patient exposure with magnification is less than that anticipated by application of the inverse square law, and in some cases there might even be no increase or an actual decrease in skin exposure.

SUMMARY

Because x rays do not originate from a point source, calculations dealing with magnification of objects which are small compared to the size of the focal spot require an understanding of the relationship between geometric magnification (m) and true magnification (M). True magnification is a function of the ratio between focal spot size and object size $(\frac{f}{d})$.

Specifications and measurements of focal spot size raise many issues. Industry standards define acceptable tolerance limits in focal spot size. Focal spot size varies with tube operating conditions, with the most marked variation being blooming with high mA, low kVp techniques. The intensity distribution of radiation from the focal spot is important in determining the resolving power of the focal spot. The pinhole technique measures the physical size of the focal spot, and this measurement is used to calculate heat loading of the tube and to calculate magnification of small objects. Resolution chart (star pattern) measurements do not measure the physical size of a focal spot, but indicate the resolving power of the focal spot.

The resolution characteristics of magnification radiography may be studied in terms of the MTF of the various components of the imaging system. Film MTF is considered 1.0. Intensifying screen MTF improves with magnification while focal spot MTF deteriorates rapidly with magnification. Magnification represents a compromise wherein deterioration of focal spot MTF and improvement in screen MTF combine to produce maximum MTF of the entire imaging system. Magnification offers advantages when high speed screens are used and object motion is present. The amount of unsharpness caused by object motion is unrelated to magnification, and depends on the velocity of motion and the exposure time. The optimum magnification for any system must be determined experimentally; with an 0.3-mm focal spot this will vary from about 1.6 to 2.0×. Quantum mottle (noise) is not increased with radiographic magnification. Patient skin dose is usually increased with magnification, but the increase is less than the inverse square law would indicate.

REFERENCES

1. Bergeron, R.T.: Manufacturers' designation of diagnostic x-ray tube focal spot size: a time for candor. Radiol. *3*, 487, 1974.
2. Bernstein, H., Bergeron, R.T., and Klein, D.J.: Routine evaluation of focal spots. Radiol. *3*, 421, 1974.
3. Bernstein, F.: Specifications of focal spots and factors affecting their size. SPIE., Vol. 56 (1975) Medical X-ray Photo-Optical Systems Evaluation, 159–163.
4. Bull, K. W.: The effects of the x-ray focal spot on primary beam magnification of small vessels. Thesis for the degree of master of science in radiological physics. The University of Texas Health Science Center at Dallas, May 1973.
5. Chaney, E.L., and Hendee, W.R.: Effects of x-ray tube current and voltage on effective focal-spot size. Medical Physics, *1*, 141, 1974.
6. Dunisch, O., Pfeiler, M., and Kuhn, H.: Problems and aspects of the radiological magnification technique. Siemens Electro Medica *3*, 114, 1971.
7. Hendee, W.R., and Chaney, E.L.: X-ray focal spots; practical considerations. Appl. Radiol. *3*, 25, 1974.
8. Milne, E.N.C.: The role and performance of minute focal spots in roentgenology with special reference to magnification. CRC Critical Reviews in Radiol. Sci. *2*, 269, 1971.
9. ———: Characterizing focal spot performance. Radiol. *3*, 483, 1974.
10. ———: Magnification radiography. Appl. Radiology and Nuclear Med. *5*, 12, 1976.
11. Rao, G.U.V., Clark, R.L., and Gayler, B.W.: Radiographic magnification: a critical, theoretical and practical analysis part I. Appl. Radiol. *2*, 37, 1973.
12. ———: part II. Appl. Radiol. *2*, 25, 1973.
13. Spiegler, P., and Breckindidge, W.C.: Imaging of focal spots by means of the star test pattern. Radiol. *102*, 679, 1972.
14. Weaver, K.E.: X-ray tube focal spots. Contained in the syllabus of the AAPM 1975 Summer School, "The Expanding Role of the Diagnostic Radiologic Physicist," Rice University, Houston, Texas July 27–Aug. 1, 1975.

CHAPTER 21

The Subtraction Technique

The subtraction technique is a photographic method used to eliminate unwanted images from a radiograph. The method does not add any information; its purpose is to make diagnostically important information easier to see. The radiographic applications of the subtraction technique were first described by a Dutch radiologist, Ziedes des Plantes, in 1935.

When two radiographs differ in only certain details, subtraction can be used to accentuate the difference. This is illustrated in Figure 21–1. Films A and B are radiographs of an assortment of lead numbers and letters. The two films are almost identical, the only difference being the addition of two letters to Film B. Because there is so much information on both

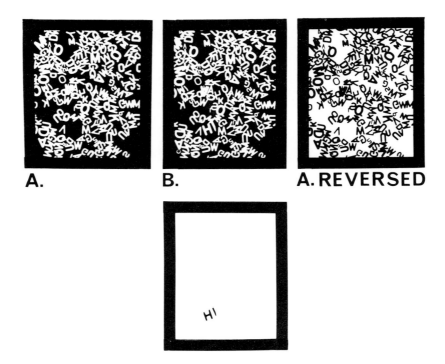

A.   **B.**   **A. REVERSED**

Figure 21–1 The first-order subtraction technique

films, it is difficult to identify this difference. However, if all the information contained in Film A could be subtracted from Film B, the two letters added to Film B would become obvious. To accomplish this, a negative of Film A is prepared ("A reversed" in Figure 21–1). Notice that the images of the letters and numbers are black in the negative. When these negative (black) images are exactly superimposed on the positive images in Film B, the images of the subtracted letters and numbers fuse with the background density. The negative (A reversed) does not contain a reversed image of the two letters which were not present in Film A; therefore, only these two letters remain visible in the final subtraction film. The subtraction technique is easily applied to angiography, in which a series of films are available which differ only in the pattern of contrast material in blood vessels. We will use cerebral angiography as an example.

Three conditions are required for the subtraction technique: (1) a **scout film,** (2) an **angiogram film with contrast material** in vessels, and (3) **no motion** of the head between the exposure of the scout film and subsequent angiogram films. Usually, the first film of a cerebral angiogram series is exposed before the bolus of contrast medium has been injected; this first film is used as a scout film. Slight patient motion is almost always present, prompted by the sensation produced by the injection of contrast material, so perfect subtraction is seldom obtained in clinical practice.

The principles of subtraction are based on the following: the scout film shows the structural details of the skull and adjacent soft tissues. The angiogram film contains exactly the same anatomical detail, if the patient did not move, plus the opacified blood vessels. If all the information in the scout film could be subtracted from the angiogram film, only the opacified vessel pattern would remain visible. Figure 21–2 illustrates the subtraction technique.

Let us consider how information can be subtracted from a radiograph. It will be

SCOUT   FIRST MASK   SECOND MASK

ANGIOGRAM   SUBTRACTION

Figure 21–2 The second-order subtraction technique

recalled that a radiograph provides diagnostically important information because of contrast, or density differences, among areas of the film. No contrast means no information. A lateral skull film usually has a density range of about 0.3 (mastoids) to 1.7 (frontal sinuses). The subtraction technique destroys this density difference by adding density to the film in a carefully controlled manner. Consider the typical lateral skull. If a density of 1.7 were added to the mastoid area, and density 0.3 added to the frontal sinus region, both would then have a density of 2. The loss of contrast would make it impossible to see any difference between the image of the mastoids and sinuses. Thus, if the correct density were added to each part of the film, all contrast would be destroyed and the image of the skull would disappear.

THE SUBTRACTION MASK

The addition of the proper amount of density to the film is accomplished by exactly superimposing a second film, which is termed the **subtraction mask,** over the original radiograph. The subtraction mask is a negative of the scout film. Where the scout film is white, the mask is black (see first mask, Figure 21–2). The mask is a contact print made from the scout film. Figure 21–3 shows how this is done. The scout film and unexposed subtraction mask film are mounted in a glass front cassette (also called a printing

light in any convenient manner. Commonly, the exposure is made with a 15-watt light bulb placed about 6 feet from the front of the glass cassette. Exposure time varies between 3 and 30 seconds, depending on the type of film used and how it is processed. Commercially available printers are usually designed for use in copying radiographs and in preparing subtraction masks and prints. Because of ease of use and uniformity of results, these printers are recommended for most reasonably busy departments. We will now deal with the question of what type of film to use to make the subtraction mask.

The subtraction mask is a negative of the scout film (look at first mask, Figure 21–2 again). It is a special type of negative. The density differences present on the negative must correspond exactly to the density differences of the scout film. In the scout film of Figure 21–2, assume the density of the mastoid area to be 0.3, the frontal sinuses 1.7, and the mid-portion of the skull 1.0. If the image on the scout film is to be completely destroyed by superimposition of the subtraction mask, the density on each part of the subtraction mask must be exactly correct. For example, assume that it is determined that the final density of the subtracted image will be 2.0 (that is, all densities will be 2.0, thus no image will be seen because there is no contrast). This will require densities on the subtraction mask to be as follows:

	DENSITY		
	Mastoid	Mid-skull	Frontal Sinus
Scout film	0.3	1.0	1.7
Subtraction Mask	1.7	1.0	0.3
Scout + Mask	2.0	2.0	2.0

frame), which is a simple wooden frame cassette available at any good photographic supply store. The purpose of the cassette is to insure perfect contact between the two films. This film sandwich is exposed to

These requirements can be met only if the film used to produce the subtraction mask has a gamma of 1. Gamma 1 means that the film will not exaggerate or lessen density differences found in the scout film, but

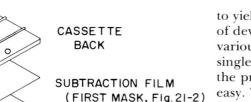

CASSETTE
BACK

SUBTRACTION FILM
(FIRST MASK, Fig. 21-2)

X RAY SCOUT FILM
(SCOUT FILM, Fig. 21-2)

GLASS FRONT
CASSETTE

Figure 21–3 The subtraction mask is a contact print made from the scout film

will produce a negative whose contrast is exactly complementary to the contrast of the scout film. In general, most films available for this purpose closely approximate this requirement, but they lack precision. The resultant image, when scout film and mask are superimposed, has little contrast, but some contrast persists. In Figure 21–2 the illustration labeled "second mask" is a photograph of the image resulting from exactly superimposing the scout film on the film labeled "first mask." As you can see, the image of most skull structures can still be seen, but contrast is sharply reduced. In the past, most subtraction masks were made using Kodak Commercial Film, Type 4127 or 6127. This film produced a transparent negative of the scout film, and it had a gamma of 1 if developed properly. Processing these films required chemicals which were different from those used in x-ray film processors, and this inconvenience limited the use of the subtraction technique. However, this problem no longer exists. Subtraction film (Du Pont Cronex subtraction and Kodak RP/SU X-OMAT subtraction) now available will produce an excellent mask when developed in an automatic x-ray film processor. These film emulsions have been designed

to yield a gamma of 1 over the wide range of developing conditions which exist in the various x-ray film processors. They are single-emulsion films, and their use makes the production of a subtraction mask very easy. The only extra equipment needed is a printing frame (glass front cassette) and a 15-W light bulb. First, the scout film and subtraction film are placed in the printing frame (Figure 21–3), exposed to the 15-W bulb for about 10 seconds at a 6-foot distance, and then the subtraction film is developed as an ordinary radiograph. The illustration in Figure 21–2 (first mask) was made with commercial film; x-ray subtraction film would have produced a similar mask with much less effort. In the literature the subtraction mask is often referred to as a diapositive. The illustration labeled "first mask" in Figure 21–2 might also be called the first diapositive.

THE SUBTRACTION PRINT

The subtraction mask can be used in several ways. It may be superimposed in exact registration on an angiogram film and the result examined directly while the study is in progress. The fact that the subtraction product can be quickly available probably will be of significant value to the angiographer. When the mask and angiogram film are superimposed, the resulting film density will be very high (about 2.0 or greater). An ordinary view box does not produce enough light to allow direct viewing of this type of subtraction. A spotlight, or special view box with brighter illumination, must be used. With direct viewing the opacified blood vessels will, of course, be seen as light (low density) structures. It is also obvious that if the patient moved between the exposure of the scout film and subsequent angiogram films, exact superimposition of the mask and angiogram will not be possible.

To produce a permanent record of the subtraction or to prepare illustrations, a print of the subtraction must be made. This is very easy to do. The subtraction

Figure 21–4   Exposing a first-order subtraction print

mask, the angiogram film with opacification of desired vessels, and an unexposed film are assembled in the glass front cassette in the order shown in Figure 21–4, and exposed to light in the same way the mask was produced.

The same film which was used to prepare the mask may be used for the print; i.e., x-ray subtraction film. Exposure must be increased 2 or 3 times because two films are now in front of the unexposed film. However, the subtraction film has a gamma of 1, and the transparent print resulting from its use will not show maximum contrast between opaque blood vessels and the background skull density. X-ray film has a high gamma (e.g., 2.5), and will produce a high-contrast print of the vessels. Because it is very light sensitive, x-ray film will require less exposure; a few trial runs will quickly determine correct exposure time. Both subtraction film and x-ray film can be processed routinely in a film processor. Therefore, both the subtraction mask and a print of the subtracted angiogram can be made within 5 to 10 minutes of the time the angiogram is first viewed. A single emulsion film designed for making the subtraction print is now available.

This technique as described will, as shown in the final subtraction film of Figure 21–2, result in a print in which blood vessels are black and the background skull density is light. If this reversal of "normal" density patterns is objectionable, a print of

the subtraction, made on subtraction film, will yield a film with white blood vessels. This step is usually omitted unless special illustrations are desired.

The final subtraction film illustrated in Figure 21–2 was actually printed on very high contrast Du Pont Ortho Type A Litho film which exaggerates contrast between blood vessels and the subtracted skull image. This is a valuable feature when clear illustrations are needed for publication, but it is seldom used in clinical situations. The Litho film cannot be processed in the x-ray film processor.

SECOND-ORDER SUBTRACTION

The technique we have described is usually termed first-order subtraction. That is, a mask is made from the scout film, then the mask and angiogram are superimposed to produce the final subtraction print. Using x-ray subtraction film to make the mask, first-order subtraction is usually adequate. However, the subtraction may be perfected if a second mask is prepared, and this is done when performing second-order subtraction. In Figure 21–2 the first mask was made as a contact print of the scout film. The second mask represents a contact print made by superimposing the scout film on the first mask. The purpose of the second mask is to destroy density differences not subtracted by the first mask. The final subtraction, using the second-order technique, requires

Figure 21–5   Exposing a second-order subtraction print

superimposing the second mask, first mask and angiogram, as shown in Figure 21–5. The combined density of these three films is high; getting the films in perfect registration is difficult and the technique requires a bright light. It is not practical to view second-order subtractions directly; a print must be made. Second-order subtraction requires considerably more effort, but the results can be spectacular, with the image of the skull all but disappearing from the final print. The subtraction product shown in Figure 21–2 is a high-contrast print of a second-order subtraction.

All the films mentioned for printing the final subtraction are transparencies. If desired, the final print can be made on photographic paper to be viewed as an ordinary photograph. Except for the preparation of illustrations for publication, this application is seldom employed.

The principle of the subtraction technique can be used to show a change in position of a structure occurring between the taking of the first and second radiographs. For example, a faintly opaque foreign body in the eye might be identified if the head were absolutely immobilized and the direction of gaze changed between two otherwise identical exposures. Because of its movement, the foreign body would theoretically be the only structure not subtracted. Successful use of the subtraction technique for foreign-body identification requires that absolutely no unwanted patient motion occur between exposures.

SUMMARY

The subtraction technique is a photographic method of eliminating (or subtracting) the unwanted images from a radiograph. Recent development of a subtraction film which can be developed in an automatic x-ray film processor has made use of the technique easy, fast, and inexpensive. First-order subtraction is usually adequate; second-order subtraction may be used when extreme enhancement of detail is desired.

REFERENCES

1. Hanafee, W., and Shinno, J. M.: Second-order subtraction and simultaneous bilateral carotid, internal carotid injections. Radiol. *86,* 334, 1966.
2. Joyce, J. W., Dalrymple; M.D., Jungkind, F. F., Scott, P. D., and Davasher, B. G.: Improved contrast in subtraction technique. Radiol. *94*, 157, 1970.
3. Oldendorf, W. H.: A modified subtraction technique for extreme enchancement of angiographic detail. Neurol. *15*, 336, 1965.
4. Oldendorf, W. H.: Subtraction and auto-subtraction techniques for reproducing radiographs. J. Biol. Photographic Assoc. *32*, 65, 1964.

CHAPTER **22**

Copying Radiographs

Making full-size copies of radiographs is now a routine procedure. Radiograph duplicating film is familiar to radiologists and offers a fast, simple, and relatively inexpensive way to copy radiographs. We will briefly examine the photographic principle (solarization) utilized in radiograph duplicating film.

Equally important to the radiologist is the ability to produce 35-mm slides of radiographs. A number of techniques have been proposed. Several of the best methods are presented in *Copying Radiographs*, published and made available to radiologists by the Eastman Kodak Company. In this chapter we will discuss a method with which the authors have had considerable personal experience and which we feel is highly satisfactory for producing large numbers of good-quality slides quickly and inexpensively. The method employs a direct positive film which, like radiograph copy film, utilizes the principle of solarization.

SOLARIZATION

We have previously discussed (Chapter 11) the fact that as light (or x-ray) exposure increases, so does the resulting developed density of the film, up to a maximum limit. If the exposure is increased considerably beyond that which produces the maximum density, a decrease in density occurs. The phenomenon responsible for this decrease in density with very high exposures is called solarization. From the standpoint of individual grains in the film emulsion, solarization means that the increased exposure has actually destroyed the developable state that had been induced by the earlier part of the exposure. Figure 22–1 shows the zones of a film's characteristic curve (toe, straight line portion, and shoulder); this curve extends into the region of solarization where increased log relative exposure produces decreased density. Remember, the exposure scale is logarithmic, so reaching the solarization region of the curve requires a huge exposure, when compared to that commonly used in photography.

The physical process responsible for solarization is still subject to debate. Current evidence favors the **rebromination hypothesis,** which we will briefly discuss.

In discussing latent-image formation, we examined in some detail the way in which

Figure 22–1 Characteristic curve extended into the region of solarization

metallic silver is deposited at latent-image centers. We also mentioned that bromine is formed when silver bromide decomposes in the photolytic process. The bromine passes from the silver halide crystal into the surrounding gelatin. Gelatin is able to neutralize the small quantities of bromine formed in normal latent-image formation. However, gelatin is easily saturated with bromine. The amount of bromine liberated during the large exposures of the solarization region cannot be destroyed by the gelatin. During such exposures, large quantities of bromine build up in the spaces between emulsion grains. When the exposure is completed, this excess bromine reacts with metallic silver at the latent-image centers on the surface of the grain. This coats the latent-image center with a layer of silver bromide which effectively isolates it from the action of the developing solution. Thus the grain, even though it contains one or more latent-image centers, will not be developed.

The important fact about the solarization process is that more light exposure produces less film density. This is just the opposite of standard photographic exposures.

The two films we are going to discuss (radiograph copy film and 35-mm direct positive film) have an emulsion that has been solarized. The emulsion may be solarized before or after it is coated on the film. The solarizing process may be done with light, but chemical treatment of the emulsion will also cause solarization. The exact processes are trade secrets. Several years ago, it was possible to solarize the emulsion of routine x-ray film. After prolonged exposure to light, the x-ray film could be used to produce a direct positive copy of a radiograph. However, the emulsions now used in x-ray film cannot be solarized satisfactorily.

RADIOGRAPH DUPLICATING FILM

Radiograph duplicating film has a solarized emulsion coated on one side of a blue-tinted polyester film base. An anti-halation coating is on the opposite side of the base.

Halation

When image-forming light passes through a film and into the air beyond it, some of the light is reflected back into the film. This reflected light spreads out beyond the boundaries of the image and causes unsharp edges. Halation may be prevented by coating the back side of the film base with a layer of gelatin that contains a dye which absorbs the reflected light to which the emulsion is sensitive. The dye used is de-colorized or washed away during film processing.

Solarized Emulsion

The emulsion of radiograph duplicating film is a solarized emulsion. It is designed to be exposed with an ultraviolet light source, such as a BLB ultraviolet, fluorescent lamp. Such lamps, mounted in a standard 14 × 17-inch radiograph illuminator, serve as a good light source. A glass front cassette (described in Chapter 21) may be used to hold the original radiograph and copy film in close contact. The emulsion side of the copy film must, of course, face the radiograph. The copy film and radiograph "sandwich," mounted in a cassette with a glass front, is exposed with light from the view box. All of this takes place in the darkroom, of course. Exposure time varies; a few trial runs are necessary. Recommended time is about 6 seconds with the view box about 2 feet from the cassette. The exposed copy film is processed like a routine x-ray film. A commercially available duplicating printer may be used. These printers are simple to operate and provide copies of uniform quality.

Since the emulsion of the copy film is solarized, light passing through the radiograph and reaching the copy film will produce a copy which looks like the original radiograph. Remember, the more light that reaches the solarized film, the less the density that is produced. Areas of low density in the original radiograph allow more light to reach the copy film and are, therefore, reproduced as areas of low density on the copy.

Densities of the duplicate may be made to differ from those of the original. If the original is too dark (too much density), a longer exposure will produce a copy with less density. Similarly, the density of the copy may be increased by decreasing the exposure.

Radiograph duplicating film is available in several sizes.

35-MM SLIDES

Camera

Most 35-mm slides are exposed with a single-lens reflex camera. This means that the exact area which is being photographed is seen through the viewfinder of the camera. An expensive camera is not necessary. Usually, the camera should be mounted on a copying stand directly above a view box. These stands can be obtained at most photo supply stores. A standard illuminator used for routine radiograph viewing provides a satisfactory light source. The standard lens on most 35-mm cameras works well, but this lens will not allow the close-up work which is important in many illustrations. However, extension tubes or positive diopter supplementary lenses provide an inexpensive means of achieving close-up capabilities. A more utilitarian lens is one which will allow both close-up and standard-distance work. Purchase of these special macro lenses is not necessary unless large volumes of work are anticipated. Positive diopter supplementary lenses simply attach to the front of the regular lens. They are easy to use, but the results are not of such good quality as that achieved with extension tubes. Extension tubes are more costly and are less convenient to use. However, they produce a better-quality close-up. At the present time, the 35-mm camera we are using

consists of a Nikkormat FTN camera body and a Micro-Nikkor Auto f/3.5, 55-mm lens, which allows focusing from about 4 inches to infinity.

Film

Three types of film are used to produce 35-mm slides of radiographs. These are (1) reversal color film, (2) negative film used with reversal processing (Kodak Panatomic-X), and (3) direct positive film. Each of these films has its own advantages and disadvantages.

Color Reversal Film

Details of using this type of film have been adequately described.[1] The film is available almost anywhere. Because short exposures are possible with some color films (such as high-speed Ektachrome), the camera can be handheld, an important feature when photographing scientific exhibits. The major disadvantage is that the slides may exhibit an abnormal tint, usually a pale green or blue, a problem which can be remedied with the proper filter. In addition, these slides are relatively expensive compared to those made with black-and-white films. In general, color films offer the advantage of convenience.

Reversal Processing

By a modification of the development process, called reversal processing, a normal emulsion can be made to yield a positive rather than a negative image. In this process, after the negative is developed, the metallic silver in the negative image is dissolved away. Then the film is reexposed to light, which makes the residual silver halide developable. The film is then redeveloped, producing a positive image.

The black-and-white film most commonly used for reversal processing in preparing slides of radiographs is Kodak Panatomic-X film.[1] It is available in cassettes of 20 and 36 exposures and may be bought in bulk form. It has a wide exposure latitude, and we have had good results using a standard x-ray view box light source with an exposure time of 2 to 5 seconds at f/16. A dark film may require an exposure time of 10 to 20 seconds.

The major disadvantage of this film is the intricate processing required. There is a direct positive developing kit available, but it requires considerable time to develop your own slides, and few commercial film processors are willing to develop Panatomic-X as a direct positive. In most cities, the film must be mailed to a processor, and the delay in receiving the finished product can be most inconvenient when the material is needed promptly. In our experience, Panatomic-X produces good slides.

Direct Positive Film

Direct positive, or direct reversal, film contains a solarized emulsion. Therefore, it produces a direct black-and-white duplicate of a radiograph when processed in a conventional manner (reversal processing is not needed).

Eastman Direct MP Film 5360[2] (MP = motion picture) is such a film. It is a fine-grain, high-resolving-power film of medium contrast. It was designed to be used for editing purposes in the motion picture industry. Herein lies its major disadvantage for those who wish to use it for making 35-mm slides, for it requires repackaging by the user. It is not available in the handy 20- and 36-exposure cassettes to which we have become accustomed. Instead, the film must be specially ordered in rolls of 1000 feet. However, empty 35-mm film cassettes are readily available, and it is quite easy to cut appropriate lengths and "roll your own" from the 1000-foot roll. Obviously, 1000 feet of film will produce several thousand 35-mm slides. Storage of this film for over 6 months requires refrigeration at 0°F. In currently available quantities, some film will usually be wasted. Perhaps this or a similar film will become available in a length better suited to the needs of the amateur photographer.

The film has several outstanding advantages. Exposure latitude is extremely large, so that exposure times are not critical. Using a standard view box for a light source, exposure time varies between 10 and 30 seconds with the lens aperture set at f/3.5. A roentgenogram of average density requires an exposure of 10 to 15 seconds. Copying drawings, charts, pictures of radiographs, etc. is also easy. We use a light source provided by four 75-W photoflood bulbs which are mounted on the copying stand (such units are commercially available). A satisfactory exposure for such prints is 12 seconds at f/3.5. Exposure latitude is so great that a change in exposure time of 2 or 3 seconds will produce no visible difference in the final product.

The other great virtue of this film is the ease with which it can be developed. Temperature and solution concentrations need not be precisely regulated. This is fortunate, for it is necessary to do your own developing. The mechanics of development can be learned in a few minutes from personnel in any photographic supply store. The exposures suggested above require the following development technique: develop in Kodak D-19 developer (diluted stock solution 1:1) for 10 minutes at normal room temperature. The developing solution should be changed after each 36-exposure roll of film is developed. In fixing, we use Kodak Rapid fixer, full strength, for 5 minutes.

The techniques suggested have evolved through trial and error in our department. The extreme latitude of exposure and processing is especially attractive in a large department where many persons are involved in producing slides, for the job does not require an expert. The processing technique is not only simple, but fast; it is possible to produce a completed slide in about an hour. The cost per slide is low; the cardboard mount costs more than the photograph!

Our experience with Eastman Direct MP Film 5360 has been gratifying. Preparation of large numbers of slides (up to 25,000 per year) has become relatively simple, and slides are routinely available in 24 hours. All processing is done in the radiology department. This method of preparing 35-mm slides can be recommended for use in any department in which many slides are needed promptly.

At the present time both Eastman Kodak and DuPont have available 35-mm films which have been designed to permit production of 2 × 2 inch slides of good quality, from radiographs or printed material, with a minimum of time and effort. The films are:

Kodak Rapid Processing Copy Film SO-185 (RPC)

Cronex DP 35 mm Black and White Film.

Both of these are slow, fine grain direct positive films. Both are available in convenient 36-exposure magazines, and the Kodak film may also be obtained in 150 feet rolls. Exposure techniques and factors are roughly the same as described for Eastman Direct MP Film 5360. Exposure latitude is great, but some experimenting and several rolls of poor slides will always be required as one first begins using these films.

The great convenience of these two films is that each can be processed in a 90-second x-ray film automatic processor to obtain a dry film as fast and almost as easy as one obtains routine radiographs. The exposed film must be taped to a film leader 8 × 10 inches or larger. The leader and film (emulsion side up) are then simply fed into the automatic processor. After processing, the film is easily cut to size and mounted as slides in one of several types of slide mounts available from almost any photographic supply dealer. Using these copy films it is possible to produce a slide ready for projection in about 10 minutes (a phenomenon which can become a nuisance when one's colleagues develop the bad habit of asking for "a little help" in preparing conferences and lectures at the last minute). A recent Kodak publication (M3-148, 12-76) titled "KODAK Rapid Processing Copy Film SO-185 (RPC) Technic Guide" contains many helpful suggestions. Technical data about the DuPont film are also available as a "Technical Data Sheet for Cronex DP 35 mm Black & White Film" (D-D-2.2). It is possible to manually process these films. Manual processing may be used to change the gamma and maximum density of these films, but such manipulation is rarely necessary unless one's hobby compels experimentation. Our continued use of MP Film 5360 is based partly on habit and a long established production routine, and partly on modest financial savings in the production of huge numbers of slides. It seems reasonable to recommend use of one of the films designed for producing 35-mm slides of radiographs for almost anyone having a need for such slides.

SUMMARY

Duplicating radiographs with radiograph duplicating film is a routine procedure requiring almost no extra equipment. The phenomenon of solarization makes this process possible.

Producing 35-mm slides of radiographs requires choice of the proper film to fit the circumstances. Reversal color film is acceptable when only a few slides are needed, and the short exposure time required by some color films offers a method of copying material when the camera must be handheld. Reversal processing of black-and-white film will also produce good slides. This film is convenient to use, but film processing is intricate. Direct positive 35-mm film is now available which is so convenient to use that this method should be considered the routine manner in which slides of radiographs are prepared.

REFERENCES

1. *Copying Radiographs.* Available from Eastman Kodak Company, Radiography Markets Division, Rochester, New York 14650.

2. KODAK Rapid Processing Copy Film SO-185 (RPC) Technic Guide. Available from Eastman Kodak Company, Radiography Markets Division, Rochester, New York 14650.

3. Technical data sheet, Eastman Direct MP Film 5360 (35-mm). Eastman Kodak Company.

4. Technical data sheet Cronex DP 35MM Black & White Film. E.I. du Pont de Nemours & Co., Inc., Photo Products Department, Wilmington, DE 19898.

CHAPTER 23

Xeroradiography

Xeroradiography is the production of a visible image utilizing the charged surface of a photoconductor (amorphous selenium) as the detecting medium, partially dissipating the charge by exposure to x rays to form a latent image, and making the latent image visible by xerographic processing. Xerography was invented by a physicist, Chester F. Carlson, in 1937. In 1944 the Battelle Memorial Institute, and in 1947 the Haloid Company (now Xerox Corporation) began laboratory investigations of this process and its potential application to industrial and medical radiographic procedures. The Xerox Corporation has developed a highly automated xeroradiographic system which has allowed radiologists to make practical clinical use of this type of x-ray imaging. It is interesting to note that medical uses of xeroradiography were investigated as early as 1952 by Dr. John F. Roach of Albany Medical College, New York.

GENERAL PRINCIPLES

Xeroradiography is a complex electrostatic process based on a special material called a photoconductor. A **photoconductor** will not conduct an electric current when shielded from radiation, but becomes conductive when exposed to radiation such as visible light or x rays. The photoconductor used in xeroradiography is **amorphous selenium.** The selenium is deposited as a thin layer on a sheet of aluminum to form the xeroradiographic plate, which is analogous to film used in conventional radiography. The plate is enclosed in a light-tight cassette.

The xeroradiographic imaging process consists of several steps:

1. A uniform charge is deposited on the surface of the selenium. This sensitizes the plate before exposure to x rays.
2. The charged plate is placed in a light-tight cassette and exposed to x rays just like a film-screen cassette. X rays reaching the plate cause the photoconductor layer to lose its charge in an amount corresponding to the intensity of the x-ray beam. The uniform charge is thus partly dissipated, and the remaining charge pattern forms the latent electrostatic image.
3. The latent electrostatic image is developed (made visible) by exposing the surface of the plate to fine charged powder particles (called "toner") which are attracted to the plate surface in proportion to the intensity of the remaining charge.
4. The powder image is transferred to paper by placing suitable paper in contact with the plate and using an electrostatic charge to attract toner away from the plate and onto the paper.
5. The powder image is fused to the

paper by exposure to heat to make a permanent record.

6. The plate is cleaned of all remaining powder (toner) and prepared for reuse. The plate is not charged during storage.

PHOTOCONDUCTION

Solid materials may be classified as **conductors, semiconductors** (of which photoconductors are a special class) and **insulators.** This classification depends on whether or not the solid is capable of sustaining a current (moving electrons) if a voltage is applied. A brief review of the structure of an atom is necessary in developing an understanding of why amorphous selenium, which is a photoconductor, is capable of forming the electrostatic latent image that is the basic physical phenomenon on which xeroradiography is based. An introduction to atomic structure will be found in Chapter 2 under the sub-heading, "Interaction of the electron beam with the target of the x-ray tube."

The atom is made up of a nucleus around which electrons are spinning in orbits. The forces existing within the atom are electrostatic forces (neglecting nuclear forces) which always exist between two electrical charges. Electron orbits represent precisely defined energy levels for the electrons, and no electron may exist at any level (or orbit) other than one of these permissible levels. Groups of permissible orbits are combined into electron shells. The number of electrons in the outer energy shells determines the chemical and electrical properties of the atom. The atomic number of selenium is 34, which means that selenium has 34 electrons: 2 in the K shell, 8 in the L shell, 18 in the M shell and 6 in the N shell, which is the outermost occupied shell for selenium. The electrons in the outermost shell are called valence (from the Latin valere, to have power) electrons because it is these electrons which determine the action of the atom when it reacts with atoms of

another element to form compounds (chemical reaction).

Electrons move in a curved orbit around the nucleus because of the electrostatic force of attraction provided by the nucleus. If the electron is provided with more energy, the orbit of the electron must change. However, the electron must obey structural laws and move into a permissible higher energy (farther from the nucleus) orbit. **Electrons cannot exist between permissible orbits.** One way that the energy of an electron is increased is by the absorption of electromagnetic radiation.

Atoms are bound together to form solids by the interaction of valence electrons. The interactions not only bond the atoms together, but also slightly change the value of permissible energy that the valence electrons may have. The energy of the valence electrons in an isolated atom is defined by the discrete energy levels. **In solids the outer discrete energy levels are replaced by energy bands, and the electrons may have any energy within the energy band (a narrow range of energies).** Inner shells may remain undisturbed by the bonding. In the isolated atom, the discrete energy levels are separated by non-permissible energy values, and electrons may not exist with non-permissible energy. The energy bands in solids may be separated by non-permissible energy values or forbidden energy bands.

In isolated atoms, the energy levels are filled to particular levels. Higher levels exist, but normally there are no electrons in these levels. Similarly, the energy bands in solids are filled to a particular level. The band with highest energy that also has electrons is called the **valence band.** The next higher band, with normally no electrons, is called the **conduction band.** The two bands may be separated by the **forbidden gap.** In considering electrical properties of solids, only these two bands are of interest. Figure 23–1 shows the relationships of the conduction and valence bands for semiconductors.

Figure 23-1 The valence, forbidden and conduction energy bands of a semiconductor

The conduction band always has more energy states than electrons, and the electrons may move from one energy state to another. Therefore, the electrons are fairly free to move when influenced by an external field in the form of a voltage (i.e., an electric current will flow). Solids which have many electrons in the conduction level are known as conductors, of which silver and copper are good examples.

The valence band is the highest energy band in which electrons normally exist. The electrons in the valence level are not free to move because nearly all the available energy states already are occupied by electrons, so an electron having no place to go must stay where it is. However, with proper addition of energy, electrons in the valence band may be elevated to the conduction band. To do this, the electron must acquire sufficient energy to bridge the gap between the valence and conduction bands. This gap is known as the forbidden energy band. It is the energy difference across this forbidden energy band that determines whether a solid acts as a conductor, an insulator, or a semiconductor.

In a conductor there is no forbidden region between the valence band and the conduction band. Insulators are those solids in which the forbidden gap is so large that electrons seldom absorb enough energy to bridge the gap.

A semiconductor is a solid which contains a small forbidden gap. However, addition of the appropriate quantity of energy will allow some electrons to bridge the forbidden gap and enter the conduction band. In a **photoconductor** the energy is provided by absorption of visible electromagnetic radiation (light). Energy added to a semiconductor will cause electrons in the valence band to enter the conduction band, and the semiconductor will then be able to conduct an electric current if an external force (voltage) is applied.

When an electron leaves the selenium atom, the atom has an excess positive charge (the atom is ionized). The area of the absent negative charge (electron) in the valence band is termed a positive hole. Thus, the action of the energy of an absorbed light photon in selenium produces an electron and a positive hole, usually termed an electron-hole pair. When an electron-hole pair is subjected to an electrical field, the two members of the pair migrate in opposite directions. The electron moves toward the positive electrode. The atom containing the positive hole does not actually move. Instead, the hole is transferred from one atom to another and the result is that the hole moves, and it moves toward the negative electrode. Later in this chapter we will discuss the migration of the electron to the positively charged selenium surface of the xeroradiographic plate and migration of the positive hole through the selenium toward the induced negative charge on the aluminum substrate of the plate.

THE XERORADIOGRAPHIC PLATE

The xeroradiographic plate is a sheet of aluminum approximately $9\frac{1}{2} \times 14$ inches in size upon which a layer of amorphous (vitreous) selenium has been deposited. In addition, there is an interface layer between the selenium and aluminum, and an overcoating protecting the selenium surface (Fig. 23-2).

Figure 23–2 Cross section of a xeroradiographic plate

Aluminum Substrate

The aluminum plate upon which the selenium is deposited is made of meticulously cleaned aluminum with an exceedingly smooth surface. Xeroradiographic sensitivity to any defect in the aluminum substrate is extremely high. Defects produce changes in the electrostatic charge in the selenium that may become visible during xerographic developing.

Interface Layer

Heat treatment of the surface of the aluminum substrate serves to form a thin layer of aluminum oxide. Although aluminum is a conductor, aluminum oxide is an insulator. The thickness of the aluminum oxide layer is not critical; a layer about 15 Å thick has been shown to be satisfactory. The purpose of this interface between the selenium and the aluminum substrate is to prevent negative charges induced in the aluminum from migrating into the selenium and dissipating the positive charge induced on the selenium surface. We will examine the nature of these induced charges shortly.

Selenium Coating

The photoconductive layer of the xeroradiographic plate is highly purified selenium in the amorphous, also called vitreous (i.e., not selenium crystals) form. It is deposited on the aluminum substrate by condensation of vaporized liquid selenium in a high vacuum. The thickness of the selenium layer is 130 microns.

Protective Overcoating

The selenium surface of xeroradiographic plates is protected by an overcoating (most other xerographic plates and drums do not have an overcoating). The material used for the overcoating is cellulose acetate, applied by dip-coating from solution to form a layer about 1 to 2 microns thick. Cellulose acetate bonds well to selenium. It has a resistance high enough to prevent lateral conduction of charges which would degrade the electrostatic latent image. Overcoating extends the life of a xeroradiographic plate by a factor of about 10.

The Photoconductive Layer

There are three properties required of the photoconductor used in xeroradiography. First, the electrical conductivity in the dark must be that of a good insulator so that a charge pattern present on the surface will be retained long enough to complete the steps of development. Second, the material must become electrically conducting during exposure to x rays so that an electrostatic image pattern can be formed on its surface by the exposure. Third, it must have mechanical properties of durability and ease of fabrication. The only photoconductor that presently fulfills these criteria for commercial use is selenium. Practically all selenium is derived as a by-product of the electrolytic refinement of copper sulfide ores, either as gaseous SeO_2 or water soluble Na_2SeO_3. Purification of the selenium is very difficult, and any residual impurity may have a significant effect on its photoconductive properties.

The most stable form of selenium is a crystalline structure. However, this form is not used in xeroradiography because it has relatively high electrical conductivity. Crystalline selenium is used in selenium rectifiers. In addition to its crystalline structure, selenium also exists in an amorphous (also called vitreous) form, and it is this form that is used as the photoreceptor in xeroradiography. The amorphous form may be considered the super-cooled form of liquid selenium, and it is formed by cooling the liquid suddenly so that crystals do not have time to form (the melting point of selenium is 216° C). In practice, amorphous selenium is deposited on the aluminum plate by condensation of vaporized liquid selenium in a high vacuum. Pure amorphous selenium is mandatory as the presence of any impurity increases the dark decay rate. **Dark decay is the reduction of plate voltage while the plate remains in darkness.** For xeroradiography this rate should not exceed 5% per minute.

The selenium layer is 130 microns thick. **Sensitivity of the plate to x rays depends upon selenium thickness and the energy (kVp) of the x-ray beam.** For x rays in the energy range usually used in medical diagnostic xeroradiography a selenium plate about 130 microns thick has been shown to exhibit maximum sensitivity. We will define sensitivity as the reciprocal of the exposure in roentgens required to reduce the charge on the plate to one-half its initial value.

Charging the Plate

The first step in the xeroradiographic process is to sensitize the photoconductor by applying a uniform electrostatic charge to its surface in the dark. Since selenium is an insulator in the dark, during charging the xeroradiographic plate can be considered to be a parallel plate capacitor in which the outer (adjacent to protective coating) selenium surface and the aluminum backing (substrate) act as the parallel plates, and the selenium itself acts as the dielectric (Figure 23–4). The device used to produce a charge on the surface of the selenium operates on the principle of corona discharge in a gas. A brief review of capacitance and corona discharge is necessary.

Capacitance

A capacitor, or condenser, consists of two sheets of conducting material, with a sheet of insulating material between them. An electrical charge is placed on each plate (one plate is positive and the other negative), and a potential difference, or voltage, exists between the two plates. The material between the plates has a strong influence on the amount of charge that can be placed on the plates. This material is an insulator or other non-conductor, and is known as the dielectric. When influenced by the electric field between the plates, the atoms of the dielectric become distorted into a configuration termed an induced dipole. Consider Figure 23–3 in which a negatively charged rod is placed near an atom. The normal atom (Fig. 23–3A) has its electron cloud centered on its nucleus. The presence of the negative rod near the atom attracts the nucleus and repels the electrons (Fig. 23–3B) so that the center of the electron cloud falls on the far side of the nucleus. The atom now appears to have a positive side and a negative side, it has become an induced dipole. Similar distortion exists in the atoms of the dielectric material between the charged plates of a capacitor.

Now consider the xeroradiographic plate. The outer surface of the selenium layer behaves like one plate of a capacitor, the aluminum backing (substrate) the other plate, and the photoconductor (selenium) as the dielectric (Fig. 23–4). If a

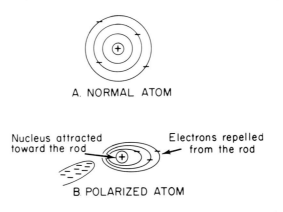

A. NORMAL ATOM

Nucleus attracted toward the rod　　　Electrons repelled from the rod

B. POLARIZED ATOM

Figure 23–3　Polarization of an atom in an electric field

Figure 23-4   Charging a parallel plate capacitor (a) and a xeroradiographic plate (b) is similar

positive charge is deposited on the surface of the selenium, the remainder of the selenium atoms are distorted into the configuration of induced dipoles. The negative pole of each atom is attracted toward the positive charge, causing the atomic layer adjacent to the aluminum substrate to present a positive charge at the selenium-aluminum interface. Polarization of selenium atoms will attract negative charges (electrons) in the aluminum substrate toward the back of the selenium layer. In other words, a negative charge has been induced in the aluminum substrate by the presence of the positive charge on the free surface of the selenium. It is obvious that these induced negative charges cannot be allowed to enter the selenium if the positive charge on the selenium surface is to be retained. It is now easier to understand the function of the interface layer between the selenium and the aluminum. The interface layer (aluminum oxide) reduces negative charge leakage from the substrate into the selenium.

Corona

If a sufficiently high potential difference (called the corona threshold voltage) is applied between a fine wire and ground, the air near the wire becomes ionized. If the voltage is positive, free electrons in the gas near the wire will move toward the wire. These electrons will get a high energy, and instead of going straight to the wire they will interact with many molecules or atoms in the air and create many additional ions. The positive ions thus created will move outward from the wire.

This movement of ions is called corona current. The corona around a wire with a positive voltage has the appearance of a uniform bluish-white sheath over the entire surface of the wire. When such a wire is placed close to the surface of the xeroradiographic plate (the distance is about $^{11}/_{16}$ inch) some positive ions repelled from the wire will be deposited on the surface of the plate. The corona threshold voltage is quite high compared with the needed positive voltage on the surface of the plate. The wire is corrosion-resistant (commonly stainless steel or aluminum) and about 3.5 mils in diameter. Corona threshold voltage for such a wire is about 4,400 volts. By comparison, the positive voltage desired on the surface of the plate ranges from about 1,000 to 1,600 volts. This creates two problems. First, overcharging the surface of the plate must be prevented, suggesting that the potential difference (voltage) on the charging wire should be kept as low as possible. Second, small variations in wire diameter or dirt on the wire will affect the threshold voltage at different points along the wire and cause nonuniformity of corona current. These variations can be minimized if the wire is operated considerably above the corona threshold voltage, at about 7,500 volts. Two devices have been developed to control the amount and uniformity of plate charging, the "scorotron" and the "corotron."

Charging Devices

The **scorotron** involves use of a control screen, or grid, that acts somewhat similar to the grid in a thyratron tube. This device consists of the corona emitting wire (or wires) and a grounded backing plate. In addition, a grid of parallel wires about $3/32$ inch apart is placed between the corona wire and the surface of the xeroradiographic plate (Figure 23–5). If the grid wires are operated at a positive potential, they will suppress the flow of positive ions from the corona wire to the surface of the plate (i.e., the positive charge on the grid will partially repel positive air ions attempting to reach the plate). The grid may be operated from about 350 to 1700 volts positive potential relative to the grounded plate. Assume that the grid is operated at +1000 volts. Initially, with no voltage on the plate surface, the entire 1000 volt potential difference will repel positive air ions from the grid to the selenium surface. As a positive voltage begins to accumulate on the plate surface, the potential difference between grid and plate will decrease. When the voltage on the plate surface reaches 1000 volts, no potential difference will exist between grid and plate and the movement of positive air ions will stop. The grid allows more precise control of plate charging. Also, since it is now grid voltage rather than voltage on the corona wire (wires) that controls plate charging, the corona wire may be operated at a voltage that produces a more uniform corona current (flow at ions). This corona voltage is usually about 7,500 volts DC, and is not under the control of the operator of the unit. The grid voltage can be regulated by local maintenance personnel to produce the contrast desired by the individual using

Figure 23–5 Cross section schematic diagram of a grid controlled corona charging device (scorotron)

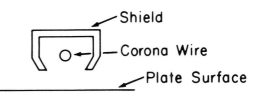

Figure 23–6 Cross section schematic diagram of a corotron

the apparatus. The influence of initial plate voltage on the developed xeroradiographic image will be discussed later.

The **corotron** is a simpler device which has the same function as the scorotron. The corotron consists of a long U-shaped channel (called the shield) with inwardly bent lips and a single corona wire. A cross section of a corotron is illustrated in Figure 23–6. The shield is usually maintained at ground potential. The corona current to the plate is controlled by the corona wire voltage, the configuration of the shield, and the location of the wire within the shield.

The plate is charged by causing it to move at a uniform rate under the stationary charging device which may be a scorotron or corotron. Since the charged photoconductor is sensitive to light as well as x rays, plate charging and all subsequent operations leading to obtaining a developed xeroradiographic image must be carried out with the plate completely shielded from light.

EXPOSING THE CHARGED PLATE

After the plate is sensitized by corona charging it must be enclosed in a cassette which is light-tight and is rigid enough to provide mechanical protection for the fragile plate. The plate-cassette combination is then used just as one would use an x-ray film in its cassette.

When the charged selenium plate is exposed to x rays (or light), **electron-hole pairs** are created (Fig. 23–7). These charged particles come under the influ-

Figure 23-7 Exposure of the charged xeroradiographic plate to x rays creates an electrostatic latent image

ence of the corona induced positive charge on the surface of the selenium, and the induced negative charge in the aluminum substrate. The electrons migrate to the plate surface and discharge the positive charge originally laid down. The positive holes "migrate" through the selenium toward the substrate where they are neutralized by the induced negative charges. The amount of discharge of the positive charges on the surface of the plate is proportional to the intensity of x rays which penetrated the patient, thus the variation of charge pattern remaining on the plate accurately reflects the pattern of attenuation of x rays caused by the patient. The remaining charge pattern on the plate is called the **electrostatic latent image.**

Conductivity Induced by X Rays

The energy gap between the valence band and conduction band (i.e., the forbidden energy band) in amorphous selenium is about 2.3 eV (electron volts). This corresponds to a wavelength of about 5400 Å, which is visible light in the green-yellow range.

$$E = \frac{12,400}{\lambda}$$

$$2.3 = \frac{12,400}{\lambda}$$

$$\lambda = \frac{12,400}{2.3} \text{ or } 5348 \text{ Å}$$

E = photon energy in electron volts

λ = wavelength in Angstroms (Å)

This calculation is a rough estimate used to illustrate the principle leading to creation of photoconductivity induced in selenium by light. Stated in another way, an electron in the valence band of amorphous selenium must absorb all the energy of a light photon of wavelength 5,400 Å in order to be elevated into the conduction band (where it will be able to move when influenced by the positive voltage on the surface of the plate). Obviously, light is absorbed very near the surface of the selenium, with 63% of attenuation occurring within 0.125μ of the incident surface.

Photoconductivity induced in amorphous selenium by x rays differs in two important ways from photoconductivity induced by light. First, the x-ray photons can penetrate further into the selenium, and their absorption may be almost uniform throughout the selenium layer. Second, the energy of an absorbed or scattered x-ray photon is transferred to a photoelectron or a recoil electron (Compton scattering), and each of these electrons will usually have enough kinetic energy to produce many more charge carrier (electron-hole) pairs along its track. One can calculate the sensitivity of selenium plates of different thicknesses of selenium by measuring the x-ray exposure required to reduce plate voltage to one-half of its original value.

Figure 23-8 Sensitivity of a selenium plate to 40 kVp x rays as a function of selenium thickness (modified from Boag[1])

This sensitivity will also vary with the quality (kVp) of the x rays. Figure 23–8 is a drawing taken from a series of curves in the literature, and shows the relative sensitivity of selenium plates of varying thickness to a 40 kVp x-ray beam. The significantly greater sensitivity of plates in the 130 to 160μ range explains the choice of 130μ as the thickness of commercially available xeroradiographic plates. While **plate sensitivity is largely a function of the thickness of the selenium layer and the kVp** at which the exposure is made, it is also true that plate sensitivity can depend on the x-ray tube type, wave form of the x-ray generator, and the amount of filtration.

The Electrostatic Latent Image

After exposure by x rays there remains on the xeroradiographic plate surface a latent image composed of variations in the positive charge representing the structure of the object examined. This is called the electrostatic latent image, and this latent image is accompanied by an electric field. The character of this electric field distribution above the latent image has a strong influence on the visible image formed when the image is developed. Since xeromammography is a well-established clinical application of xeroradiography, we will use this examination as a prototype to illustrate some basic principles. Typically, a xeroradiographic plate used for mammography will be charged to a positive potential of about 1,625 volts. After exposure, some areas of the plate will be almost completely discharged (i.e., areas outside the breast tissue), while other areas will retain almost all the 1,625 volts (i.e., under a large calcified fibroadenoma).

Electric Field Distribution Above the Latent Image

Since the development of the electrostatic latent image depends on the attraction of charged toner particles to the surface of the plate, knowledge of local electric field strengths is necessary to a good understanding of the development process. This subject is highly complex, but for practical purposes we can confine our attention to two aspects of the electric fields existing above the latent image. First, the field has both a vertical and a horizontal component. Second, the field strength declines rapidly as one moves away from the charged surface.

Consider a plate which has been exposed so that a narrow strip retains its full initial charge (i.e., no x rays have reached the plate in that area), and the area on each side of the strip has been completely discharged. The lines of force existing above the plate will be similar to those shown in Figure 23–9 in which lines drawn close together represent stronger electrical fields. Notice that the lines of force become further apart rapidly as distance from the plate surface increases by only a few microns. A negative charge at A which is placed directly above the charged strip will be attracted to the plate surface only by a nearly vertical force pulling it straight down to the surface of the plate. If the negative charge were located directly over the discharged portion of the plate, but near the charged area, (B), both a vertical and a horizontal force act on the particle and cause it to pursue a curved path as it is attracted to the edge of the charged area. Because of this horizontal force compo-

Figure 23–9 Electric field configuration above a narrow charged strip (modified from Boag[1])

nent, negatively charged particles will be "stolen" from the area adjacent to a charged zone on the plate. We will use this concept to explain the phenomena of edge enhancement and deletion that are encountered in the developed xeroradiographic image.

Sensitometry of the Electrostatic Latent Image

Xeroradiography is unique in that the response of the plate to x-ray exposure can be measured independently of the development process. To do this, the plate is usually exposed using an aluminum step wedge just as film sensitometry is done. Then an electrometer is positioned over the plate and the voltage remaining on the plate under the center of each step of the wedge can be measured (this must be done in the dark). The results can be plotted as a discharge curve giving the voltage remaining on a plate after exposure through a given thickness of the aluminum step wedge. Such a curve is illustrated in Figure 23–10, in which response for variation in x-ray tube kVp is plotted. In this illustration plate voltage may be considered the

Figure 23–11   Effect of mAs on the electrostatic latent image (modified from Thourson[7])

equivalent of film density in the more familiar film characteristic curve. Notice that these curves have a toe, straight line portion, and shoulder, similar to x-ray film characteristic curves. Notice also that **the effect of increasing kVp is to decrease the slope of the straight line portion of the curve (decrease contrast).** This is an important difference compared to an x-ray film characteristic curve. The characteristic curve of a film is established by the manufacturer; inherent film contrast cannot be changed by the radiologist.

The effect of changing mAs (kVp constant) is illustrated in Figure 23–11. **Increasing mAs shifts the curve to the right** (i.e., more mAs more completely discharges the plate under each step of the wedge) without making any significant change in the slope of the straight line portion of the curve. This result should be easily understood based on knowledge of the effect of mAs and x-ray film exposure.

Xeroradiographic Undercutting

Xeroradiographic undercutting is caused by ionization of the air in the space

Figure 23–10   Effect of kVp on the electrostatic latent image (modified from Thourson[7])

between the selenium surface of the xeroradiographic plate and the lid of the cassette. This ionization can be caused by interaction of x rays directly with air molecules, or it may be caused by high speed electrons being able to escape from the selenium and enter the air space. This results in the presence of positive and negative air ions in the dark space between the selenium surface and the cassette lid. At the same time these air ions are being created, the x-ray exposure has caused some areas of the selenium plate to be discharged more than others (i.e., the electrostatic latent image has been formed). Assume that a test exposure has been made in which part of the cassette has been covered by a lead bar that prevents any x rays from reaching the selenium plate (Fig. 23–12 A). This will cause an abrupt step in charge density on the plate surface, with charge varying from virtually zero to almost the initial voltage on the plate. Across this step strong electrostatic fields will exist in the air space immediately above the plate. Since the initial charge on the plate surface is positive, the electrostatic forces

will cause negative air ions to be deposited on the edge of the high plate charge and tend to neutralize the charge. This **deposition of negative ions would tend to "move" the edge of the electrostatic image toward the shielded side of the plate** (Fig. 23–12 B), and in extreme cases could actually **cause the image to become considerably smaller** than the object being imaged. To eliminate this problem, a DC voltage is applied between the cassette lid and the aluminum backing of the plate. This will cause any air ions formed to move in a direction perpendicular to the plate so that they cannot be pulled from any area into the charge field at the edge of an image. If the cassette lid is made positive, negative air ions can be attracted away from the plate surface. In practice, the potential difference (voltage) applied between the cassette lid and aluminum plate substrate is about 450 volts. The problem of xeroradiographic undercutting is rarely serious in medical xeroradiography, but can occur frequently in industrial radiography at the border of totally absorbing metal parts.

Figure 23–12 Xeroradiographic undercutting

Because of the highly localized nature of the electrostatic fields at the edge of a sharp charge difference, the results of xeroradiographic undercutting tend to move the charge pattern toward the center of the more highly charged area. Notice that this differs from the more familiar concept of edge unsharpness on film radiographs, which causes a sharp edge to become less sharp but does not move the position of the edge.

DEVELOPMENT

Development of the xeroradiographic image may be defined as the selective deposition of imaging material on a surface in response to electrostatic forces. Development consists of attracting small charged dust particles, called **toner**, to the electrostatic latent image on the selenium surface of the plate. The most commonly used toner in xerographic copy machines is charcoal with a particle size of about 1 micron. However, xeroradiography requires use of a pigmented thermoplastic material of dark blue (called Type 5B by Xerox Corporation) or blue-green (Type 5) color. Particle size is in the general range of a mean diameter of a few microns.

Powder-Cloud Development

The terms powder-cloud development and aerosol development are synonyms. This is the form of development used in xeroradiography. It is fast, relatively simple, and **provides the edge enhancement** which is so characteristic and desirable in the developed image. Also, the powder-cloud method is the form of development which is least damaging to the selenium surface.

The exposed xeroradiographic plate is placed on top of a dark box into which an aerosol of charged toner particles is sprayed through a nozzle (Fig. 23–13).

Aerosol Generation and Toner Charging

If pressurized gas (commonly nitrogen gas) is used to force toner through a small-bore tube, an aerosol of toner particles is created. An aerosol is a suspension of small liquid or solid particles in a gaseous medium. Aerosol particles have random movement. It has been found that a conventional paint spray gun will produce satisfactory aerosols from dry powders. Agglomeration of toner into unacceptably large particles is prevented because of the turbulent flow produced when the aerosol passes through the small-bore nozzle.

Figure 23–13 Powder-cloud development chamber

The electric charge on the toner particles is produced by friction between the toner and the wall of the nozzle. This process is called triboelectrification (from the Greek "tribein," meaning "to rub"), or contact electrification. Charging particles by contact electrification involves complex processes, and a discussion of the physics involved is beyond the scope of this text. Toner particles with both a positive and a negative charge are produced in roughly equal numbers, and it is possible to attract either the positive or negative particles to the surface of the selenium. "Positive" developing involves attracting negatively charged toner particles to the remaining positive charge on the surface of the selenium.

The Development Process

Xeroradiographic development consists of attracting the charged toner particles to the configuration of residual positive electrostatic charges on the selenium surface. The plate containing the electrostatic latent image is clamped onto the top of a powder cloud chamber (Fig. 23–13), and toner is introduced into the chamber as an aerosol. Diffusion air is also introduced into the chamber to create air turbulence. The toner cloud contains both positive and negatize particles of pigmented thermoplastic, but particles of only one polarity are used to form the image. To get a "positive" image a positive voltage is applied to the aluminum backing of the plate to attract only negatively charged toner. It is necessary to use this positive voltage applied to the plate back (termed the back-bias voltage) to attract negatively charged toner particles close enough to the plate to allow the electrostatic forces of the latent image to act on the toner. There are now two electrostatic forces influencing the motion of the particles: the uniform electric field of the back-bias voltage, and the non-uniform field due to the latent image. For typical positive development the back-bias potential is +1,750 volts DC. Conversely, a "negative" image can be produced by ap-plying a negative bias voltage to the back, −2,750 volts DC is a typical value, and attracting positive toner to the plate. This is done by moving one switch in the development processor. In the positive mode, positive toner particles are repelled by the positive potential on the plate and are directed to the grounded bottom of the powder cloud chamber.

We must now examine what happens to the negatively charged toner particles (all examples will be for positive development) as they approach the surface of the selenium in the region of an image representing a high contrast edge. For example, we might consider a step wedge image in which an abrupt change in charge on the selenium surface of 100 volts is produced (e.g. +900 vs. +1,000 volts) by the abrupt change in x-ray exposure at one step. Examination of this high contrast edge will help in understanding the concepts of edge enhancement and deletion. **Edge enhancement** arises from the electric field pattern associated with any abrupt change in charge density on the surface of the plate. The negatively charged toner particle in the powder cloud moves toward the plate under the influence of both the back-bias voltage and the latent image electric field. Although a uniform flow of toner approaches the plate, the electrostatic latent image electric field will cause significant change in "flow" as toner gets very near (i.e., 100 microns) the plate surface. Near an abrupt step in charge the electrostatic lines of force actually form closed loops, and charged toner particles moving along these lines of force are thrown toward the side of highest charge and excluded from the other side. The increase in toner deposited on the more highly charged side of the edge will be at the expense of toner deposition on the lower charge side. At some distance from the edge, in either direction, the influence of the edge gradient is greatly diminished and the uniform back-bias field dominates to cause more even deposition of toner.

Deletions can also be explained in terms

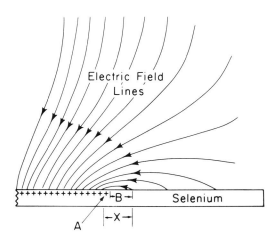

Electric Field Lines

Selenium

A |-B-| |-x-|

Figure 23-14 Deletions are caused by electric field lines of force

of the electric field distribution. In Figure 23-14 it can be seen that if toner particles strictly followed the lines of force, no toner would be deposited in the region marked "X." However, air turbulence in the development chamber causes some toner to break through the "shield" formed by the lines of force. But toner that does penetrate will be attracted only to the highly charged side of the edge. This causes development to occur completely to the edge of the area of higher charge (A, Fig. 23-14), but still leaves the region immediately adjacent the edge (B, Fig. 23-14) undeveloped. This undeveloped region is called a deletion. While small deletions may sometimes be desirable, a large deletion may result in loss of information in the deletion zone.

There is a relationship between edge enhancement (or edge contrast), initial xeroradiographic plate voltage, the back-bias voltage, and the size of a deletion. The size of a deletion depends upon the voltage contrast (voltage difference) at an edge, and the magnitude of the back-bias voltage. Large contrasts lead to large deletions, while increasing the bias voltage reduces deletion width. If the back-bias voltage is too high, low contrast detail in other parts of the image may be obscured. A lower

initial plate voltage will reduce overall image contrast, and this will also reduce deletion width. However, for the low contrast encountered in mammography, higher initial plate voltage is usually used.

TO REVIEW:

	CONTRAST	DELETION WIDTH
High Back-bias	Low	Small
High Plate Voltage	High	Large
High Contrast Image	High	Large
Low Contrast Image	Low	Small

The Development Electrode

The development electrode (Figure 23-13) is an electrode placed in front of the plate during powder cloud development, and given a voltage of appropriate sign (+ voltage for "positive" development) to superimpose a uniform helping field in the direction of the plate for the toner particles of desired charge. **One of the major effects of the development electrode is to cause a visible image to be developed in uniformly exposed regions of the electrostatic latent image.** Otherwise, these areas would go undeveloped. For example, use of a development electrode with xeromammography will make imaging of skin and large soft tissue areas of the breast possible. Additionally, the development electrode can be used to influence edge enhancement and the width of deletions such as surround dense breast calcifications. The developing electrode is actually a grid (series of wires) placed close (1.5 to 2.5 mm) to the surface of the plate. The potential applied to the grid is usually +500 volts DC.

We will use a specific example to explain the way in which a development electrode influences the electrostatic field of the latent image. Assume a selenium plate with an initial surface charge of +1625 volts has been exposed so that a large area (e.g. a 2 cm² area of normal dense breast tissue) retains a uniform charge of +1200 volts. Close to this large area, there is a small area (e.g. a $50\mu^2$ area under a breast calcification) in which the plate receives little x-ray exposure and retains +1500 volts

Figure 23–15   Effect of the development electrode

charge. Figure 23–15A diagrams the electric field which exists above both these areas (it is assumed that the space between these two areas has been completely discharged). Above the small area there is a strong electric field, but the electric field strength and potential have decreased significantly at a distance of 1.5 mm from the surface of the plate (we will assume that +600 volts remains). Above the broad area the electric field is weak, and the potential drop is minimal so that at 1.5 mm most of the original potential persists. The voltage above each area must fall to zero volts at the opposite side of the development chamber (this side of the chamber is grounded to keep it at zero volts potential, see Figure 23–13) but the potential drop over the small charged area is very fast near the plate while the potential over the large area drops rather evenly from the plate to the grounded development chamber bottom. To summarize: (1) the electric field strength above the small area is strong and drops rapidly with distance from the plate, and (2) the electric field strength above the large area is weak, and drops slowly. Charged toner particles approaching the surface of the plate in Figure 23–15A would be strongly attracted to the narrow area, and to the edge of the broad area, but would have little attraction to the central part of the broad area. Thus, edge enhancement and deletions would be maximal, but there would be little visualization of structures in broad areas of

relatively uniform exposure (e.g. normal breast tissue or skin).

Now let us place a development electrode 1.5 mm from the surface of the plate, and place a potential of +500 volts on the development electrode. What effect does this electrode have on the electric field above the $50\mu^2$ and the 2 cm² areas of the plate? Above the small area ($50\mu^2$), almost no effect. Above the large area (2 cm²) there will be a marked increase in strength of the electric field, shown by the increased number of lines of force drawn in Figure 23–14B. We must explain why this happens.

The electric field (E) between two parallel plates is equal to the voltage (V) divided by the distance (d) between the plates, provided d is small compared to the area of the plates:

$$E = \frac{V}{d}$$

If the distance (d) can be made smaller, the electric field (E) will increase if voltages are the same. Without the development electrode in place, the potential above the 2 cm² field falls to zero across the entire distance from the surface of the plate to the grounded bottom of the development chamber (i.e., distance "d" is large, so $\frac{V}{d}$ is small). The addition of a development electrode with a +500 volt potential, 1.5 mm from the surface of the plate will force the voltage above the 2 cm² field to drop from +1,200 to +500 volts over a small (1.5 mm) distance. This causes a large potential difference (V) to occur in a short distance (d), so the expression $\frac{V}{d}$ is now large, and the electric field (E) between the plate and development electrode has become much stronger. Conversely, the strength of the electric field above the small ($50\mu^2$) area is minimally affected because a strong electric field (E) associated with a rapid potential drop (V) existed without the development electrode being present.

The important concept is the change the development electrode has caused in the electric field above each area. The development electrode has little effect on the field near fine detail, but greatly increases the strength of the electric field over more uniformly charged areas. Properly used, **the development electrode allows satisfactory detail to be developed in broad exposure areas without sacrificing information in areas of fine detail.**

SENSITOMETRY OF THE DEVELOPED IMAGE

We have previously explored the way in which kVp affects the contrast present in the electrostatic latent image. It is now necessary to consider the characteristics of the developed optical density of the xeroradiographic print. Figure 23–16 shows developed optical density as a function of plate voltage, using positive development and a plate initially charged to +1625 volts. Notice that there is little change in developed optical density, or contrast, across the entire range of voltage in the electrostatic latent image. This provides a system with **great latitude**, in that all variations in plate voltage can be developed, but the resulting image would have so little contrast that it would be of almost no diagnostic value. More important than this total density range is the **contrast** (change in optical density) **across an image edge.** Because of the edge en-

Figure 23–16 Developed optical density as a function of plate voltage (positive development)

Figure 23–17 Densitometer scans across step edges of different voltage contrast

hancement, inherent in xeroradiography, the developed optical density on the high voltage side of the edge falls above the general density level of the plate (positive development), while the density on the low voltage side of the edge falls below the general density level. A density peak and valley exist at the edge. The perceptibility of an edge depends on the difference in optical density (contrast between the high density peak and the low density valley) that exists at an edge. This density difference is a function of the voltage contrast that exists at the edge in the electrostatic latent image, more voltage contrast resulting in greater density difference. Figure 23–17 shows examples of densitometer scans across step edges of various voltage contrasts. You will recall that it is possible to measure voltages on the selenium plate before the electrostatic latent image is developed. In Figure 23-17 the average optical density is about 0.5, and at edge gradients developed optical density falls above and below the average density. Because of edge enhancement, a voltage difference of only 1 volt across an edge can be detected in the developed image.

QUALITY OF THE XERORADIOGRAPHIC IMAGE

The quality of the developed xeroradiograph may be evaluated by its resolving power (line pairs per mm) and its modulation transfer function (MTF).

The inherent resolution of the latent image on the surface of a selenium plate is high, with resolution as high as 2000 line pairs per millimeter being reported in laboratory experiments using liquid developer. When powder cloud development is used, the size of the toner particles sets a limit on resolving power. For toner with a mean particle diameter of 5 microns, this limit is thought to be about 50 line pairs per mm. Other factors, such as the charge on the toner particles and the thickness of the selenium layer, have some influence on resolution. The inherent resolving power of both the selenium plate and the powder cloud development process are not limiting factors in resolution in the xeroradiographic image as it is used for medical diagnosis. Limitations imposed by the focal spot of the x-ray tube and patient motion are the two major factors in limiting resolving power.

The modulation transfer function of xeroradiography is quite different from that of film. Curves comparing the MTF of xeroradiography and film have been pub-

Figure 23–18   Comparison of the modulation transfer function of film and xeroradiography (similar to Kilgore, Gregg and Rao[4])

lished, and such a diagram is presented in Figure 23–18. Notice that for xeroradiography, the low spatial frequencies are poorly reproduced, while frequencies near one line pair per mm are greatly accentuated. Film has its best response at lower spatial frequencies (i.e., the less information to be recorded, the better job film can do). The upper limit of both film and xeroradiography MTF curves is about the same because this represents a limit imposed by factors other than the film or xeroradiographic plate (i.e., x-ray tube focal spot and patient motion). The unusual shape of the MTF curve of a xeroradiograph is compatible with clinical observations that large homogeneous structures, such as areas of normal dense breast tissue, are difficult to image. Stated another way, **xeroradiography may be said to exhibit enhanced fine structure contrast and subdued broad area contrast.**

Exposure Latitude

Xeroradiography exhibits broad exposure latitude compared to x-ray film exposure. Experimental data show that xeroradiography will produce satisfactory image resolution over a wider range of kVp selections than will film. Stated another way, it may be said that with xeroradiography the resolution capability is less sensitive to exposure, and a single exposure will produce good image resolution in all portions of a breast (thick and thin areas). Using film, obtaining good resolving power of the image under thin breast areas often requires a significantly different kVp than is required to produce a similar image under thick breast areas. With xeroradiography an appropriate kVp that produces satisfactory resolution in all portions of the image is more easily found. Another illustration of this concept of broad exposure latitude of xeroradiography is that objects such as blood vessels will exhibit equal contrast over wide variations in breast thickness.

IMAGE TRANSFER AND FIXING

It is necessary that the powder image on the surface of the xeroradiographic plate be transferred to paper, and fixed there to form a permanent image. An electrostatic transfer process is used. The paper is coated with a slightly deformable layer of plastic such as a low-molecular weight polyethylene material. When this paper is pushed against the powder image under relatively high pressure, the toner particles become slightly embedded in the plastic.

After development, the plate is removed from the development chamber and prepared for this transfer process by being passed over a pre-transfer corotron which has a negative charge. This negative corona loosens the attraction between toner particles and the selenium surface of the plate, and gives the toner a negative charge to prepare it for the transfer process. The plate then comes in contact with the paper over a transfer corotron and the image is transferred to the paper. The transfer corotron has a positive charge which attracts the negatively charged toner to the paper. The paper is also mechanically pressed against the powder image. After the image is transferred, the paper is peeled off the plate, and the loosely held

powder image is made into a permanent bonded image by heating the paper to a temperature of about 475° F. The heat softens the plastic coating on the paper and allows toner particles to sink into and become bonded to the plastic. The toner particles do not melt or flow. After fixing, also called fusing, the imaging portion of the xeroradiographic process is completed, and the completed image is delivered from the processor ready for viewing. With positive development, areas which received little x-ray exposure (such as dense breast calcification) will appear dark blue on the print, and areas receiving heavy x-ray exposure will appear light blue. If a charged plate is inadvertently exposed to room light and then developed (positive), the paper will be almost devoid of toner. Conversely, a charged but unexposed plate will produce a uniformly deep blue print if it is subjected to positive development.

PLATE CLEANING AND STORAGE

After transfer of the toner to paper, some toner remains on the plate surface. All toner must be removed before the plate can be used again. After the transfer process is completed, the plate is exposed to a light source (electro-luminescent strip) that reduces the bond holding residual toner to the plate. Next a preclean corotron exposes the plate to an alternating current which serves to neutralize the electrostatic forces holding toner to the plate. A cleaning brush then mechanically brushes the residual toner from the plate.

Relaxation (Plate Fatigue)

Relaxation is done to prevent faint "ghost" images from appearing (this phenomenon is sometimes called plate fatigue). Absorption of x rays in the selenium causes an alteration in the physical state of the selenium atoms that causes some photoconductivity to persist for as long as several hours after exposure. If the plate were charged for a new exposure without allowing it to rest for several hours, this residual photoconductivity would cause some discharge in the dark and create a faint "ghost" image of the previous exposure to appear when the plate was developed. This rest period can be reduced to only 2 or 3 minutes if the plate is relaxed by heating it to a temperature of 140° F for 150 seconds. The cleaned and relaxed plate is then held in the storage compartment of the conditioner module of the xeroradiographic system, at a temperature of 89° F, until needed for another exposure.

The life of a xeroradiographic plate is of the order of several thousand exposures. Exposure to x rays or light does not shorten the life span. The main cause of plate failure is physical damage caused by handling and the cleaning process.

THE AUTOMATIC XERORADIOGRAPHIC SYSTEM

Processing of a xeroradiographic plate takes place in two units which have been termed the Conditioner (prepares the plates for exposure) and the Processor. Refer to Figure 23–19, which is a diagram of these two units. Following processing, cleaned plates are stored in a box (1) in the processor unit. The box can hold as many as 6 plates. When this storage box is inserted into the input station of the conditioner, the plates are extracted one at a time and transported to the relaxing oven (2). The relaxed plates are stored in the storage unit (3) for an indefinite period of time. When a sensitized plate is needed, an empty cassette is inserted into the cassette station of the conditioner (5). This causes a plate to be removed from the storage area and passed under the charging device (4). Immediately after charging, the plate is moved into the cassette (5) and is ready for use. The conditioner requires about 15 seconds to charge a stored plate and place the plate in a cassette.

After exposure, the cassette (5) is placed in the processor where development, transfer and cleaning take place. The ex-

CONDITIONER

PROCESSOR

1. Plate storage box
2. Relaxation oven
3. Plate storage compartment
4. Plate charging
5. Cassette
6. Plate transport mechanism
7. Development chamber
8. Pre-transfer station
9. Paper storage and feeder
10. Transfer station
11. Fusing oven
12. Paper print tray
13. Pre-cleaning station
14. Plate cleaning station

Figure 23–19 Diagram of the automatic xeroradiographic processing system (modified from McMaster and Hoyt[5])

posed plate is extracted from the cassette and transported (6) to the back of the processor unit where it is sealed to the top of the development chamber (7). During development, a sheet of paper is transported from the paper storage tray (9) to the transfer station (10). The developed plate passes the pre-transfer station (8), then proceeds to the transfer station (10) where the image is transferred from the plate to the paper. The paper is then pulled away from the plate and into the fusing oven (11) where the image is fixed to form a permanent image. The paper then proceeds to the output tray (12). At the same time the paper is being processed, the plate passes through the precleaning (13) and cleaning (14) stations. The clean plates may be stored in the storage box (1) until 6 plates have accumulated, or transferred back to the conditioner before the box is full. The processor is able to produce a completed print in about 2 minutes. In many processors it is possible to begin transport of a plate to the developing chamber while another plate is in the transfer and cleaning areas, thus speeding the rate of processing of multiple plates.

The front of the conditioner of the Xerox 125 conditioner has a control knob labeled "B", "C" and "D". This control changes the initial plate voltage, and corresponds to approximately 975 volts (B), 1300 volts (C), and 1625 volts (D). The "D" setting is generally used in xeromammography because high contrast is desirable.

The front of the Xerox 125 processor has two control knobs, labeled "Mode" and "Density". The Mode knob determines whether a positive or negative print is obtained. The density knob is used only with the negative mode, and determines the number of bursts of powder which will be introduced into the development chamber during plate development. The stations on the density knob are labeled "B", "C", and "D", and correspond to 10 (B), 18 (C) and 26 (D) powder bursts. In the positive mode, development is accomplished with 10 powder bursts.

PATIENT EXPOSURE FROM FILM AND XERORADIOGRAPHIC MAMMOGRAPHY

A comparison of patient exposure during mammography using industrial film (Kodak AA), the DuPont Lo-Dose system and xeroradiography has been reported.[6]

The Du-Pont Lo-Dose System, introduced in 1973, consists of a single-emulsion film and a high definition intensifying screen packed in a vacuum cassette. Both film systems were exposed using a molybdenum target x-ray tube, and the xeroradiographic plates were exposed using both a molybdenum tube and a tungsten-target tube (three phase generator). Average exposure, in Rads per view for each system using a molybdenum tube was:

AA film (30 kVp)	10.1	(range 3.5–16.8)
Lo-Dose (30 kVp)	1.3	(range 0.2– 5.0)
Xeroradiography (38 kVp)	5.6	(range 1.2–11.2)

Using a tungsten tube, average xeroradiography exposures were:

Cephalo-caudad	2.7	(range 2.2–3.6)
Lateral	3.0	(range 2.2–3.6)

SUMMARY

The summary is contained in the beginning of this chapter under the heading "General Principles."

Xeroradiography is a radiographic method which has imaging characteristics which are different than those of film and include:
1. Edge enhancement
2. Subdued broad area response
3. Deletions
4. Broad exposure latitude

This system is useful for imaging low contrast objects defined by sharp edges. Because of subdued broad area response and edge enhancement, object latitude is large and a single image can contain useful information over a wide range of object thicknesses.

REFERENCES

1. Boag, J. W.: Xeroradiography. Phys. Med. Biol., *18*, 3, 1973.
2. ————: Electrostatic Imaging. AAPM Summerschool. The Expanding Role of the Diagnostic Radiologic Physicist, 1975, p. 159.
3. Dessaver, J. H., and Clark, H. E.: *Xerography and Related Processes*. London: Focal Press., 1965.

4. Kilgore, R. A., Gregg, E. C., and Rao, P. S.: Transfer Functions for Xeroradiographs and Electronic Image Enhancement Systems. Opt. Engr. *13*, 130, 1974.
5. McMaster, R. C., and Hoyt, H. L.: Xeroradiography in the 1970's. Mater. Eval. *29*, 265, 1971.
6. Rothenberg, L. N., Kirch, R. L. A., and Snyder, R. E.: Patient Exposures from Film and Xeroradio-graphic Mammographic Techniques. Radiol. *117*, 701, 1975.
7. Thourson, T. L.: Xeroradiography. Proc. Soc. of Photo-optical Eng. *56*, 225, 1974.
8. Wolfe, J. N.: *Xeroradiography of the Breast*, Springfield: Charles C Thomas. 1972, pp. 3–17.
9. Xerox Corporation Training Manual, Chapter III, Principles of Xeroradiography.

CHAPTER 24

Computed Tomography

At the Annual Congress of the British Institute of Radiology, in April of 1972, Mr. G. N. Hounsfield, a senior research scientist at EMI Limited in Middlesex, England, announced the invention of a revolutionary new imaging technique, which he called computerized axial transverse scanning.[6] The basic concept was quite simple, a thin cross section of the head, a tomographic slice, was examined from multiple angles with a pencil-like x-ray beam. The transmitted radiation was counted by a scintillation detector, fed into a computer for analysis by a mathematical algorithm, and reconstructed as a tomographic image. The image had a remarkable characteristic, one never before seen in an x-ray image—it demonstrated a radiographic difference in the various soft tissues—blood clots, gray matter, white matter, cerebrospinal fluid, tumors, and cerebral edema all appeared as separate entities. The soft tissues could no longer be assigned the physical characteristics of water. The computer had changed that concept.

Computed tomography has had many names, each referring to at least one aspect of the technique. Some of the more popular names are as follows:

1. Computerized axial tomography (CAT)
2. Computer aided tomography (CAT)
3. Computerized transverse axial tomography (CTAT)
4. Reconstructive tomography (RT)
5. Computed transmission tomography (CTT)
6. Computed (computerized) tomography (CT)

Computed (computerized) tomography (CT) is currently the preferred name and the one which we will use in this text.

Like most great discoveries, computed tomography (CT) was the end product of years of work by numerous investigators. An Austrian mathematician, J. Radon, working with gravitational theory, proved in 1917 that a two- or three-dimensional object could be reproduced from an infinite set of all of its projections.[17] Thus, the mathematical concept was established 55 years before the production of a commercial CT scanner. Workers in several unrelated fields (electron microscopy, astronomy, optics, etc.) were all struggling with a similar problem. In 1956, R. N. Bracewell, working in radioastronomy, constructed a solar map from ray projections.[1] W. H. Oldendorf[16] (1961) and A. M. Cormack[3] (1963) understood the concept of computed tomography and built laboratory models, but both lacked either the foresight or resources to develop a production unit. D. E. Kuhl[8] (1968) built a successful mechanical scanner for nuclear imaging, but he did not extend his work into diagnostic radiology. It remained for Hounsfield to put a CT system together and demonstrate its remarkable ability.

The field of computed tomography is changing more rapidly than any other area in radiology. Numerous companies have built, or are building models to compete with the EMI-Scanner. The hardware and computer programs are changing from day to day. These constant changes make it difficult to describe computed tomography in a way that will still be meaningful after several years. The description is made more difficult by the fact that the mathematical principles are beyond the knowledge of the authors and scope of this text. To avoid the problem of constant change, we will use the one unit that will never change, the original EMI-Scanner as the

prototype to describe the basic principle. By necessity, the discussion of the software, or mathematics, will be exceedingly superficial.

BASIC PRINCIPLE

The basic principle behind computed tomography is that **the internal structure of an object can be reconstructed from multiple projections of the object.** The principle is illustrated in Figure 24–1. The object (A) is made up of multiple square blocks, five of which have been removed to form a central cross. Projections could be obtained by passing an x-ray beam through the blocks and measuring the transmitted radiation. However, for the sake of simplicity, we will represent the ray projections by the number of blocks in each row. The horizontal sums (called ray

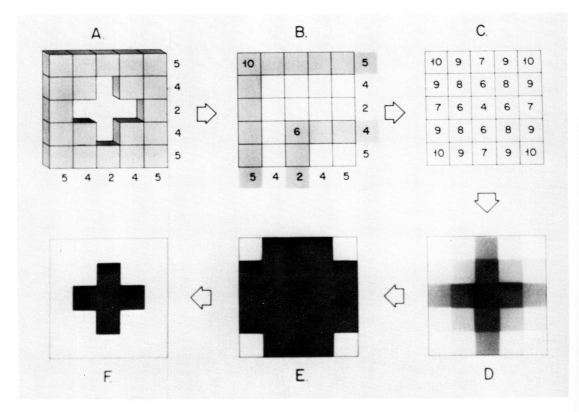

Figure 24–1　The basic principle of computed tomography

projections) are shown on the right, while the vertical ray sums are shown below the object. All of the horizontal and vertical ray sums are added, like the two shown in B, to produce a numerical reconstruction of the object (C). The numbers included in the reconstruction are 4, 6, 7, 8, 9, and 10. A gray scale value is then assigned to the numbers to produce an image like the one shown in D. The image can be manipulated to highlight certain areas, i.e. contrast can be adjusted. For example, the gray scale can be narrowed to include only black and white, and applied at any point along the numerical sequence. In E, the scale is centered at the 9–10 level. Blocks with the number 10 are white and all other blocks are black. A perfect reproduction is achieved in F by centering the black-white scale at the 6–7 level.

In x-ray computed tomography the method of forming the ray projections is different than in our illustration, and the number of projections and picture elements is much greater, but the principle is exactly the same. The ray projections are formed by scanning a thin cross section of the body with a narrow x-ray beam and measuring the transmitted radiation with a sensitive radiation detector, the same as the ones used to detect the disintegrations of radionuclides. The detector does not form the image. It merely adds up the energy in all of the transmitted photons. The numerical data from multiple ray sums are then computer processed to reconstruct an image.

DATA ACCUMULATION

Data gathering techniques have progressed through four distinct stages, called generations, in the first 5 years of clinical CT scanning. In a human society, a generation lasts between 20 and 30 years, and the younger generations tend to care for their elders. Computed tomographic units reproduce much more rapidly than humans, and younger generations have little regard for their elders. Each new genera-

tion of scanner has pushed the older generations into relative obsolescence. In view of the staggering cost of CT scanners, this is a frightening situation. Obviously, future designs must be engineered for easy updating to accommodate technological advances. Before going through the various generations, the original EMI-Scanner will be used as the prototype to show how data are accumulated.

The Original EMI-Scanner

The original EMI-Scanner was designed specifically for evaluation of the brain. In this unit, the head was enclosed in a water bath between the x-ray tube above and a pair of detectors below, as shown in Figure 24–2. A third, a reference detector, intercepted a portion of the beam before it reached the patient. A rigid scanner gantry maintained the relative position of the

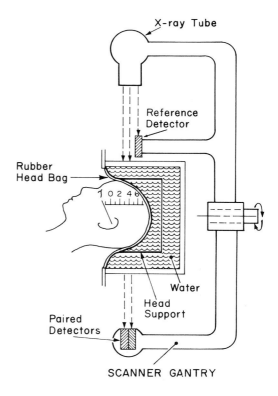

Figure 24–2 The scanner gantry

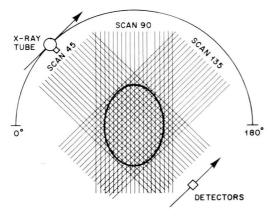

Figure 24–3 First generation scanner (the original EMI unit)

x-ray tube and detectors and assured their proper alignment. The x-ray beam was collimated to the exact size of the two side-by-side detectors.

The patient remained in one position throughout the scan. The gantry moved through two different types of motion, one linear and the other rotary, as shown in Figure 24–3. The linear motion was repeated over-and-over 180 times. Between each of these 180 linear movements, the gantry rotated one degree. Thus, the total rotary motion encompassed a 180° semicircle. The axis of rotation passed through the center of the patient's head. In Figure 24–3, the linear motions are called "scans." Only 3 of the 180 linear motions are shown, i.e. numbers 45, 90 and 135. The x-ray beam was "on" throughout the linear movement and "off" during the rotary movements. The transmitted radiation was measured 160 times during each linear movement. The total number of transmission measurements was the product of the number of linear measurements (160) and rotary steps (180), which was 28,800 in the original EMI-Scanner. The total scan time was between 4.5 and 5 minutes. Each scan pass simultaneously examined two tomographic sections, one for each of the paired detec-

tors. Multiple tomographic sections were required for most patients, frequently as many as 10. Each pair of tomographic sections took 5 minutes, so the total scan time for a clinical study was approximately 25 minutes (5 minutes × $^{10}/_2$ tomographic sections), plus a few minutes to reposition the patient in the gantry between sections.

The x-ray tube and paired detectors moved continuously and in unison during the linear scanning movement. They did not stop for the 160 transmission readings. The transmission readings represented a composite of the absorption characteristics of all of the elements in the path of the beam. In the original EMI-Scanner, the CT image was reconstructed and then displayed on an 80 × 80 matrix in two different formats: a paper printout of CT numbers and a visual image on a cathode ray tube. The CT numbers were proportional to the linear attenuation coefficient. They will be discussed in more detail later. Each square in the image matrix was called a **pixel** and it represented a tiny elongated block of tissue which was called a **voxel.** Figure 24–4 shows the sizes of the x-ray field (A), distance between transmission

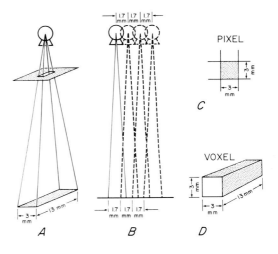

Figure 24–4 Comparison of the width of the x-ray beam (A) distance between detectors (B), pixel size (C), and voxel size (D) of the original EMI-Scanner

readings (B) and sizes of the pixel and voxel for the original EMI-Scanner. The x-ray field (A) was collimated to 3 × 13 mm (the actual length was 26 mm, which produced two parallel slices per scan, one for each of the paired detectors). This field moved across the 27-cm wide water bath making 160 transmission measurements, one every 1.7 mm (270 mm ÷ 160). The data from these measurements were computer processed and presented in multiple little squares (pixels), each representing 3 × 3 mm of patient cross section. The CT number for each pixel represented the average attenuation coefficient for all of the elements in a block of tissue (voxel) 3 × 3 × 13 mm in size. The size of the pixel was determined by the computer program and not by the dimensions of the x-ray beam. The same transmission data could be computer processed for any pixel size. With a modified program, the original EMI data could be displayed with either 1.5 or 3 mm pixels. The length of the voxel, 13 mm in Figure 24–4, was determined by the width of the x-ray beam. This dimension could not be changed once the transmission data had been collected. It could only be changed by recollimating the x-ray beam and repeating the scan.

An oil-cooled stationary anode tube was used in the original EMI-Scanner. Its nominal focal spot size was 2.25 × 12 mm. The tube was operated by a three phase generator at 120 kVp and 33 mA. The x-ray beam was heavily filtered with a half value layer of 6 mm of aluminum (0.22 mm of copper).[9] The mean, or effective energy of the 120 kVp beam when it reached the detectors, was 70 keV.[14] Beam size was restricted by a pair of slit-like collimators, one near the·tube and the other near the detectors. The detectors were sodium iodide scintillation crystals coupled to photomultiplier tubes. The reference detector furnished an exposure factor to compensate for moment-to-moment variations in x-ray output.

A large difference in attenuation between adjacent areas, such as air surrounding the head, makes computations more difficult, so the patient's head was incorporated into a box-like water bath in the original EMI unit to ease data analysis within the computer. A slip ring between the rubber head cap and water bath allowed the bath to rotate independently of the head.

Scanning Motions

Like human generations, CT generations are not accurately defined. The most agreed upon standard is probably the type of motion that is used to gather the transmission readings. At the present time, the fall of 1977, four generations are already clearly defined and a fifth generation is in its planning stages.

1. **First Generation.** The original EMI unit was a first generation scanner. It employed a pencil-like x-ray beam and a single detector, that is one detector per tomographic section. The x-ray tube-detector movements were both linear and rotary.

2. **Second Generation.** One of the major objectives of second generation scanners, and all later generations, was to shorten the scanning time for each tomographic section. Faster scanning times facilitate patient handling and improve equipment utilization. If a CT unit is sufficiently fast, a whole scan can be accomplished while the patient holds his breath, a necessity for body scanning, where respiratory motion tends to destroy image quality. The increased speed was accomplished by abandoning the single detector and pencil beam of the original EMI-Scanner and adopting a fan-shaped beam and multiple detectors like the ones shown in Figures 24–5, 6 and 7. The fan beam is a cross between a conventional x-ray beam and the pencil beam of the original EMI unit. As viewed from the side, the fan beam looks like a conventional x-ray beam. In the other view, parallel to the page in the illustration, the beam is

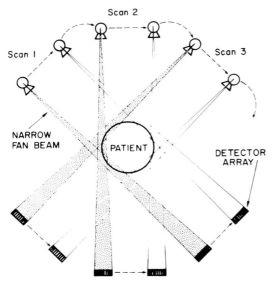

Figure 24–5   Second generation scanner

graphic section in between 10 and 90 seconds, depending upon the manufacturer.

3. **Third Generation.** Third generation scanners employ a much wider fan beam and many more detectors than a second generation unit. A typical configuration for a third generation scanner is shown in Figure 24–6. The fan beam is wide enough to encompass the entire width of the patient. The number of detectors may be in the 300 range (quite variable with different manufacturers). In the illustration, the x-ray beam is shown in three different positions, but the gantry actually rotates

collimated to the width of the detectors so it actually has the shape of an open fan.

Figure 24–5 shows the physical makeup and the movements of a typical second generation scanner. The number of detectors in the fan beam array varies from one manufacturer to another. Only a few detectors are shown in the illustration, but there may be as many as 30. The movements of the x-ray tube-detector array are both linear and rotary, just like a first generation scanner, but the rotary steps are larger. The 30 detectors gather more data per linear scan, so fewer linear movements are needed to gather an adequate data base. Instead of moving 1° at the end of each linear scan, the gantry rotates through a greater arc, up to 30°, and the process is repeated at greater than 1° intervals. The number of repetitions is determined by the number of detectors in the detector array. With 30 detectors, the linear movements only have to be repeated 6 times rather than the 180 linear movements of the original EMI unit. Second generation scanners produce a tomo-

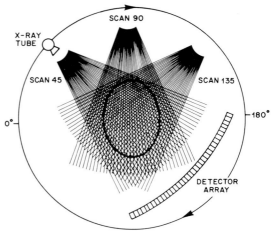

Figure 24–6   Third generation scanner

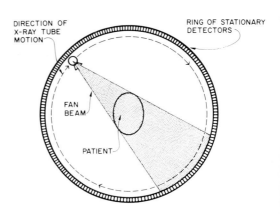

Figure 24–7   Fourth generation scanner

through a complete 360° circular movement. There are no linear-type movements with third generation scanners. Each rotation completes one tomographic section. The scanning gantry does not stop to make readings. The gantry moves continuously, and the computer program is designed to compensate for this movement. Scan times for third generation scanners range from 2 to 10 seconds.

4. **Fourth Generation.** Figure 24–7 shows the configuration of a fourth generation scanner. A ring of detectors completely surrounds the patient. Only the x-ray tube moves and the detectors remain stationary. The tube rotates through a 360° arc with a wide fan beam. As the fan beam revolves, it activates the detectors that fall in its path. Fourth generation scanners are no faster than third generation units. Their major advantage is easier detector calibration, a subject that we will discuss later.

At the present time, the fall of 1977, the fastest scan times are around 2 seconds. This represents a reduction in time by a factor of over 100, from 4 to 5 minutes in 1972 to 2 seconds in 1977. If the next five years are as fruitful, then CT scan times will be the same as the exposure times used in conventional radiography. However, this seems unlikely with current units because of the massive size of the scanning gantry. Future progress will more likely come from a fifth generation scanner, probably one with multiple x-ray tubes surrounding the patient. A scanner of this type will have no moving parts. The x-ray tubes will be fired sequentially at a ring of fixed detectors, and tomographic sections will be completed in a few milliseconds.

The advantage of a fan beam-multiple detector array is speed. Obviously, multiple detectors can gather data faster than a single detector. One of the principal disadvantages of the fan beam is an increased amount of scattered radiation. At the high energies used for computed tomography, usually 120 kVp, Compton scattering is a

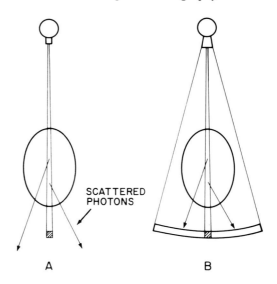

Figure 24–8   Pencil beam scanner (A) is less likely to record scattered radiation than fan beam scanner (B)

common basic interaction. The total number of Compton reactions is nearly the same for pencil beam and fan beam scanners, but the scattered photons are more likely to be recorded by a fan beam unit. Figure 24–8 shows the comparison diagrammatically. In A, two scattered photons are generated by a narrow pencil beam, but both miss the detector and go unrecognized. In B, the same two scattered photons, generated from the same volume of tissue, strike a detector and are recorded as noise. The problem of scatter radiation is exaggerated by the illustration for two reasons. First, the likelihood of a photon striking the detectors depends upon the solid angle between the point of origin of the scatter radiation and the detectors. The scattered photons shown in the illustration may have been scattered into, or out of the page, and thus they would go undetected. Secondly, the detectors in a fan beam array have their own individual collimators. Most scattered photons are absorbed by these collimators.

X-ray Tubes

Ideally, the radiation source for computed tomography would supply a monochromatic x-ray beam, i.e. one made up of photons all having the same wavelength. With a monochromatic beam, image reconstruction is simpler and more accurate. Early experimental models used radionuclides to supply such a beam, but radiation intensities were too low to be clinically useful. Conventional x-ray tubes are being used in all commercial scanners at the present time. Earlier models used oil cooled, fixed anode, relatively large (2 × 16 mm) focal spot tubes at energies of about 120 kilovolts (constant potential)[12] and 30 mA. The beam was heavily filtered to remove low energy photons and increase the mean energy of the radiation.

Most of the newer fan beam units have a diagnostic-type x-ray tube with a rotating anode and a much smaller focal spot, in some units down to 0.6 mm, and generate x rays in short bursts, or pulses. These tubes are air cooled and operate at much higher currents, up to 600 mA. They are oriented in the gantry with their long axis (cathode-anode) perpendicular to the fan beam to avoid asymmetry in x-ray output because of the heel effect. In a third generation scanner, more than 300 separate radiation pulses may be delivered during the circular motion required to produce one tomographic section. The tube moves continuously, even though the radiation is pulsed. The computer is programmed to compensate for the motion. Each pulse lasts 2 to 3 msec, so the tube is actually producing radiation for a little less than 1 sec for each scan (3 msec/pulse × 300 pulses = 0.9 sec). With a 5-sec scan time, the actual exposure occupies approximately 20% of the total time. The advantages of a pulsed system are:

1. Much larger quantities of radiation can be delivered in a short time, so scan times are less.
2. Smaller focal spots allow much more accurate collimation, which results in lower patient exposures, especially with multiple slices (discussed in more detail later).
3. The electronic circuitry can be recalibrated between pulses so that x-ray output is more accurately controlled.
4. The pulse length can be accurately regulated to optimize counting statistics and detector response.

Collimators

The x-ray beam is collimated at two points, one close to the x-ray tube and the other at the detector(s). Perfect alignment between the two is essential. The collimator at the detector is the sole means of controlling scatter radiation. Each detector has its own collimator. The collimators also regulate the thickness of the tomographic section, i.e. the voxel length. Most units employ section thicknesses of 3 to 13 mm. Some have provisions for variable thickness, for example, in the original EMI-Scanner you could select a section thickness of either 8 or 13 mm. Pixel size is determined by the computer program and not the collimator. The computer can use the input data to print out an image on any size matrix.

Detectors

The CT detectors measure the energy deposited in them. As you will recall from Chapter 5, the energy in a beam is the product of the number and energy of the individual photons. The detectors are the same as those used to detect radionuclide scintillations. Radionuclide detectors are usually "gated" to detect only a narrow range of photon energies. More, or less energetic photons, those falling outside of the gate, are ignored. When all primary photons have the same energy (a monochromatic beam), gating is an excellent way of discriminating against (ignoring) scatter radiation, since the scattered photons are all less energetic than the primary photons. However, gating is impractical for CT detectors. To begin with, the beam is heterochromatic (polychromatic), so it contains a whole spectrum of energies, and the gate would have to be quite wide. Secondly, photons only lose a small amount of energy during a Compton scattering in the CT energy range. A 75 keV photon, which is near the mean energy of most CT beams, only loses 0.7 keV when it undergoes a 30° scattering. At 74.3 keV it would still fall within the gate and would be erroneously recorded as a primary photon. Consequently, the detector collimator is used as the sole means of controlling scatter radiation. The tube collimator decreases the overall size of the scattering medium and thus the number of scattered photons. The detector collimator eliminates most of the small residuum.

Characteristics of Detectors

The most important characteristics of detectors are their cost, efficiency, stability and responsiveness.[12]

1. **Cost.** Detector costs are a major reason for the high cost of CT scanners, especially fan beam units which may have as many as 600 detectors.

2. **Efficiency.** Efficiency refers to the percentage of the energy absorbed from the beam. Ideally, detector efficiency should be 100%. Then the entire beam would be captured, which would improve counting statistics and minimize patient exposures. Later we will see that the computer must correct for the heterochromatic nature of the beam. The correction is more difficult with less than 100% efficiency, because many of the higher energy photons go through the sensor undetected.

3. **Stability.** Stability refers to the consistency and reproducibility of detector response from moment to moment. Detectors are constantly recalibrated to insure their stability. In first generation linear scanners, detectors are calibrated at the end of each linear run, or 180 times for each tomographic section. Second genera-

tion scanners are also calibrated at the end of each linear movement. Third generation scanners may only be calibrated once per day, so detector stability is much more important with these units. When the response of one third generation detector strays from the norm, ring-like artifacts are produced in the tomographic image. Fourth generation scanners are calibrated twice during one rotation: first along the leading edge of the moving fan beam and later along the trailing edge.

4. **Responsiveness.** Response time refers to the length of time it takes for a detector to receive, record and discard a signal. A detector should respond instantaneously to a signal and then just as quickly discard that signal and be ready for the next one. Afterglow, or phosphorescence after the signal has passed, is a serious problem with some detectors. It is most pronounced when an unattenuated portion of the beam strikes the detector. The water bath was incorporated into the original EMI-Scanner to cope with this problem.

Other desirable features are a linear response over a wide range of beam intensities and energy levels, freedom from noise and a compact size.

Types of Detectors

Two types of detectors are currently being used in CT scanners: scintillation crystals coupled to photomultiplier tubes and gas filled ionization chambers. Figure

Figure 24–9 Scintillation crystal-photomultiplier tube detector

24-9 shows a scintillation crystal-photomultiplier type detector. The crystal in the illustration is sodium iodide, which we will use as a prototype. When a scintillation crystal absorbs an x-ray photon, the interaction produces light (a scintillation). The amount of light is proportional to the energy of the x-ray photon, i.e. high energy photons produce more light than low energy photons. The surface of the scintillation crystal is coated with a highly reflective material so that most of the light from a scintillation eventually reaches the immediately adjacent photomultiplier tube.

We described photomultipliers in Chapter 3 (page 44) so we will only briefly review them at this time. A photomultiplier tube consists of an evacuated glass envelope containing an anode, cathode and several intermediate electrodes called dynodes. The cathode is coated with a photoemissive surface, so it is called a photocathode. When the photoemissive surface is struck by light from the scintillation crystal, the surface emits electrons in numbers proportional to the intensity of the light. The electrons are called photoelectrons, but they are no different than any other electrons, the "photo" simply referring to the manner in which they were liberated. The dynodes are coated with a material that emits secondary electrons when struck by another electron. The first dynode has a higher voltage (-2 in the illustration) than the photocathode and each subsequent dynode has a higher voltage (less negative) than the one preceding it. Thus, electrons are propagated down the tube in a step-wise fashion from one dynode to another. At each step the number of electrons is multiplied. Only a single light photon and photoelectron are shown in the illustration, but the actual numbers are much greater. Many light photons are produced with each scintillation and each light photon produces one or more photoelectrons. Only three dynodes are shown, but there may be as many as ten. At each dynode the number

of electrons is multiplied and the degree of multiplication is the same for every electron. Therefore, the strength of the output signal (an electric current) is proportional to the strength of the input signal (light from scintillations), but the output signal is greatly amplified.

The principal advantage of scintillation crystal detectors is their efficiency. A 2.5-cm thick sodium iodide crystal is almost 100% efficient in the diagnostic energy range. However, sodium iodide crystals have an important disadvantage. The disadvantage is afterglow, or phosphorescence, after encountering high radiation intensities. Afterglow is an especially serious problem in scanners that do not have a water bath surrounding the patient. In fact, sodium iodide detectors cannot be used without a water bath. Because of this problem with afterglow, two other crystals are now being used by some CT manufacturers: **calcium fluoride** and **bismuth germinate.** These two crystals do not have the afterglow problems of sodium iodide. Calcium fluoride is a little less efficient (62% for a 2.5-cm and 86% for a 5-cm crystal at 70 keV) than sodium iodide. Bismuth germinate combines the desirable features of high efficiency and no afterglow. All scintillation crystal-photomultiplier detectors have a non-linear response for different radiation intensities. This limits the range of x-ray intensities over which they can be used.

The second type of radiation detector, a **gas filled ionization chamber,** is shown in Figure 24-10. It is much simpler than a scintillation type detector. An ionization chamber has only two electrodes, an anode and a cathode. The cathode is plated onto the inner wall of the chamber. The anode is a wire running through the center of the chamber. Gas molecules in the chamber are ionized by interactions with the x-ray beam. The ions are then attracted to the appropriate electrodes by a voltage between the electrodes. The magnitude of the voltage is adjusted so that the number

COLLIMATOR   PROPORTIONAL COUNTER

Figure 24–10   Gas filled ionization chamber detector

of ionizations is proportionate to the intensity of the x-ray beam. The voltage is not as high as that of a Geiger counter. The voltage in a Geiger counter is high enough to produce an avalanche effect, i.e. the ions from one interaction acquire enough energy as they move towards the electrodes to produce other ionizations and completely discharge the chamber. The voltage in CT ionization chambers is accurately adjusted so that the resultant current is proportional to the energy of the absorbed x rays.

The principal disadvantage of ionization chambers is their inefficiency. Because of the relatively low density of gases, compared to solids, many x-ray photons pass through the chamber undetected. This problem is at least partially overcome in three ways: (1) by using xenon, the heaviest of the inert gases; (2) by compressing the xenon to 25 atmospheres to increase its density; and (3) by using a long chamber to increase the number of molecules along the path of the beam. The voltage between the electrodes must be high enough to instantaneously remove

ion pairs before they can recombine and be lost to the detector system. The principal advantage of gas detectors is a linear response unaffected by changes in beam intensity (no afterglow) over a wide range of energies. They are also easier to manufacture in small sizes. The disadvantages of gas chambers are reduced efficiency and some problems with stability.

IMAGE RECONSTRUCTION

In computed tomography a cross-sectional layer of the body is divided into many tiny blocks like the ones shown in Figure 24–11 and then each block is assigned a number proportional to the degree that the block attenuated the x-ray beam. The individual blocks are called voxels. Their composition and thickness, along with the quality of the beam, determine the degree of attenuation. The linear attenuation coefficient (μ) is used to quantitate attenuation. The mathematics are really quite simple. We will start by describing the simplest case—a single block of homogeneous tissue (an isolated voxel) and a monochromatic beam of x rays:

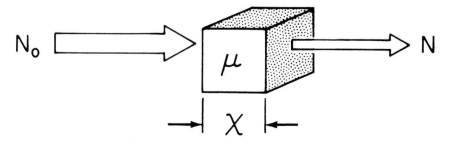

**TISSUE SECTION
REPRESENTED IN
COMPUTER MATRIX**

Figure 24–11   The tissue section represented in the computer matrix

The value of μ, the linear attenuation coefficient, can be calculated with the equation for exponential attenuation which was described earlier in Chapter 5.

$$N = N_0 e^{-\mu x}$$

In this equation, e is the base of the natural logarithm (2.718). The number of initial photons (N_0), transmitted photons (N) and thickness' (x) can all be measured. The linear attenuation coefficient (μ) is the only unknown in the equation.

If two blocks of tissue with different linear attenuation coefficients are placed in the path of the beam, the problem immediately becomes more complex:

Now the equation has two unknowns, μ_1 and μ_2, and it is written as follows:

$$N = N_0 e^{-(\mu_1 + \mu_2)x}$$

The values of μ_1 and μ_2 cannot be determined without additional information. At least one additional equation is required, and the equation must contain the same two unknowns. Additional equations can be obtained by examining the blocks from different directions. In this case, we will also increase the number of blocks in our example to four, so that each reading represents the composite of two blocks:

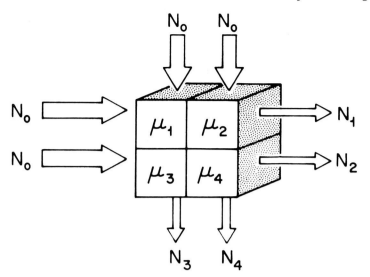

We have gone from two to four unknowns, but we can now construct four different equations as follows:

$$N_1 = N_0 e^{-(\mu_1 + \mu_2)x}$$
$$N_2 = N_0 e^{-(\mu_3 + \mu_4)x}$$
$$N_3 = N_0 e^{-(\mu_1 + \mu_3)x}$$
$$N_4 = N_0 e^{-(\mu_2 + \mu_4)x}$$

This array looks formidable, but the equations can all be simultaneously solved for the value of the linear attenuation coefficient with the aid of a computer. Exactly the same principle applies to computed tomography, but the number of unknowns is much larger. For example, in the original EMI-Scanner, the matrix in the computer contained 80 × 80 or 6,400 separate picture elements. Each transmission measurement records the composite of 80 separate linear attenuation coefficients:

To solve this equation, we must have transmission readings taken from at least two different directions just as we did for the simple example above. The number of separate equations and unknowns now becomes 6,400. The original EMI unit took 28,800 readings (160 linear readings × 180°) and a fan beam scanner may take as many as 90,000 readings (300 pulses ×300 detectors). An equation, like the one shown above, can be reconstructed for each of these readings. Even though Radon understood the mathematical principles in 1917, he could not put his knowledge to practical use. The mathematics were so tediously long that before computers it would have taken years to construct a single image.

Two correction factors are incorporated into the CT program. The first is a correc-

The equation is longer and looks more awesome, but it has exactly the same format.

$$N = N_0 e^{-(\mu_1 + \mu_2 + \mu_3 + \dots \mu_{80})x}$$

tion for the heterochromatic (polychromatic) nature of the beam. As heterochromatic radiation passes through an absorber, filtration increases its mean energy. The linear attenuation coefficient changes with energy as shown in Figure 24–12. The illustration compares the linear attenuation coefficients of water for 70 keV monochromatic and 120 kVp hetero-

chromatic beams. The initial mean energy of the heterochromatic beam is 70 keV. The monochromatic linear attenuation coefficient (μ) is constant, but the heterochromatic μ strays down on the graph as filtration increases its mean energy from 70 to 75 keV. The CT program must be written to compensate for this stray and bring the calculated μ back to a straight line.

The second program correction is a weighting factor to compensate for the differences between the size and shape of the scanning beam and the picture matrix. Figure 24–13 shows the problem geometrically. In A, the parallel rays of a linear type scanning motion exactly coincide with the size and square shape of the picture elements. In B, the scanning rays cross the picture elements obliquely. A weighting factor (WF) is used to compensate for the difference in size between the actual elements and that seen by the beam. In these examples, the weighting factor would be 1 in A and less than 1 in B.

Figure 24–12 The linear attenuation coefficient of a heterochromatic beam decreases as filtration increases its mean energy

Figure 24–13 When only a portion of a pixel is included in the scanning beam, a weighting factor (WF) is used in the mathematical reconstruction

Algorithms for Image Reconstruction

An algorithm is a mathematical method for solving a problem. Thousands of equations must be solved to determine the linear attenuation coefficients of all of the pixels in the image matrix. Several different methods, or algorithms are in current use. They all attempt to solve the equations as rapidly as possible without compromising accuracy. The original EMI-Scanner took 4 to 5 minutes to process the data for a single CT section. This long processing time seriously limited the number of patients that could be handled in a working day. More recent algorithms are much faster and can display a picture immediately after the tomographic section is completed. We have tried to make the discussion more pictorial than mathematical, since the actual mathematics go beyond the intended scope of this text. Most of our description of mathematical principles is taken from an excellent article by Brooks and DeChiro that appeared in Radiology in December of 1975.[2] The following three mathematical methods of image reconstruction are described:

1. Back-projection
2. Iterative methods
3. Analytical methods

The object of all of the methods is to produce an accurate cross-sectional display of the linear attenuation coefficients of each element in the image matrix.

Back-Projection

Back-projection, sometimes called the summation method, is the oldest means of

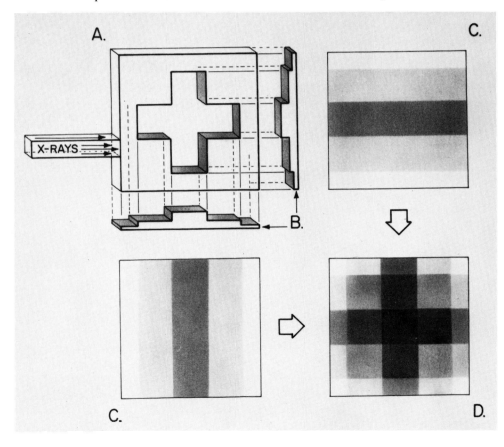

Figure 24–14   Image reconstruction by back-projection

image reconstruction. None of the commercial CT scanners use back-projection, but it is the simplest method to describe so we will use it as a prototype. The principle is shown schematically in Figure 24–14. The illustration demonstrates a two-dimensional reconstruction of a cross cut from the center of a solid block. The block is scanned (A) from both the top and left sides by a moving x-ray beam to produce the image profile shown in B. The image profiles look like steps. The height of the steps is proportional to the amount of radiation that passed through the block. The center transmitted the most radiation, so it is the highest step in the image profile. The steps are then assigned to a gray scale density which is proportional to their height. These densities are arranged in rows, called rays, as shown in C. The width of the rays is the same as the width of the steps in the profile. In the illustration, the ray length is equal to the height of the original object, but in an actual clinical situation, where the image was displayed on a television monitor, these heights and

widths could be any convenient size. When the rays from the two projections are superimposed, or back-projected (D), they produce a crude reproduction of the original object. In practice, many more projections would be added to improve image quality, but the principle is the same.

All points in the back-projected image receive density contributions from neighboring structures. The result of these contributions is dramatized in Figure 24–15. The black dot in A represents a radiodense material, such as a drop of Pantopaque. The radiodense material severely attenuates the beam and produces localized spikes in the image profiles. Back-projection of the rays from these spikes produces a star pattern like the one shown in B. A great number of projections will obscure the star pattern, but the background density remains as noise to deteriorate the quality of the CT image.

Iterative Methods

An iterative reconstruction starts with an assumption, for example, that all points in

Figure 24–15   Star pattern from back-projection of a dense object

the matrix have the same value, and compares this assumption with measured values, makes corrections to bring the two into agreement, and then repeats the process over and over until the assumed and measured values are the same or within acceptable limits. There are three variations of iterative reconstructions depending upon whether the correction sequence involves the whole matrix, one ray or a single point.

1. **Simultaneous reconstruction.** All projections for the entire matrix are calculated at the beginning of the iteration, and all corrections are made simultaneously for each iteration.

2. **Ray-by-ray correction.** One ray sum is calculated and corrected, and these corrections are incorporated into future ray sums, the process being repeated for every ray in each iteration.

3. **Point-by-point correction.** The calculations and corrections are made for all rays passing through one point and these corrections are embodied in ensuing calculations, again the process being repeated for every point.

Figure 24–16 illustrates a ray-by-ray iterative reconstruction for a four element square. Horizontal, vertical and diagonal ray sums are shown in the adjacent blocks. In the first step, the two horizontal ray sums (16 and 6 in the hatched blocks) are divided equally among the two elements in the ray. If the ray sums had represented ten elements, the sum would have been

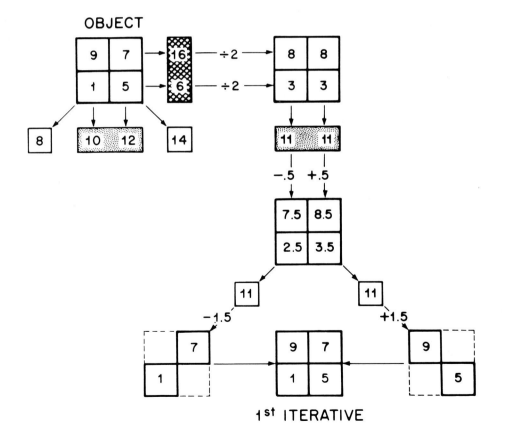

Figure 24–16 Iterative ray-by-ray reconstruction of a four element object

divided equally among all ten elements. Next, the new numbers in the vertical row are added to produce the new ray sums (11 and 11 in the shaded blocks) and compared with the original measured ray sums (also in shaded blocks). The difference between the original and new ray sums ($10 - 11 = -1$ and $12 - 11 = +1$) is divided by the number of elements in the ray ($-1 \div 2 = -.5$ and $+1 \div 2 = +.5$). These differences are algebraically added to each element ($8 - .5 = 7.5$, $3 - .5 = 2.5$, $8 + .5 = 8.5$ and $3 + .5 = 3.5$). The process is repeated for diagonal ray sums to complete the first iteration. In this example, the first iteration produces a perfect reconstruction. With more complex data, iterations may have to be repeated six to twelve times to reach an acceptable level of agreement between the calculated and measured values. The first 80 × 80 matrix EMI-Scanner used an iterative reconstruction, but most manufacturers are now using one of the analytical methods.

Analytical Methods

Analytical algorithms differ from iterative methods in that exact formulas are utilized for the analytical reconstructions. These formulas are frighteningly complex to most radiologists, although mathematicians say they are really quite simple. We will only attempt a pictorial explanation of the two popular analytic methods, which are two-dimensional Fourier analysis and filtered back-projection.

Two-Dimensional Fourier Analysis. The basis of Fourier analysis is that any function of time or space can be represented by the sum of various frequencies and amplitude of sine and cosine waves. Figure 24–17 shows three functions, i.e. projections of a phantom skull containing bone, air and calcium. The ray projections are shown with squared edges, which is the most difficult wave form to reproduce. The actual projected images would be more rounded than those shown, which would simplify a Fourier reconstruction.

Figure 24–17 Projection of a skull phantom

Figure 24–18 shows progressively improving Fourier reconstructions. A single cosine wave of the appropriate height (amplitude) and length (frequency) makes a first approximation of the square wave and each subsequent addition improves the reproduction. The last reconstruction represents the sum of eight cosine waves, but only the first four steps are shown. This type of mathematical manipulation is easily and quickly processed in a computer. The reconstruction is a little more complex for a two-dimensional image such as a CT section, but the basic principle is the same.

Filtered Back-Projection. Filtered back-projection is similar to back-projection except that the image is filtered, or modified to exactly counterbalance the effect of sudden density changes, which causes blurring (the star pattern) in simple back-projection. The projected information is filtered much like light is filtered by a polarizing lens. Certain frequencies are eliminated, those responsible for blurring, in order to enhance more desirable frequencies. Figure 24–19 is a two-dimensional filtered back-projection of a square object. The density of the projected rays is adjusted to compensate for the star effect,

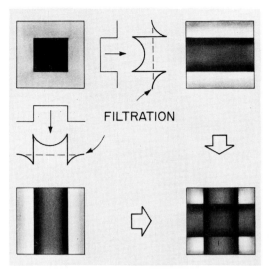

Figure 24–19 Filtered back-projection of a square object

Figure 24–18 Fourier reconstruction of a square wave form. (Courtesy of Robert C. Murry, M.S., University of Texas Health Science Center at Dallas)

i.e. the inside margins of dense areas are enhanced while the centers and immediately adjacent areas are repressed. The net effect is an image more closely resembling the original object than could have been achieved with back-projection alone. Image quality is further improved with each additional projection. Most computed tomographic units are using a Fourier reconstruction or filtered back-projection.

Comparison of Mathematical Methods

No general agreement exists as to which mathematical method is superior, and indeed, a system's superiority under one set of circumstances may disappear under new circumstances. In terms of speed, analytical reconstructions are clearly faster than iterative methods. A projection can be processed immediately after recording, so the entire reconstruction can be displayed seconds after completion of the last projection. Iterative reconstructions may take several minutes to process after scan completion. Both methods are equally accurate if the projection data are complete. With incomplete data, i.e. insufficient to fully determine the image, iterative methods are superior. Analytical methods must do time-consuming interpolations to fill in missing data, while iterative methods simply average adjacent points. Thus, with incomplete data, analytical methods are slowed while iterative methods are actually made faster than they would be with complete data.

CT Numbers

Ideally, linear attenuation coefficient calculations should be precisely correct, both in absolute value and in relative value from pixel to pixel. Computers are designed for maximum relative accuracy, which is the more important of the two for imaging purposes. The relative accuracy of the original EMI-Scanner was 1 part in 200, or ±0.5%. As we shall see later, the degree of accuracy is limited primarily by patient exposure and pixel size, and not by equipment design. Therefore, accuracy is approximately the same in the newer generations of scanners as it was in the original EMI unit.

After the CT computer calculates a relative linear attenuation coefficient for each pixel, the number is normalized to a reference material (water), magnified to a larger whole number (integer) and reported as a new number, called a CT number. The densest body tissue, compact bone, and least dense body tissue, air, are assigned the values of +1 and −1, times a magnifying constant. The size of this constant was 500 in the original EMI-Scanner, but it could be any number large enough to express the accuracy of the scanner in whole numbers. Since the original EMI accuracy was 1 part in 200, a magnifying constant of 500 left a generous margin for technical improvements. Nevertheless, some of the newer units have an even more expanded scale employing a magnifying constant of 1000. The mathematical manipulations involved in the derivation of a CT number are shown in the following equation:

$$\text{CT Number} = K \frac{\mu_p - \mu_w}{\mu_w}$$

K = magnifying constant
μ_p = linear attenuation coefficient of pixel in question
μ_w = linear attenuation coefficient of water

You can see from this equation that the CT number of water is 0, regardless of the size of the magnifying constant. With a mag-

Table 24–1. CT Numbers and Linear Attenuation Coefficients for Various Body Tissues with a Magnifying Constant of 500 (120 kVp—effective 70 keV)

ABSORBER	CT NUMBER	LINEAR ATTEN. COEF. (cm⁻¹)*
Bone (dense)	+500	0.380
Intracranial soft tissues	+25 to +5	0.200 to 0.192
Water	0	0.190
Fat	−50	0.171
Air	−500	0

*These linear attenuation coefficients were calculated from the CT numbers, except for water, which was taken to be 0.190

nifying constant of 500, the CT number of dense bone is +500 and air is −500. All other tissues are intermediate in value as shown in Table 24–1. The computer will print out the CT numbers for any, or all elements in the matrix, upon request. Knowing the magnifying constant of the computer, the linear attenuation coefficient can be calculated from the above equation. Magnifying the scale does not improve the accuracy of a scanner. An accuracy of 1 part in 200 (±0.5%) is ±2.5 CT numbers with a magnifying constant of 500 and ±5 CT numbers with a magnifying constant of 1000. All three of these plus-or-minus numbers represent exactly the same degree of accuracy.

Image Display

A CT image can be displayed in two basic modes: (1) As a paper printout of CT numbers, or (2) as a gray scale image on a cathode ray tube or television monitor (Figure 24–20). The paper printout is time consuming and is used primarily to evaluate scanner performance, and not as an imaging method. Figure 24–21 shows the type of gray scale that is used to construct the visual image. The CT num-

Figure 24–20 Gray scale CT television image (Courtesy of Kenneth R. Maravilla, M.D., University of Texas Health Science Center at Dallas)

bers in the illustration are for a unit with a magnification constant of 500. At full scale, dense bone with a CT number of +500 is assigned a gray scale level of peak white and air at −500 the level of black. The contrast difference between the intermediate structures, like brain and cerebrospinal fluid, may be too small to demonstrate at full scale, because the CT numbers of these structures are so close together. However, the contrast of the video image can be adjusted to augment minor differences in specific areas, the one capability which sets CT apart from every other radiographic imaging technique.

As a general rule, conventional roentgenograms cannot show a density difference of less than 10%. The CT numbers for intracranial soft tissues range from +5 to +25 (Table 24–1), a total of 20 CT

Figure 24–21 EMI gray scale display with adjustable window width and level

numbers on a scale of 500. This represents a difference between the least dense and most dense of 4% (20 ÷ 500 = 0.04 × 100% = 4%). This difference can be demonstrated by coning down to a narrow portion of the CT scale as shown in Figure 24–21. In the illustration, the gray scale is adjusted so that the CT numbers between −5 and +55, a total of 60 numbers, covers the whole range of gray from black to white. Viewed in this way, −5 and all lower numbers are black, while +55 and all higher numbers are white. The result is greatly increased contrast within the preselected range. In this example, the contrast difference betweeen the most dense and the least dense intracranial soft tissue structures changes from 4% to 33% (20 ÷ 60 = .33 × 100% = 33%). The range of CT numbers that is selected for gray scale amplification is called the window width (60 CT numbers in Figure 24–21). Window width can be adjusted in various increments from full scale to a single unit. The size and number of the increments is determined by the manufacturer. For example, the options on a theoretical unit may include the following window widths: 1, 8, 16, 32, 64, 128, 256, 512. The operator could select one of these widths and center it to a specific level, called the window level. In the example shown in Figure 24–21, the window level is +25 (halfway between −5 and +55). When the window width is set at 1, all points in the image matrix are either black or white.

IMAGE QUALITY

Image quality is not accurately defined for computed tomography. We will attempt to use the same terms and definitions described in Chapter 13 for the radiographic image. Image quality (clarity) is the visibility of diagnostically important structures in the CT image. The factors that affect quality are all interrelated, so when we discuss one, we will frequently refer to the others. The more important factors are defined below under three separate headings:

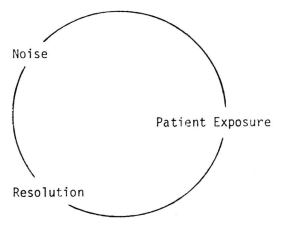

These three factors are intimately tied together, but we will discuss them separately. All of the other factors affecting image quality will be included under these three headings.

Quantum Mottle (Precision–Noise)

Precision in computed tomography is a measure of background, or matrix uniformity. If a perfectly homogeneous object like a water bath is examined with a CT scanner, all elements in the picture matrix should have exactly the same CT number. Deviations from uniformity represent statistical fluctuations, which is called quantum mottle. We will use the terms quantum mottle and noise interchangeably. **A lack of precision, or the presence of mottle, is the limiting factor in CT performance at the present time.** The number of photons for each ray projection is precariously close to the statistical limit of acceptability for an intracranial scan where subject contrast is minimal. Figure 24–22 shows anticipated statistical fluctuations as a function of the number of counts in a ray projection. Counts of 100, 1000, 10,000 and 100,000 are shown as paired bar graphs, each bar in the pair representing one standard deviation above and

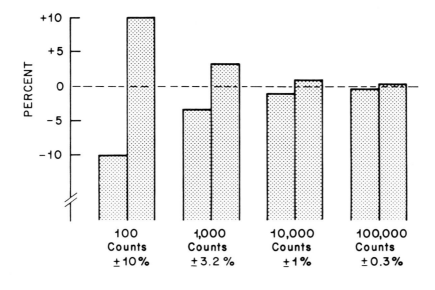

Figure 24–22   Decreasing statistical fluctuations with increasing count rates

below the anticipated value. The counts are normalized to demonstrate the decrease in percent fluctuation. At 100 counts, the statistical fluctuation is ±10%, or from 90 to 110 counts. As the number of counts increases, the percent fluctuation decreases. At 10,000 counts, one standard deviation is 100 counts ($10,000^{\frac{1}{2}} = 100$), which is a percentage fluctuation of ±1% ($100 \div 10,000 = 1\%$). The advertised accuracy of the original EMI-Scanner is ±0.5%. With a 4.5 minute scan time, approximately 100,000 photons[13] were recorded for each ray in the projection. The illustration shows a statistical fluctuation of ±0.3% at 100,000 counts, which is consistent with the claims of the manufacturer. However, if the number of counts is decreased to any significant degree, there must be a concomitant decrease in precision and increase in mottle.

Precision cannot be improved by a more accurate mathematical reconstruction. In fact, mottle becomes more visible as the accuracy of the reconstruction improves. This principle is shown diagrammatically in Figure 24–23, a bar graph similar to the one shown earlier in Figure 24–22. The

heights of the shaded bars depict the actual number of counts in two adjacent ray projections of a water phantom. Since the phantom is homogeneous, the difference in the counts between the two bars represents noise (statistical fluctuations). Employing an iterative algorithm, after the first iteration, the two bars are almost the same height, and if the image were displayed at this time, the noise would be smoothed out and the image would appear quite homogeneous. Each iteration more closely approximates the reconstructed image to the original data, until finally after many iterations, the two are nearly identical. The image will then show the noise more accurately than the earlier reconstruction. **Most of the noise in current CT images is from statistical fluctuations and not related to the mathematical reconstruction.**

The number of counts per picture element is determined by numerous factors including the quantity and quality of the x-ray beam, the number and efficiency of the detectors, the amount of absorber in the path of the beam, the number and volume of the picture element, and the scan

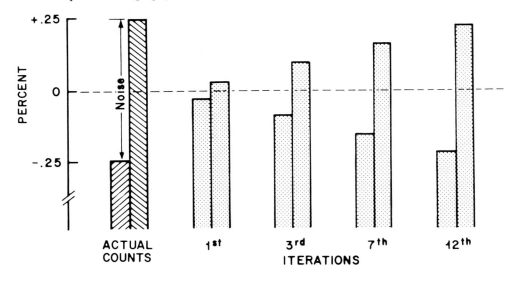

Figure 24–23   Accurate reconstructions bring out statistical fluctuations (noise)

time. Motion has a devastating effect on image quality in computed tomography, so shorter scan times are a noble objective, especially in body work where respiratory motion is a problem. However, for any given scanner and voxel size, scan times can only be shortened at the expense of precision. When high quality images are essential, scan times may have to be lengthened to produce a statistically more accurate reconstruction.

Counting statistics are intimately related to voxel size. **A voxel is a volume element, as opposed to a pixel which is a picture element.** A pixel is a flat surface without thickness. The image is displayed on a television monitor as thousands of tiny pixels, each representing a specific tiny cross-sectional area in the patient. The stated size of a pixel, i.e. 3 × 3 mm, refers to their size in the patient. Their actual size in a video image is determined by the size of the television monitor. A given size pixel will appear larger on a large TV monitor than it would on a smaller monitor, but in both cases it would represent the same size area in the patient. A voxel adds the third dimension to the area represented by the

pixel, so the voxel is a volume element. A 1 mm square pixel might represent a 5 or 10 mm thick section; the first would be a 5 mm³ and the second a 10 mm³ voxel. Diminishing voxel size decreases the number of counts per each element, assuming that other factors remain constant. Table 24–2 shows the size of some EMI voxels with volume factors and patient exposure factors normalized to the original 3 × 3 mm pixel (80 × 80 matrix) and the 13-mm thick section of the original EMI-Scanner. Assuming that the counting statistics (precision) are kept constant, the superior resolution of the smallest size (18 mm³) voxel can only be realized with a 6.4 fold increase in patient exposure. An important point to keep in mind when selecting techniques is that precision is better (and noise is less) with an 80 × 80 matrix than with a 160 × 160 matrix for any given patient exposure.

Matrix size, field size and pixel size are all interrelated as shown in Figure 24–24. Matrix size is the number of points in a picture matrix, for example, 6,400 (80 × 80) in A and 25,600 (160 × 160) in both B and C. The name **matrix size** is firmly

Table 24–2. Relationship Between Voxel Size and Patient Exposure

VOXEL SIZE (mm)	VOLUME (mm³)	VOLUME FACTOR	PATIENT EXPOSURE FACTOR*
3 × 3 × 13	117	1.0	1.0
3 × 3 × 8	72	.62	1.6
1.5 × 1.5 × 13	29.3	.25	4.0
1.5 × 1.5 × 8	18	.15	6.4

*For comparable counting statistics

Figure 24–24   Comparison of field size (×, 2×), matrix size (80 × 80, 160 × 160) and pixel size (1.5 mm, 3 mm)

entrenched in the CT literature, but it is a confusing name, since the "size" refers to the size of a unitless number and not a physical size. **Field size** (× and 2× in the illustration) refers to the outside dimensions of the CT slice, for example 27 × 27 cm in the original EMI-Scanner. Field size dictates the maximum size anatomic part that can be examined. In the illustration, the smaller field size shown in A and B might be used for head scans, while the larger size in C could accommodate a larger part and might be used for body scans. Note that the matrix size is the same in B and C and the pixel size is the same in A and C.

Continuing with Figure 24–24, if exactly the same precision (counting statistics) was required for the pixel in all three blocks, the patient exposure would have to be increased four times in going from the 80 × 80 to either of the 160 × 160 matrices, since there are four times as many pixels in the larger matrix. As we shall discuss next, resolution is a function of pixel size. With equal exposures per voxel, resolution would be better in B than in A because the pixels are smaller in B. Resolution would be equal in both A and C, because both have the same size pixels.

Resolution

Resolution, pixel size, quantum mottle and subject contrast are so intimately tied

Figure 24–25   Resolution improves with a large matrix (smaller pixels)

together that it is difficult to talk about one without referring to the other three. **With high subject contrast and good precision, resolution is approximately 1½ times pixel size,**[10] i.e., a 3 × 3-mm pixel should be capable of resolving objects with a diameter of 4.5 mm. Figure 24–25 demonstrates the effect of pixel size on resolution. In A, the letters EMI are displayed on a 32 × 32 matrix (1024 pixels). The large M is easily seen but the smaller E and I cannot be recognized. With the 80 × 80 matrix (6400 pixels) shown in B, the quality of all of the images improves, but the images of the smaller E and I improve more than the image of the large M. The unobtainable goal is shown in C, a matrix with an infinite (∞) number of points. Pixel size determines resolution for high contrast objects, so theoretically, image quality improves with a large matrix, i.e. smaller pixels.

Perhaps high contrast should be more accurately defined. In computed tomography, the difference between plexiglass and water is considered high contrast and their linear attenuation coefficients differ by approximately 12% at an effective energy of 70 keV.[8] With this sort of contrast, resolution is pixel size limited. The differences between air and water, or water and bone are enormous by CT standards. For example, a tiny fleck of calcium in a pineal gland, a fleck too small to be seen on a radiograph, may be easily seen on a CT scan. **The calculated linear attenuation coefficient for a pixel is a weighted average of all materials in the pixel.** Photoelectric attenuation is so much greater for calcium than for water, that a small amount of calcium weights the average towards the higher linear attenuation coefficient of calcium. With even a small amount of calcium, a whole picture element appears white. This effect is called **partial volume averaging.** The predominance of calcium over water has a deleterious effect on imaging in some circumstances. Figure 24–26 shows how the skull can obscure large areas of brain, especially in the more superficial cuts

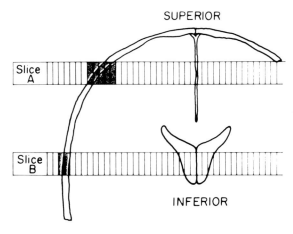

Figure 24–26   Apparent increase in skull thickness when a slice (A) cuts the bone obliquely

where the tomographic slice traverses the calvarium obliquely. In slice A, 5 picture elements contain bone (shaded pixels) while only 2 contain bone in slice B. In the shaded area the brain is hidden from view by the calvarium.

Low contrast resolution, or perhaps visibility is a better term, is more dependent upon noise and object size than on pixel size. **The more homogeneous the background, the better the visibility of low contrast images.** The noiser the background, the larger the low contrast image must be before it can be detected. The only way that resolution can be improved for low contrast objects is with better counting statistics which produces a more homogeneous background. Low contrast resolution is studied quantitatively by comparing two plastics, such as lexan and plexiglass, whose linear attenuation coefficients differ by approximately 1%.[10] At this level of subject contrast, resolution is limited to objects 6 to 10 mm in diameter. With a 1 cm object, a subject contrast of 1% and a fixed patient exposure, visibility may be better with 3-mm pixels than it is with 1.5-mm pixels because the counting statistics are better with the larger pixels. The comparison is shown diagrammatically in Figure 24–27. The illustration represents a portion of a CT matrix, uniformly radiated to 10,000 counts per unit element (i.e. small squares). The number of counts in the smaller squares will vary statistically by 1%. This is the same percentage as the subject contrast and the object will be obscured in this noisy background. With the larger pixels, the statistical fluctuation is only 0.5%, and the 1% subject contrast should be visible against this more uniform background.

Low contrast resolution can be improved if subject contrast is enhanced. Some iodine-containing compounds are preferentially concentrated in certain tissues of the brain. Since iodine has a much higher atomic number than elements normally found in the brain, even small traces sig-

Figure 24–27   Statistical fluctuations are less with larger pixels

nificantly enhance contrast in selected areas. It is now common practice to intravenously inject iodinated compounds as part of a routine CT brain scan study.

Spatial Uniformity

Spatial uniformity refers to the accuracy of readings over one area of the matrix relative to another area. The count rate for a perfectly uniform object (water phantom) should be the same over all areas of the matrix. Breaks in uniformity can be detected by plotting the counts for a single line as shown in Figure 24–28. The arrow in A shows the matrix line plotted in B. With good spatial uniformity (B) almost all of the points fall within ±2 standard deviations (S.D.). The plot from a scanner with

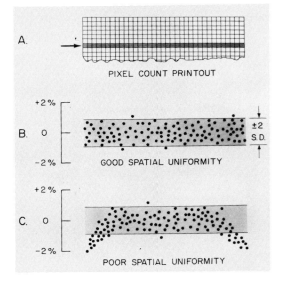

Figure 24–28 Spatial uniformity (Modified from E. C. McCullough and J. T. Payne[10])

poor spatial uniformity is shown in C. Counts fall below 2 S.D. at the margins of the field. Non-uniformity can be caused by beam hardening, detector flaws (non-linearity or afterglow) or a poor mathematical reconstruction.

Size Adjustability

The original EMI-Scanner was designed specifically for head work, a wise decision, since the head could be easily immobilized, did not undergo any significant physiologic motion (like breathing) and was reasonably small. The next step was to build a unit with a larger format, adaptable to any area of the body. Ideally, pixel size, field size, section thickness, matrix size and speed (scanning times) should all be independently adjustable. Then a radiologist could select the precision (noise) and resolution (pixel size) needed to cope with a clinical situation.

PATIENT EXPOSURE

One of the more pleasant surprises with the original EMI-Scanner was the relatively small patient exposure. The radiation dose to the skin for a complete head examination (3 scans, or 6 slices at 4.5 minutes per scan) was 1.6 rads maximum and 1.0 rads mean.[4] Exposures were higher than this for a 3 or 4 film standard radiographic examination where the volume of irradiated tissue was also larger.

Theoretically, each small increment of tissue in a CT scan is exposed only during the time that the slice containing the increment is being tomogrammed. At other times, the increment is exposed only to scatter radiation, which is minimal because of the narrow beam. Since the scan fields do not overlap, the absorbed doses are not compounded. This theory is only partially true. Many CT units have relatively large focal spots and as a result, prepatient collimation cannot sharply delineate the margins of the beam. Adjacent slices are partially exposed to stray radiation with each scan and the cumulative dose is substantial. The exposure to the center of the head increases from 2.7 to 6.4 rads (2.4 times) in going from a 1 to a 5 slice study with an EMI-CT 5000 Scanner set at 70 sec (slow speed).[10]

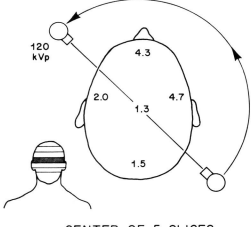

CENTER OF 5 SLICES

Figure 24–29 Radiation dose from computerized tomography (Modified from E. C. McCullough and J. T. Payne[10])

Doses are not uniform with CT scans, at least not when the gantry only rotates through 180°. The distribution from an EMI-CT 5000 is shown in Figure 24–29. The scanner is a body unit that was not designed specifically for head work. The doses are for a 10-inch field and a 20-sec (fast) scan time. The gantry in this unit only moves through a 180° arc, so the doses are much higher on the side of the head that is adjacent to the x-ray tube. The dose distribution is symmetrical with a fan beam unit that rotates through a 360° arc.

ARTIFACTS

Under artifacts, we will discuss a variety of technical problems that may arise during computed tomography. The first is a major aberration that occurs at the interface between two objects with linear attenuation coefficients differing by greater than 60%. Iterative reconstructions "undershoot" the density of soft tissues (brain and cerebrospinal fluid) at junctions with bone, producing a lucent 2- to 6-mm ring adjacent to the bone. The same phenomenon occurs at air-soft tissue interfaces (pneumocephalus) but with "overshoot," i.e. a ring of apparently greater density. The aberrations are less troublesome with a larger (160 × 160) matrix and analytical rather than iterative reconstructions.[13]

Motion Artifacts

Patient motion has a devastating effect on image quality. This was the primary reason for developing a body unit that could complete a scan during the time that a patient could hold his breath. Two types of patient motion produce artifacts. The first is a rotary, and/or back-and-forth motion in which all elements in the CT slice remain in the beam throughout the exposure, but the elements change their orientation with respect to each other. The resulting scan contains black and white vertical bands for side-to-side motion and diagonal bands for rotary motion. This type of motion artifact is not as damaging

Figure 24–30 Motion artifacts. (Courtesy of Kenneth R. Maravilla, M.D., University of Texas Health Science Center at Dallas)

to image quality as the second type in which elements move completely out of the beam for a portion of the exposure. This type motion is most devastating when high contrast objects such as bone or air move in-and-out of the beam, as shown in Figure 24–30. They are especially likely to occur in the posterior fossa because of the close proximity of the petrous pyramids.

High Density Foreign Material Artifacts

The linear attenuation coefficients of metals (tantalum clips, missiles from penetrating injuries, droplets of Pantopaque) are much higher than those of any body tissue, including bone. A small metal fragment produces a star pattern (Figure 24–31), and the star effect is accentuated by any motion. The only way to avoid the problem with current mathematical reconstructions is to change the angle of the slice to exclude the foreign body, which may also exclude a pathologic abnormality. A similar pattern is produced by gas, for example the residual of air from a ventriculogram, but the effect is less spectacular.

Figure 24–31   Star artifact from a metallic clip. (Courtesy of Kenneth R. Maravilla, M.D., University of Texas Health Science Center at Dallas)

Detector Artifacts

Artifacts from errors in detector calibrations and balance are common. The character of the artifact depends upon the design of the particular scanner. Rotating fan beam scanners produce ring artifacts similar to those shown in Figure 24–32. The illustration greatly exaggerates the problem. At the time this image was made, we were calibrating our fan beam unit by scanning a water phantom. The detectors were badly out of balance and the multiple concentric rings are the consequence of this imbalance.

Geometric Oversights

The CT tomographic slice does not have parallel sides as we have implied to this point.[5] Figure 24–33 shows the geometric configuration of an EMI slice with 2 detectors, each 13 mm in height and each recording a separate slice from a single focal spot (nominal 12 mm). The beginning of

Figure 24–32   Ring artifact from a third generation scanner. (Courtesy of Kenneth R. Maravilla, M.D., University of Texas Health Science Center at Dallas)

Figure 24–33   Configuration of the original EMI beam showing overlap (shaded) and skip areas (cross-hatched)

the scan (0°) is shown in A, the end of the scan (180°) in B, and the superimposition of the two in C. The two scan slices partially overlap (shaded area in C) and record some areas twice. The top surface of the upper slice and bottom surface of the lower slice are concave in their centers and flared at their peripheries. This configuration does not lend itself well to stacking. Consecutive slices are shown in Figure 24–33D. If scanned as drawn, the cross hatched area would be completely excluded from both slices.

SUMMARY

Computed tomography is a radiographic technique for producing cross-sectional tomographic images by first scanning a slice of tissue from multiple angles with a narrow x-ray beam, then by calculating a relative linear attenuation coefficient for the various tissue elements in the section, and finally by displaying the reconstruction as a gray scale image on a television monitor. Two basic scan patterns are used: repetitive linear scanning through a 180° arc with one or several detectors; and fan-beam scanning with a delta-shaped beam and a large array of either rotating detectors, or a stationary ring of detectors. The fan beam offers the advantage of greater speed and more uniform patient exposures, and the disadvantages of greater cost, more scatter radiation and a more complex mathematical reconstruction.

In the original EMI-Scanner, mathematical reconstructions were done with iterative methods, but now reconstructions are usually done with analytical techniques, using either two-dimensional Fourier analysis, filtered back-projection, or a combination of the two. Analytical methods start computations as soon as the first ray projection is scanned, so they are fast and the reconstruction may be completed a few seconds after all of the data are collected. The mathematical reconstruction is a display (on paper as numbers or on a cathode ray tube as a gray scale) of CT numbers, which are proportional to the linear attenuation coefficients of the tissues in the tomographic section. A relatively high energy, heavily filtered heterochromatic beam is used in all current commercial scanners, but a monochromatic beam would be superior, since the mean energy of a monochromatic beam is not affected by filtration and linear attenuation calculations would be more accurate. Transmission counts are measured on either scintillation crystal detectors which have a high counting efficiency, but suffers from non-linear response and afterglow; or pressurized xenon detectors which have a linear response and do not suffer from afterglow, but are less efficient.

Contrast levels can be adjusted to augment specific areas in the image. All CT scanners have an arbitrarily expanded scale of relative linear attenuation coefficients called CT numbers. Dense bone is assigned the highest value, air the lowest value (usually a negative number) and water a value of 0. In the original EMI-Scanner, dense bone was +500, water 0 and air −500. The difference in the linear attenuation coefficients of soft tissues, excluding fat, is about 4% with fresh blood clots among the densest and cerebrospinal fluid the least dense. This 4% difference is easily demonstrated when a normal or pathologic anatomic structure is sufficiently large and appropriately located. The most serious factor limiting image quality is statistical noise. This problem can be partially solved by increasing scan times (more radiation) and picture element (pixel) size, but both of these alternatives are objectionable. Increasing scan times increases patient exposures and increasing pixel size decreases high contrast resolution.

REFERENCES

1. Bracewell, R.N.: Strip integration in radioastronomy. Aust. J. Phys. *9,* 198, 1956.

2. Brooks, R.A., and DiChiro, G.: Theory of image reconstruction in computed tomography. Radiol. *117,* 561, 1975.

3. Cormack, A.M.: Representation of a function by its line integrals, with some radiological applications. J. Appl. Phys. *34,* 2722, 1963.

4. EMI-Scanner: A new perspective on brain tissues. EMI Limited, Middlesex, England, 1973.

5. Goodenough, D.J., Weaver, K.E., and Davis, D.O.: Potential artifacts associated with the scanning pattern of the EMI scanner. Radiol. *117,* 615, 1975.

6. Hounsfield, G.N.: Computerized transverse axial scanning (tomography). Brit. J. Radiol. *46,* 1016, 1973.

7. ———: Picture quality of computed tomography. Amer J. Roentgenol. *127,* 3, 1976.

8. Kuhl, D.E., and Edwards, R.Q.: Reorganizing data from transverse section scans of the brain using digital processing. Radiol. *91,* 975, 1968.

9. McCullough, E.C., Baker, H.L., Houser, O.W., and Reese, D.F.: An evaluation of the quantitative and radiation features of a scanning x-ray transverse axial tomography: The EMI Scanner. Radiol. *111,* 709, 1974.

10. McCullough, E.C., and Payne, J.T.: Performance evaluation: CT-scanners. Presented at the International Symposium & Course on Computerized Tomography (CT), San Juan, Puerto Rico, 1976.

11. McCullough, E.C., Payne, J.T., Baker, H.L., Hat-tery, R.R., Sheedy, P.F., Stephens, D.H., and Gedgaudus, E.: Performance evaluation and quality assurance of computed tomography scanners with illustrations from the EMI, ACTA, and Delta scanners. Radiol. *120,* 173, 1976.

12. McCullough, E.C., and Payne, J.T.: X-ray transmission computed tomography. Medical Physics *4,* 85, 1977.

13. New, P.F.T., and Scott, W.R.: *Computed Tomography of the Brain and Orbit.* Baltimore; Williams & Wilkins, 1975.

14. Phelps, M.E., Gado, M.H., and Hoffman, E.J.: Correlation of effective atomic number and electronic density with attenuation coefficients measured with polychromatic x-rays. Radiol. *117,* 585, 1975.

15. Phelps, M.E., Hoffman, E.J., and Ter-Pogossian, M.M.: Attenuation coefficients of various body tissues, fluids, and lesions at photon energies of 18 to 136 keV. Radiol. *117,* 573, 1975.

16. Oldendorf, W.H.: Isolated flying spot detection of radiodensity discontinuities displaying the lateral structural pattern of a complex object. IRE Transactions on Biomed Electronics. Vol. BMW 8, no. 1, 1961.

17. Radon, J.: Berichte uber die Verhandlungen der koniglich Sashsischen Gesellschaft der Wissenschaften zu Leipzig. Mathematisch—Physische Klasse. *69,* 262, 1917.

CHAPTER 25

Ultrasound

X rays were put to practical use the moment they were discovered, and improvements in equipment and techniques progressed rapidly during the first few years. In contrast, ultrasound has been notoriously slow in its medical evolution. The technology for producing ultrasound and the characteristics of sonic waves have been known for many years. The first major attempt at a practical application was made in the search for the sunken Titanic in the North Atlantic in 1912. The search was unsuccessful. A few early attempts at applying ultrasound in medical diagnosis met with the same fate. Techniques were not sufficiently developed, especially imaging techniques, until the mas-

sive military research effort that accompanied World War II. Sonar (**SO**und **N**avigation **A**nd **R**anging) was the first important successful application. Successful medical applications began shortly after the war in the late 1940s and early 1950s. Since then progress has been rapid, especially in the last decade with B-mode imaging and even more recently with the addition of gray scale presentations.

A simplified overview of a sonic imaging system is shown in Figure 25–1. The vital ingredients are (1) a transducer, (2) an ultrasonic beam and (3) a display method, usually a cathode ray tube (CRT) or television monitor. The transducer serves a dual function as both a transmitter and re-

Figure 25–1 An ultrasonic imaging system

ceiver. Sound is transmitted in approximately 1000 short bursts (pulses) each second. During the time interval between pulses, the transducer functions as a detector, sensing the returning echoes from the previous pulse. An operator, frequently a physician, positions the transducer on the patient, moves it about to produce the appropriate echoes over the region of interest, and simultaneously manipulates the CRT controls to optimally display the image. A permanent photographic record is made of this image. In its current state of development, the interplay between the patient, operator and instrument is much more complex than it is in diagnostic radiology, where a technician can select a technique, push a button, and have a reasonably good chance of success. Ultrasonic imaging is more of an art than x-ray imaging. The operator must have a thorough enough knowledge of anatomy to interpret the images as they appear. Then he can adjust the controls and position the transducer to show subtle abnormalities that could not be demonstrated without this interplay.

THE CHARACTERISTICS OF SOUND

A sound beam is similar to an x-ray beam in that both are waves transmitting energy. One of the more important differences is that x rays pass readily through a vacuum while sound requires a medium for its transmission. The velocity of sound depends upon the nature of the medium. A useful way to picture matter (the medium) is as a series of spherical particles, representing either atoms or molecules, separated by tiny springs as shown in Figure 25–2. When the first particle is pushed (B), it moves and compresses the attached spring exerting a force on the adjacent particle. This sets up a chain reaction, but each subsequent particle moves a little less than its neighbor. The tension, or pressure applied to the spring is greatest between the first two particles and less between any two down the line. If the driving force reverses its direction, the particles also reverse their direction. If the force vibrates to-and-fro like a cymbal, the particles respond by oscillating back-and-forth. The particles in a sound beam behave in the same manner, i.e. they oscillate back-and-forth, but over a short distance of only a few microns in liquids and even less in solids.

While the individual particles move only a few microns, you can see from Figure 25–2 that the effect of their motion is transmitted through their neighbors over a much longer distance. During the time, or almost the same time, that the first particle moves through a distance **a,** the effect of the motion is transmitted over a distance **b.** The velocity of sound is determined by the rate at which the force is transmitted from one molecule to another.

Longitudinal Waves

Ultrasonic pulses are transmitted through liquids as longitudinal waves. The molecules of the conducting liquid move

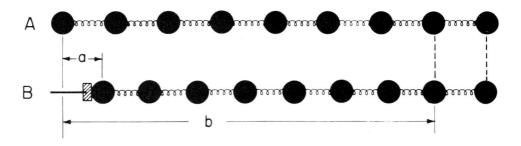

Figure 25–2   Propagation of a sound wave

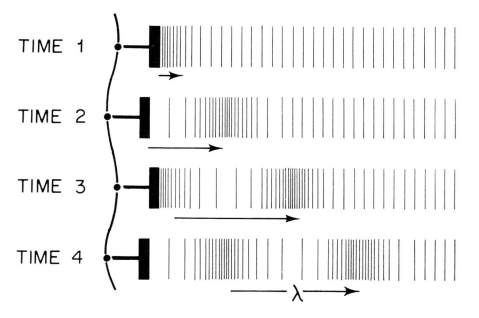

TIME 1

TIME 2

TIME 3

TIME 4

λ

Figure 25–3   Birth of a sound wave

back-and-forth producing bands of compression and rarefaction, shown diagrammatically in Figure 25–3. The wavefront starts at time 1 in the illustration when a vibrating drum compresses the adjacent material. A band of rarefaction is produced at time 2 when the drum reverses its direction. Each repetition of this back-and-forth motion is called a cycle, and each cycle produces a new wave. **The length of the wave is the distance between two bands of compression, or rarefaction**, and is represented by the symbol λ. Once the sound wave has been generated, it continues in its original direction until it is either reflected or absorbed. The motion of the vibrating drum, plotted against time, forms the sinusoidal curve shown along the left side of Figure 25–3. Ultrasound, by definition, has a frequency of greater than 20,000 cycles per second. The sonic beams used in diagnostic imaging have frequencies from 1,000,000 to 20,000,000 cycles/second. One cycle/second is called a Hertz; a million cycles/second is a megaHertz—abbreviated MHz.

The Velocity of Sound

In the medical ultrasound range, **the velocity of transmission of sound is independent of frequency and depends primarily on the physical make-up of the material through which the sound is being transmitted.** The important characteristics of the transmitting medium are its (1) compressibility and (2) density. Table 25–1 shows the velocity of sound in some common materials including several types of body tissue. The materials are listed in order of increasing speed of transmission, and you can see that sound travels slowest in gases, at intermediate velocity in liquids and most rapidly in solids. It should be noted that all body tissues, except bone, behave like liquids, and therefore they all transmit sound at about the same velocity. A velocity of 1540 meters per second is used as an average for body tissue.

Compressibility

The velocity of sound is inversely related to the compressibility of the conducting material; that is, the less compressible a material, the more rapidly it transmits sound. Sound waves move slowly in gases because the molecules are far apart and easily compressed. They behave as though they are held together by loose springs. A particle must move a relatively long distance before it can affect a neighbor. Liquids and solids are less compressible because their molecules are closer together. They need only move a short distance to affect a neighbor, so liquids and solids propagate sound more rapidly than gases.

Table 25–1. Velocity of Sound in Various Materials

MATERIAL	VELOCITY (m/sec)
Air	331
Fat	1450
Mercury	1450
Castor Oil	1500
Water (50°C)	1540
"HUMAN SOFT TISSUE"	1540
Brain	1541
Liver	1549
Kidney	1561
Blood	1570
Muscle	1585
Lens of eye	1620
Skull—bone	4080
Brass	4490
Aluminum	6400

From Wells, P. N. T.[13]

Density

Dense materials are composed of massive molecules, and these molecules have a great deal of inertia. They are difficult to move, or stop once they are moving. Since the propagation of sound involves the rhythmic starting and stopping of particulate motion, we would not expect a material made up of large molecules (i.e. large in mass), such as mercury, to transmit sound at as great a velocity as a material composed of smaller molecules, such as water. Mercury is 13.9 times denser than water, so we would expect water to conduct sound much more rapidly. Nevertheless, you can see from Table 25–1 that water and mercury transmit sound at fairly similar velocities. The apparent discrepancy is explained by the greater compressibility of water, which is 13.4 times as compressible as mercury.[3] The loss in mercury's ability to transmit sound rapidly because of its greater mass is almost exactly balanced by a gain because of its lesser compressibility. As a general rule, this same principle applies to all liquids, i.e. density and compressibility are inversely proportional. Consequently, all liquids transmit sound within a narrow range of velocities.

The relationship between wavelength and wave velocity is as follows:

$$C = f\lambda$$

C = velocity of sound in conducting media (cm/sec)

f = frequency (cycles/sec)

λ = wavelength (cm)

Figure 25–4 The wavelength of sound decreases as its frequency (MHz) increases

In the ultrasonic frequency range, the velocity of sound is constant in any particular medium. When the frequency is increased, the wavelength must decrease. This is shown diagrammatically in Figure 25–4. In A, the vibrator has a frequency of 1.5 MHz. Assuming the medium to be water which propagates sound at a velocity of 1540 m/sec (154,000 cm/sec), the wavelength will be:

$$154,000 = 1,500,000\lambda$$

$$\lambda = 0.1 \text{ cm or } 1.0 \text{ mm}$$

Therefore, 1.0 mm is as far as the wave can propagate in the time available before a new wave starts. In B, the frequency is doubled to 3.0 MHz, but the waves move away at the same velocity, so their length is halved to 0.5 mm.

Intensity

The intensity of sound, or loudness in the audible range, is determined by the length of oscillation of the particles conducting the waves. The greater the oscillations, the more intense the sound. Figure 25–5 diagrammatically illustrates high and low intensity longitudinal waves of the same frequency, wavelength and velocity. The compression bands are more compacted in the high intensity beam. The harder the vibrator is struck, the more energy it receives and the wider its vibrations. These wider excursions are transmitted to the adjacent conducting media and produce a more intense beam. In time, the vibrations diminish in intensity, although not in frequency, and the sound intensity decreases producing a lower intensity beam. Ultrasonic intensities are expressed in watts (power) per square centimeter. The mathematical expression that relates intensity to particle velocity, wave velocity and medium density is rather complex and of no practical importance in radiology, so we will not attempt to explain it in this text.

Relative Sound Intensity

Sound intensity is measured in **decibels.** A decibel is a relative unit and not an absolute one. Simply defined, a decibel (dB) is one-tenth of a bel (B). A **bel** is a comparison of the relative power of two sound beams expressed logarithmically using the base 10. For those who may have forgotten, we will briefly review logarithms. Starting with the number 10 and raising it to various positive and negative powers, we get a series of numbers as follows:

10 Raised to a Power	Corresponding Number	Log (base 10)
10^4	10,000	4
10^3	1,000	3
10^2	100	2
10^1	10	1
10^0	1	0
10^{-1}	.1	−1
10^{-2}	.01	−2
10^{-3}	.001	−3

1.5 MHz — HIGH INTENSITY — 1mm

1.5 MHz — LOW INTENSITY — 1mm

VIBRATION AMPLITUDE

Figure 25–5   Larger amplitude of vibration produces denser compression bands and a higher intensity sound

Table 25–2. Comparison of Relative Intensity, Bels, Positive and Negative Decibels, and Percent of Sound Remaining in Beam

BELS (B)	DECIBELS (dB)	RELATIVE INTENSITY	NEGATIVE DECIBELS (−dB)	PERCENT OF SOUND REMAINING IN BEAM
0	0	1	0	100
1/10	1	1.26	−1	79
2/10	2	1.59	−2	63
3/10	3	2.00	−3	50
4/10	4	2.51	−4	40
5/10	5	3.16	−5	32
6/10	6	3.98	−6	25
7/10	7	5.01	−7	19
8/10	8	6.31	−8	16
9/10	9	7.94	−9	13
1	10	10	−10	10
2	20	100	−20	1
3	30	1,000	−30	.1
4	40	10,000	−40	.01
5	50	100,000	−50	.001
6	60	1,000,000	−60	.0001

For example, 10 raised to the 4th power is 10,000. The log of 10,000 is 4. Notice that there is no zero in the center column. The log of zero is undefined. The number 10 raised to the 0 power is 1, and not 0 as one might expect at first glance.

Returning to our definition of a bel, it is a logarithmic comparison of the relative intensity of two sound beams. Table 25–2 summarizes the relationships between the bel, decibel and intensity (or power) of an ultrasonic beam. Note that increasing intensity from 1 bel to 2 bels increases relative intensity by a factor of 10. The number of decibels is obtained by multiplying the number of bels times 10. If an ultrasonic beam has an original intensity of 10 watts/cm², and the returning echo 0.001 watts/cm², their relative intensity will be:

$$\log \frac{10}{.001} = \log 10,000 = 4 \text{ bels or } 40 \text{ decibels}$$

Decibels may have either a positive or negative sign. Positive decibels indicate a gain in power, while negative decibels express a power loss. Ultrasound loses power as it passes through tissue, so in the above example, the intensity of the returning echo relative to the original beam is really a minus 40 dB. Table 25–2 shows a column of negative decibels and the percentage of sound remaining in the beam at the new decibel level. In our example, the intensity of the returning echo (−40 dB) is only 0.01% that of the original intensity.

TRANSDUCERS

The general make-up of an ultrasonic transducer is shown diagrammatically in Figure 25–6. The most important component is a thin (approximately 0.5 mm) **piezoelectric crystal** element located near the face of the transducer. The surfaces of the crystal are plated with gold or silver electrodes. The outside electrode is grounded to protect the patient from electrical shock, and its outside surface is coated with a water tight electrical in-

Figure 25–6   Ultrasound transducer

sulator. The inside electrode abuts against a thick backing block that absorbs sound waves transmitted back into the transducer. The housing is usually a strong plastic. An acoustic insulator of rubber or cork prevents the sound from passing into the housing. A large variety of sizes and shapes of transducers are available to perform specific functions, but they all have this general design.

The Characteristics of Piezoelectric Crystals

Piezoelectric materials are made up of innumerable **dipoles** arranged in a geometric pattern as shown in Figure 25–7. A dipole is a distorted molecule that appears to have a positive charge on one end and a negative charge on the other. The positive and negative ends are arranged so that an electric field will cause them to realign and thus change the dimensions of the crystal (B). The illustration shows a considerable change in thickness, but in actual practice the change is only a few microns. Notice that no current

flows through the crystal. The plating electrodes behave as capacitors and it is the voltage between them that causes the electric field, which in turn causes the crystal to change shape. If the voltage is applied in a sudden burst, or pulse, the crystal vibrates like a cymbal which has been struck a sharp blow, and generates sound waves. The backing block quickly dampens the vibrations to prime the transducer for its second function, which is to detect returning echoes.

As the sound pulse passes through the body, echoes reflect back towards the transducer from each tissue interface. These echoes carry energy and they transmit their energy to the transducer causing a physical compression of the crystal element. This compression forces the tiny dipoles to change their orientation, which induces a voltage between the electrodes. The voltage is amplified and serves as the ultrasonic signal for display on an oscilloscope or television monitor. Incidentally, the compression force and associated voltage are responsible for the name

Figure 25–7   An electric field realigns the dipoles in a piezoelectric crystal

piezoelectricity which means "pressure" electricity.

Some naturally occurring materials possess piezoelectric properties, for example, quartz, but most of the crystals used in medical ultrasound are man-made ceramics. The exact make-up of these materials is usually an industrial secret, but most are some form of barium titanate and lead zirconate titanate. Piezoelectric crystals can be designed to vibrate in either the thickness or radial mode as shown in Figure 25–8. Medical crystals are designed to vibrate in the thickness mode. However, they still vibrate to a lesser extent in the radial mode, so the receiving amplifier is gated to tune out all frequencies except those from the thickness mode.

Curie Temperature

Ceramic crystals are made up of innumerable tiny dipoles as stated above, but in order to possess piezoelectric characteristics, the dipoles must be arranged in a specific geometric configuration. To produce this polarization, the ceramic is heated to a high temperature in a strong electric field. At the high temperature, the dipoles are free to move and the electric field brings them into the desired alignment. The crystal is then gradually cooled while subjected to a constant high voltage. As room temperature is reached, the dipoles become fixed and the crystal then possesses piezoelectric properties. The Curie temperature is the temperature at which this polarization is lost. Heating a piezoelectric crystal above the Curie temperature reduces it to a useless piece of ceramic, so obviously, transducers should never be autoclaved. The approximate Curie temperatures for several crystals are as follows:

Quartz .... 570° C
Barium titanate .... 100° C
Lead zirconate titanate ...... 350° C

Resonant Frequency

The thickness of a piezoelectric crystal determines its natural frequency, which is called its resonant frequency. Crystal thickness is analogous to the length of a pipe in a pipe organ. Just as a long pipe produces a low pitch audible sound, a thick crystal produces a low frequency ultrasound. The surfaces of a piezoelectric crystal behave like two identical cymbals, facing each other but separated in an open space. When one cymbal is struck, its vibrations set up sound waves that cause the

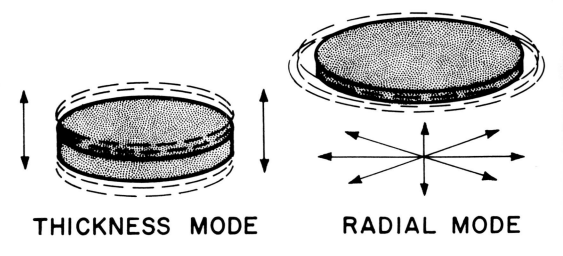

THICKNESS MODE   RADIAL MODE

Figure 25–8   Modes of vibration of a piezoelectric crystal

other cymbal to vibrate. Vibrations are maximum in the second cymbal when the space separating the two is equal to ½ of the wavelength of the sound. At this separation the sound waves from, and vibrations of, the two cymbals are exactly synchronized. The sound from one reinforces the vibrations of the other. A vibrating piezoelectric crystal transmits sound in both directions from each surface. The internally transmitted waves cross the transducer to synchronize with vibrations from the other side, just like the two cymbals in our analogy. When a crystal is struck with a single sharp voltage spike, it vibrates at its natural frequency, which is determined by its thickness. The natural frequency is that which produces internal wavelengths twice the thickness of the crystal.

A crystal can be forced to vibrate at the frequency of any alternating voltage, but the intensity of this sound is much less than it would be for a comparable voltage at the crystal's natural frequency. If the frequency of an applied alternating voltage were exactly the same as the natural frequency of the crystal, the vibrations would increase in intensity until the crystal disintegrated, like the Biblical walls of Jericho. **In medical sonography, the crystal is usually subjected to a single voltage pulse and allowed to vibrate at its natural fre-**

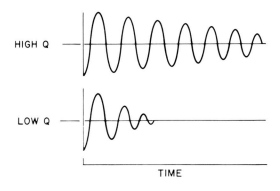

Figure 25–9 Ring down-time of a high Q and low Q transducer

quency. The fact that piezoelectric crystals have a natural frequency has considerable practical importance. With an x-ray machine, the wavelength, or kilovoltage, can be adjusted by simply turning a few dials on a control panel. We do not have this freedom with ultrasonic imaging. A frequency change requires another transducer, one designed for the desired frequency. Only a few different sizes and frequencies are needed to handle most clinical situations, which is fortunate since transducers are rather expensive.

Transducer Q-Factor

The Q-factor refers to two characteristics of piezoelectric crystals: the purity of their sound and the length of time that the sound persists. A high Q transducer produces a nearly pure sound made up of a narrow range of frequencies, while a low Q transducer produces a whole spectrum of sound covering a much wider range of frequencies. Almost all of the internal sound waves of a high Q transducer are of the appropriate wavelength to reinforce vibrations within the crystal. When an unsupported high Q crystal, i.e. a crystal without a backing block, is struck by a short voltage pulse, it vibrates for a long time producing a long continuous sound. The time interval between initiation of the wave and complete cessation of vibrations is called the ring down-time or Q-factor. Figure 25–9 shows the ring down-time for high Q and low Q crystals. The Q-factor can also be defined mathematically in terms of the purity of the sound, but we will not attempt to explain this definition.

A long continuous sound is unsatisfactory for sonic imaging. **The transducer is both a transmitter and a receiver**, but it cannot send and receive at the same time. When continuous sound is being transmitted, the associated vibrations in the crystal produce continuously fluctuating voltages between the electrodes. If the internally generated sound waves are stronger than the returning echoes, as they may be, the returning signal is lost in the noise of the system. Another reason why continuous sound is undesirable for imaging is that depth resolution is determined by the length of the sonic pulse. Depth resolution will be defined later in this chapter. The length of the sonic pulse, called the **spatial pulse length,** is the number of waves times their wavelength. The sonic pulse from an unsupported high Q crystal is long because the sound persists for a long period of time. The Q factor of a crystal can be altered by external forces, especially by the material in the backing block of the transducer. **A backing block is incorporated to quench the vibrations and shorten the sonic pulse.** If the wavelength of sound from a transducer is 0.5 mm and the pulse is quenched after two wavelengths, then the spatial pulse length is 1 mm. Ideally, the ultrasonic pulse should be a single wavelength. Backing blocks are made of a combination of tungsten and rubber powders in an epoxy resin. The ideal backing material should accept all of the sound waves that reach it, i.e. not reflect any back into the crystal, and then completely absorb the energy from these waves. As a general rule high Q crystals are more efficient transmitters and low Q crystals are more efficient receivers.

THE CHARACTERISTICS OF AN ULTRASONIC BEAM

A single vibrating point sends out waves in all directions much like those produced by a pebble thrown into a quiet pond; the waves move away from their point of origin as concentric circles. If two pebbles simultaneously land side-by-side, they each cause ring-like waves, and these waves may either reinforce or cancel each other depending on their phase when they meet. This is shown diagrammatically in Figure 25–10. At time A, two waves are approaching each other from opposite directions. At B, they are touching but not overlapping. One-half cycle later, the valley of one has reached the crest of the other and they

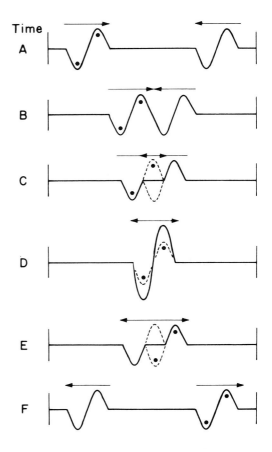

Figure 25–10 Interactions between two sound waves traveling in opposite directions

cancel each other. Another one-half cycle later at D, the crest and valleys are exactly superimposed reinforcing themselves and doubling the height and depth of the peaks and valleys. Another one-half cycle later, the waves have separated and finally go on their own way as two separate waves moving in the opposite direction.

Piezoelectric crystals behave as a series of vibrating points and not as the piston-like surface that we have implied in previous discussions. The wave fronts are not uniform, at least not close to the crystal. This is shown diagrammatically in Figure 25–11. The crystal is depicted as five vibrating points, each point producing multiple

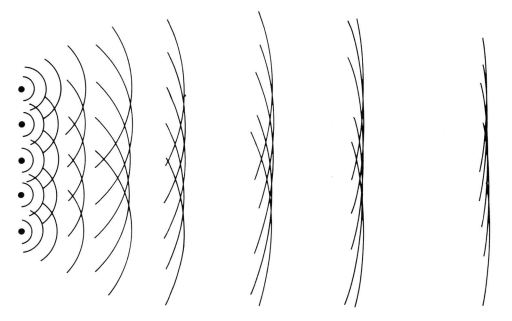

Figure 25–11   Superimposition of waves to form a wavefront

concentric rings, or waves that eventually form a continuous front as they reinforce each other along a line parallel to the face of the crystal. The distance at which the waves become synchronous depends on their wavelengths. The shorter the wavelength, the closer the front forms to the surface of the transducer.

The intensity of ultrasound varies both from one side of the beam to the other, and longitudinally along the length of the beam. Numerous ingenious methods have been employed to demonstrate these variations. The more common ones are summarized in Figure 25–12. The simplest way of depicting a beam is that shown in A, where the beam is drawn as a parallel bundle for a certain distance beyond which it disperses. The parallel component is called the near, or **Fresnel** (pronounced Fre-nel) **zone.** The diverging portion of the beam, that beyond **x′**, is called the far, or **Fraunhofer zone.** The notation **x′** is used to identify the transition point between the Fresnel and Fraunhofer zones.

Figure 25–12 B shows a schematic Schlieren photograph of a sonic beam, the same beam shown in A. When sound passes through a transparent medium, such as water, it changes the refractive index of the medium. This change can be photographed with the proper lighting arrangement. The sound in the illustration originates from four point sources. The waves from these points reinforce and cancel each other in phase: the initial four beams become three, then two, and finally a single wave front at x′, the transition zone.

Figure 25–12 C is produced by plotting the intensity of the beam along its central longitudinal axis. The plot shows the same variations in beam intensity that are shown photographically in B. The black and white areas of B appear as peaks and valleys in C.

These illustrations all describe a continuously emitted sound beam, which is a little different than the pulsed beam used for imaging. The transition from continu-

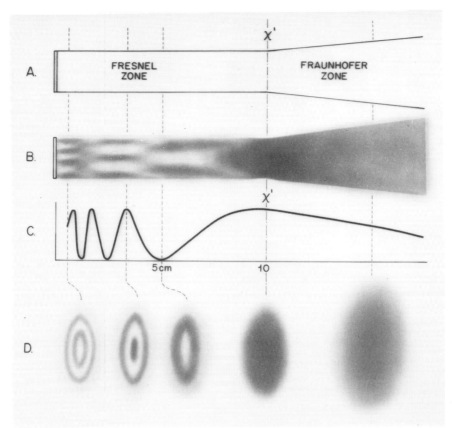

Figure 25–12   Methods of displaying a sonic beam

Table 25–3.   The Length of the Fresnel Zone for Various Size Transducers and Frequencies*

FREQUENCY MHz	LENGTH OF FRESNEL ZONE (cm)				
	DIAMETER OF TRANSDUCER (cm)				
	0.5	1.0	1.5	2.0	2.5
1.0	.37	1.6	3.4	6.5	10
1.5	.58	2.4	5.1	9.7	15
2.0	.79	3.2	6.8	13.0	20
2.5	1.01	4.0	8.5	16.0	25
5.0	2.01	8.1	17.0	32.0	50
7.5	2.97	11.9	25.0	48.0	75

*Based on a sound velocity of 1540 m/sec

ous to pulsed beams is easy to picture with the aid of Figure 25–12 D, which is a cross-sectional photographic display. The sonic pulse changes its character as it moves away from the transducer. It passes in rapid succession through each of the stages shown in the illustration. The pulse becomes homogeneous at the transition point. Beyond the transition point, the pulse remains homogeneous but increases in diameter and decreases in intensity.

The length of the Fresnel zone is determined by the diameter of the transducer, and the wavelength of the ultrasound.

$$X' = \frac{r^2}{\lambda}$$

X′ = length of the Fresnel zone (cm)
r = radius of the transducer (cm)
λ = wavelength (cm)

Table 25–3 shows the length of the Fresnel zone for various wavelengths and transducer diameters. The zone is longest with a large transducer and high frequency sound and shortest with a small transducer and low frequency sound. For those who have difficulty interpreting tables, the same type data are visually displayed in Figures 25–13 and 14. In Figure 25–13, the size of the transducer is constant at 1.5

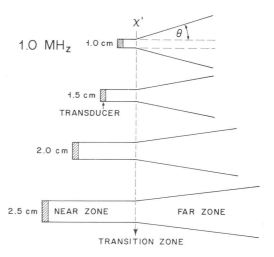

Figure 25–14 Elongation of the near zone with increasing transducer size

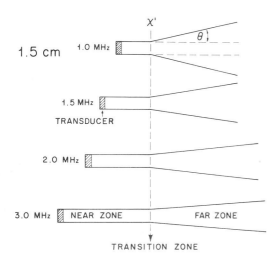

Figure 25–13 Elongation of the near zone with increasing frequencies

cm, and the frequency of the sound is increased in stages from 1 to 3 MHz. The near zone increases in length with increasing frequency. In Figure 25–14, the frequency is fixed at 1 MHz and the size of the transducer is increased in stages from 1 to 2.5 cm. Again, the near zone increases in length with larger transducers.

High frequency beams have two advantages over low frequency beams: depth resolution is superior, and the Fresnel zone is longer. It would seem logical to use high frequencies for all imaging. However, high frequencies have a major drawback related to penetration. **Tissue absorption increases with increasing frequency**, so a relatively low frequency beam is required to penetrate thick parts. It would also seem logical to increase the size of the transducer to keep the beam coherent for sufficient depth to reach the point of interest. However, while larger transducers improve coherence, they deteriorate side-to-side resolution. This dilemma is at least partially resolved with focused transducers which we will discuss later. The amount of dispersion in the far zone is shown diagrammatically in the uppermost illustration in Figure 25–14. The size of the angle is determined as follows:

$$\sin \theta = 1.22 \, \frac{\lambda}{D}$$

θ = dispersion angle of far zone
λ = wavelength (mm)
D = diameter of transducer (mm)

The equation is rather simple to use with mathematical tables or a calculator with trigonometric functions. For example, the dispersion angle for a 10-mm transducer and a wavelength of 1 mm (a frequency of 1.5 MHz) is as follows:

$$\sin \theta = 1.22 \, \frac{1.0}{10} = 0.122$$

$$\theta = 7°$$

If the wavelength is shortened to 0.5 mm (a frequency of 3 MHz), and the transducer size kept at 10 mm, the dispersion angle is 3.5°.

INTERACTIONS BETWEEN ULTRASOUND AND MATTER

The types of interactions between sound and matter are similar to those of light and include the following: (1) reflection, (2) refraction, and (3) absorption.

Reflection

In x-ray imaging, the transmitted radiation blackens the film and creates the actual image. Attenuated radiation creates defects or holes in the transmitted beam, and thus contributes to image formation, but in a passive way. Scattered radiation fogs the film and is detrimental to image quality. With ultrasound, however, the image is produced by the reflected portion of the beam. Transmitted sound contributes nothing to image formation, but transmission must be strong enough to produce echoes at deeper levels. The percentage of the beam reflected at tissue interfaces depends upon: (1) the tissue's acoustic impedance, and (2) the beam's angle of incidence.

Acoustic Impedance

Acoustic impedance is a fundamental property of matter. The impedance of a material is the product of its density and the velocity of sound in the material.

$$Z = pc$$

Z = acoustic impedance (Rayls)
p = density (gm/cm³)
c = velocity of sound (cm/sec)

For example, the acoustic impedance of water is the velocity of sound in water (154,000 cm/sec) times the density of water (1 gm/cm³), or:

cm/sec × gm/cm³ = gm/cm² sec
154,000 × 1 = 154,000

This is an inconveniently large number, so it is divided by 100,000 (the same as multiplying by 10^{-5}) to reduce it to a more convenient size. Thus, the unit for acoustic impedance in the cgs system, the Rayl, is defined as gm/cm² sec × 10^{-5}. **The velocity of sound is fairly constant over a wide range of frequencies so a substance's acoustic impedance is a constant.** Table 25–4 lists the acoustic impedance of various materials including several body tis-

Table 25–4. Acoustic Impedance of Various Materials

MATERIAL	ACOUSTIC IMPEDANCE (RAYLS—gm/cm² sec × 10^{-5})
Air	0.0004
Fat	1.38
Water (50°C)	1.54
Brain	1.58
Blood	1.61
Kidney	1.62
Liver	1.65
Muscle	1.70
Lens of eye	1.84
Skull—bone	7.80
Aluminum	18.00
Mercury	19.7
Brass	38.0

From Wells, P. N. T.[13]

sues. As sound waves pass from one tissue plane to another, the amount of reflection is determined by the difference in the impedances of the two tissues. The greater the difference, the greater the percentage reflected. Notice that the difference between most body structures is fairly small, the two exceptions being air and bone. A soft tissue-air interface reflects almost the entire beam, and a soft tissue-bone interface a major portion of it. The sum of the reflected and transmitted portions is 100%. For example, if 90% of a beam is reflected, 10% will be transmitted. At a tissue-air interface, more than 99.9% of the beam is reflected, so none is available for further imaging. For this reason, transducers must be directly coupled to the patient's skin without an air gap. Coupling is accomplished with a slippery material such as mineral oil for contact scanning or with a water bath when the transducer cannot be placed directly on the patient.

Angle of Incidence

The amount of reflection is determined by the angle of incidence between the sound beam and the reflecting surface. The higher the angle of incidence, i.e., the closer it is to a right angle, the less the amount of reflected sound. Below a certain critical angle, the entire beam is reflected. The angles of incidence and reflection are equal, just as they are for visible light. When a sound beam strikes a smooth interface that is perpendicular to the beam, the amount of reflection is given by the following equation:

$$R = \left(\frac{Z_2 - Z_1}{Z_2 + Z_1}\right)^2 \times 100$$

R = percent of beam reflected
Z_1 = acoustic impedance of medium I
Z_2 = acoustic impedance of medium II

For example, to determine the percentage of a sonic beam reflected in going from the chest wall to the lung, substitute the acoustic impedance of lung and chest wall (muscle) from Table 25–4 as follows:

$$R = \left(\frac{1.70 - .0004}{1.70 + .0004}\right)^2 \times 100 = 99.9\%$$

As you can see, the number .0004 is so small that for practical purposes it can be ignored, and the beam is almost totally reflected giving an intense echo, but leaving no beam for further imaging. At a kidney-fat interface, the amount of reflection is as follows:

$$R = \left(\frac{1.65 - 1.38}{1.65 + 1.38}\right)^2 \times 100$$

$$R = \left(\frac{0.27}{3.03}\right)^2 \times 100 = 30\%$$

Approximately 30% of the beam is reflected at a kidney-fat interface. The skull is intermediate between the soft tissues and air. At a skull-brain interface, approximately 81% of the beam is reflected. The preceding equation applies only to perpendicular reflections.

Refraction

When sound passes from one medium to another, its frequency remains constant, but its wavelength changes to accommodate a new velocity in the second medium. This concept is shown diagrammatically in Figure 25–15. In the illustration, the velocity of sound is twice as fast in the first medium as in the second. Each wave is shown as a single horizontal line and reflection is ignored. When the waves reach the surface of the second medium, they are slowed to half speed, but they keep coming at the same frequency. Their spacing, or wavelength, must be reduced by one-half to accommodate the decrease in velocity.

Exactly the same thing happens when the sound beam strikes the second medium at an angle, but the change in wavelength necessitates a change in direction. The reason for the direction change is shown in Figure 25–16. At time 1, a wave front approaching from a 45° angle just barely makes contact with the second medium. As it progresses, straddling the two media, one edge is traveling at a different velocity than the other. The wave front remains

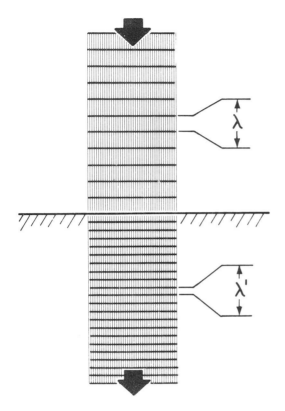

Figure 25–15 The wavelength of sound shortens when its velocity decreases

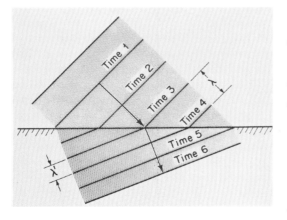

Figure 25–16 Refraction of sound waves

continuous, but one edge lags behind the other until the beam finally emerges in the second medium with a different wavelength and direction. This bending of waves as they pass from one medium to another is called **refraction.** Exactly the same process occurs in optics. Since the beam could be traveling in either direction, the arrows can be reversed in the illustrations to demonstrate the change that occurs when velocity increases in the second medium.

The angles of reflection and refraction are shown in Figure 25–17. The angle of refraction is governed by **Snell's law** which is as follows:

$$\frac{\sin \theta_i}{\sin \theta_t} = \frac{V_1}{V_2}$$

θ_i = incident angle (see Figure 25–17)
θ_t = transmitted angle
V_1 = velocity of sound for incident medium
V_2 = velocity of sound for transmitting medium

Absorption

Absorption is the conversion of sound into heat. The mechanisms involved in absorption are rather complex, and our explanation will be greatly simplified. Three factors determine the amount of absorption: (1) the frequency of the sound; (2) the viscosity of the conducting medium; and (3) the "relaxation time" of the medium.[3] We will discuss frequency last since it is affected by the other two factors.

If we picture sound as vibrating particles, the importance of viscosity is obvious. Particle freedom decreases, and internal friction increases with increasing viscosity. This internal friction attenuates the beam, or decreases its intensity, by converting sound into heat. The mechanism is relatively unimportant for low viscosity materials such as water, but most body tissues are quite viscous and frictional losses are significant.

The relaxation time is the time that it takes for a molecule to return to its original position after it has been displaced. It refers to the resilience of a material. Two

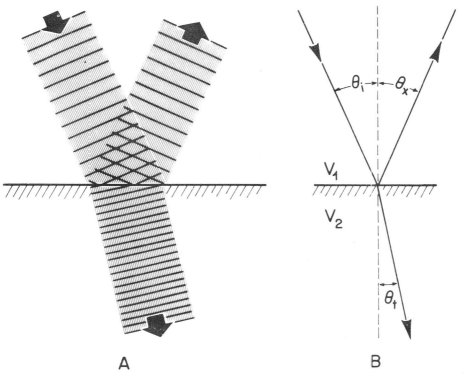

Figure 25–17   Refraction and reflection of sound waves

substances with the same viscosity may have different relaxation times. The relaxation time is a constant for any particular material. When a molecule with a short relaxation time is pushed by a longitudinal compression wave, the molecule has time to return to its resting state before the next compression wave arrives. A molecule with a longer relaxation time may not be able to completely return before a second compression wave arrives. When this happens, the compression wave is moving in one direction and the molecule in the opposite direction. More energy is required to reverse the direction of the molecule than was needed to move it originally. The additional energy is consumed as heat.

In body tissues, absorption is directly proportional to frequency. Doubling frequency doubles absorption and halves the

intensity of the transmitted beam. The frequency of sound affects the amount of absorption that is caused by the viscosity of a material. The higher the frequency, i.e. the more often a particle moves back-and-forth in a given time, the more its motion is affected by the drag of a viscous material. Frequency also affects the amount of absorption that is caused by the relaxation time. At low frequencies, molecules have sufficient time to relax between cycles, but as frequencies increase, the relaxation time consumes a greater and greater proportion of the total cycle. These effects are already appreciable in the lower range of diagnostic frequencies (1 MHz), and they continue to increase at higher frequencies.

Only rather fragmentary data are available to quantitate the absorption of ultrasound. An absorption coefficient is usually employed. This coefficient is identical

Table 25–5. Absorption Coefficients for Various Materials at a Frequency of 1 MegaHertz

MATERIAL	ABSORPTION COEFFICIENT (decibels/cm)
Lung	41
Skull—bone	20
Air	12
Muscle (across fiber)	3.3
Lens of eye	2.0
Kidney	1.0
Castor oil	0.95
Liver	0.94
Brain	0.85
Fat	0.63
Blood	0.18
Aluminum	0.018
Water	0.0022
Mercury	0.00048

From Wells, P. N. T.[13]

in concept to the linear attenuation coefficient that we described for x rays in Chapter 5. The unit for the absorption coefficient is decibels/cm of thickness at a frequency of 1 MHz. The stipulation of 1 MHz is essential because absorption is frequency dependent. At 2 MHz, the absorption coefficient is twice as large. Table 25–5 lists absorption coefficients for various materials. A 1-cm thick slice of kidney, with an absorption coefficient of 1 dB/cm absorbs 1 dB of sound. Table 25–2 shows that minus 1 dB represents an absorption of 21% of the beam and that 79% of the beam remains. A 1-cm thick slice of lung absorbs 41 dB which reduces intensity by a factor of more than 10,000, leaving less than 0.01% of the beam remaining.

ULTRASONIC DISPLAY

The ultrasonic image is an electronic representation of data generated from returning echoes, and displayed on a T.V. monitor. The image is assembled, one bit at a time, much like a television image. Each returning echo generates one bit of data, and many bits together form the electronic image. The evolution of sonic imaging began slowly from a static one-dimensional base (A-mode), improved somewhat when a component of motion was added (TM-mode), made a giant leap forward with two-dimensional imaging (B-mode), and reached its current zenith with gray scale imaging. These advancements can all be attributed to refinements in electronic instrumentation. Further refinements are being made every year, and undoubtedly, other major improvements will occur before this book is published.

A-Mode

In the A-mode, echoes are displayed as spikes projecting from a baseline as shown in Figure 25–18. The baseline identifies the central axis of the beam. Spike height is proportional to echo intensity, strong echoes producing large spikes. A series of sonic pulses is used for A-mode imaging but for simplicity, we will begin with a single pulse. When a voltage pulse strikes a transducer, an echo spike is generated on the monitor to mark the beginning of the sonic pulse. As the pulse passes through the patient, sound is reflected to the transducer from each tissue interface. The depth of the interface recorded on the display is proportional to the time that it takes for the echo to return. Using a sound velocity of 1540 m/sec in average soft tissue, it is a simple mathematical task to convert time into distance. At a velocity of 154,000 cm/sec, sound travels 1 cm in 6.5 microseconds (μsec). However, an echo must make a round trip, so when the echo takes 13 μsec to return, it is displayed at a depth of 1 cm.

If the tissue planes are in a fixed position, and the transducer is held stationary between pulses, as is customary, then the echo spikes from subsequent pulses will fall in the same positions as those from the

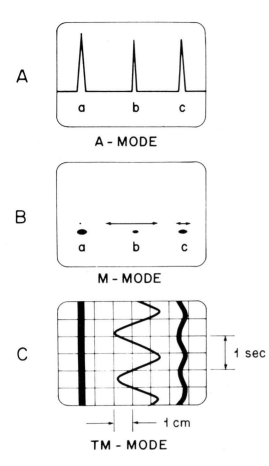

Figure 25–18 A-mode and TM-mode displays

initial pulse. No memory is built into the display mechanism so it discards previous pulses as it receives new ones. A permanent record is made by photographing the electronic display. The A-mode shows only one dimension, depth. It is of limited value but is still used in echoencephalography for midline localization.

TM-Mode

In the A-mode, if the echoes are produced by moving structures, then the echo spikes will also move. If the echoes shown in Figure 25–18 (A-mode) had originated from the anterior chest wall (a), the posterior leaflet of the mitral valve (b), and the

posterior heart wall (c), the echoes from the moving structures would move back-and-forth along the baseline. At any moment, they might appear as shown in the illustration. However, a moment later the mitral valve and heart wall would be in a different position, the mitral valve moving more than the heart wall. For the TM-mode, the spikes are converted into "dots" as shown in Figure 25-18 (M-mode). The dots move back-and-forth as indicated by the arrows. The M-mode is an intermediate mode that cannot be meaningfully recorded. To make a permanent record, the motion must be recorded over a period of time. This is accomplished by moving the line of dots to the top of the scope and then gradually dropping them to the bottom. A record of the sweep is made with a camera using an exposure time longer than the sweep time. Such a record is shown in Figure 25–18 (TM-mode). Since this is a time-motion study, it is referred to as the TM-mode. The sweep time in the illustration is 3 sec. If a longer sweep time is used, more beats are recorded and they are compacted from top to bottom, but their back-and-forth excursions remain unchanged. The obvious disadvantage of this method is the short time that can be recorded. A longer record can be made with an electronic strip chart recorder that can also simultaneously display several other parameters such as the ECG. A strip chart record can be as long as the operator desires, and this method is increasing in popularity for echocardiography which is where the TM-mode is most useful.

B-Mode

Sonography came of age as an imaging technique with the B-mode. The other modes produced valuable information, but they were only useful in limited areas. The B-mode greatly expanded the role of ultrasound as a diagnostic tool, especially in abdominal diseases. **The B-mode produces a picture of a slice of tissue.** Echoes are displayed as dots, similar to the TM-mode, but in contrast to the TM-mode, the transducer is moved so that the sound beam traverses a plane of the body. The electronic display, either an oscilloscope or television monitor, records and retains all of the bits of data that are fed into it. A persistence feature in the display scope allows it to retain images, as in stop-action T.V., and then discard the image upon command. The transducer is like the handle of a saber with the ultrasonic beam as the blade. The blade images a sagittal section when it cuts through the length of the body, and a transverse, or cross section when drawn from side-to-side. The images are similar to what we would see if the section could be exposed and viewed face-on.

In assembling the image, the localization of one echo relative to another is accomplished with a small computer which is fed information by an arm containing three joints as shown in Figure 25–19. The computer calculates the alignment of the baseline by the number of degrees in the three joints. Echo depth is determined by the time delay, as in the A-mode. When the transducer moves from one position to another, from A to B in the illustration, the computer recalculates the angles and time delays to properly position returning signals in the display. Even though the echoes arise from two completely different transducer positions (A and B), the computer correctly interprets them as originating from one point (P). Many thousands of these calculations and echoes produce an image that appears on the scope as a cut section. Various manufacturers employ different methods for measuring the three angles, but usually a fine thread is looped over pulleys at each joint and the angles are calculated from the length of thread moving past a fixed point.

Gray-Scale Imaging

B-mode scanning took a major step forward with the advent of gray-scale imaging in 1974. Prior to that time, a bit of anatomical information, an echo, was displayed via an all-or-none mechanism. If an echo was rather weak, it could be rejected and not displayed, thus appearing as a void or white dot, or it could be accepted and displayed as a black dot. There was nothing between black and white. With gray-scale imaging, a weak echo is displayed as a light gray and a stronger one as a darker gray, or black. Before being displayed on the T.V. monitor, the echoes are recorded on a television scan converter. The target of the converter consists of a matrix of approximately one million tiny silicon dioxide diodes arranged in a square matrix. The diodes are tiny capacitors that collect and store an electrical charge in an array that corresponds to the spatial position of the returning echoes. Only the maximal echoes from a particular area are displayed. They are assigned a shade of gray determined by their intensity. The scan converter can store over 30 shades, but only approximately 10 are used for the display on the T.V. monitor, since the eye cannot detect finer gradations. However, in some units the operator can select 10 shades from either the light or darker component of the 30 shades.

Controls

The number and intensity of echoes from any particular area are extremely vari-

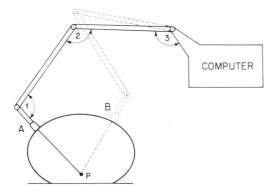

Figure 25–19 Computer localization of transducer alignment

able, and setting the scanner to optimally demonstrate one area frequently detracts from image quality in another area. Multiple controls are built into ultrasonic units, all designed to regulate the intensity of echoes from various depths. Usually several controls are manipulated simultaneously, so there is no logical sequence for discussion. The following is a list of the controls that may be available, although they may not all be provided by a single manufacturer.

1. Time gain compensator
2. Delay
3. Intensity
4. Coarse gain
5. Reject
6. Near gain
7. Far gain
8. Enhancement

The echoes from deep structures are much weaker than those from closer structures. The two may differ by a factor of one million. If an echo from an object close to the surface produces a 10-cm spike, as displayed in the A-mode, the echoes from deeper structures may be a mere .001 mm, less than the thickness of a hair. Obviously, something must be done to remedy this situation and most of the controls are designed for just that purpose. The **time gain compensator (TGC)** is the most important control. Its function is shown diagrammatically in Figure 25–20. The echoes from deep structures are severely attenuated and produce small spikes (B). The TGC is depicted in C as a sloping line, and the height of the slope is added to that of the pulses. The result, shown in D, is a series of pulses of similar amplitude. The slope of the TGC adjusts the degree of amplification. The slope is shown as a straight line, but it is actually exponential, since the deeper echoes require more of a boost than it would appear from the illustration. They may actually be amplified more than a thousand times. The delay control regulates the depth at which the TGC begins to augment weaker signals.

Three controls govern amplitude across the entire display without discrimination for, or against, a particular depth. The first is the **intensity control** which determines

VIDEO SIGNAL

TIME GAIN COMPENSATION

COMPENSATED VIDEO SIGNAL

Figure 25–20 Time gain compensation

the potential difference across the transducer, i.e. the strength of the voltage pulse. Increasing intensity produces a more energetic ultrasonic beam and thus stronger echoes at all levels. The second amplitude control is the **coarse gain** which regulates the height of echoes from all depths. Increasing the coarse gain control

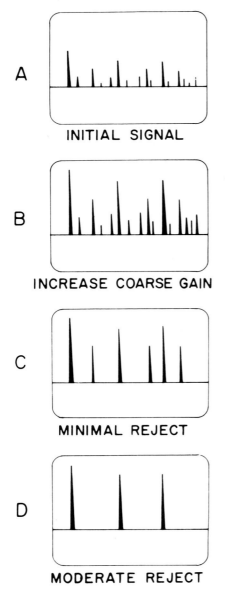

Figure 25–21   Coarse gain and reject controls

against echoes from a particular depth, it does discriminate against those below a minimum amplitude. This is shown diagrammatically in Figure 25–21 C and D. Reject cleans up the image by removing small useless signals. Selective rejection of weaker signals enhances the clarity of the stronger ones.

A **delay control** regulates the depth at which the time gain compensator begins to augment the weaker signals (Figure 25–22). Obviously the strong superficial echoes do not require amplification by the time gain compensator. In fact, they may have to be dampened. This is accomplished with the **near gain control** which is poorly named, since it is used primarily to diminish, and not enhance near echoes. The distance over which near gain operates is controlled by the delay.

Two additional means may be used to supplement distant echoes, that is, those originating deep in the tissues: the **far gain** and the **enhancement controls.** Far gain is similar to near gain only at the opposite end of the time gain compensator curve. It is used to enhance all distant echoes. The enhancement controls augment a localized portion of the TGC curve as shown in Figure 25–22. It gates a specific depth and

enhances all echoes proportionately as shown in Figure 25–21. The initial echoes (A) are all enhanced to near double their amplitude by increasing coarse gain (B). The third amplitude regulator is the **reject control,** and it is a little different from the other two. While it does not discriminate

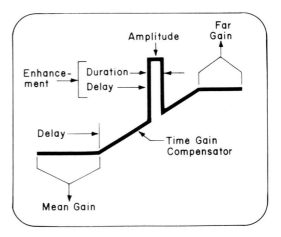

Figure 25–22   Various controls for the sonic display

enhances echoes within the gate to any desired level. For example, the gate can be set to "frame" the near and far extremes of mitral valve motion, then echoes from this specific region will be amplified to better delineate the valve.

The interplay between all of these controls is extremely complex and it is impossible to learn their effect upon imaging from a book. To quote Dr. Roger Sanders, "The relationship between the time gain compensation, the output and transducer frequency is so complex and variable that it defies description and is far better understood if the trainee acts as an apprentice to an experienced sonographer."[11]

Pulse Rate

Pulse rate and frequency are different and unrelated. Frequency refers to a characteristic of the sound, that is, the number of times that conducting particles vibrate back-and-forth per second, usually between 1 and 20 MHz in medical sonography. **Pulse rate refers to the number of separate little packets of sound that are sent out each second** as shown in Figure 25–23. Each sonic pulse is short (only a few wavelengths) and its duration varies with the Q-factor of the transducer. Between pulses, the transducer serves as a receiver. A commonly used rate is 1000 pulses/sec. At this rate, the total time available for each pulse is 1/1000 sec. Approximately 1/1000 of this time is devoted to transmission, so the transducer is a receiver almost 1000 times longer than it is a transmitter.

The pulse rate determines the total number of echoes returning to the trans-

Table 25–6. Maximum Part Thickness That Can Be Imaged at Various Pulse Rates

PULSE RATE (per sec)	MAXIMUM PART THICKNESS (cm)*
1,000	75
3,000	25
6,000	12.5
10,000	7.5

*Based on a velocity of sound of 150,000 cm/sec; the sound must travel twice as far as the thickness to complete a round trip.

ducer in a unit of time. Doubling the rate from 1000 to 2000 pulses/sec will double the number of echoes returning to the transducer each second.

Obviously a high pulse rate is desirable, but too high a rate creates another problem. The transducer cannot send and receive at the same time. As the pulse rate increases, the receiving time decreases. If the receiving time is too short, echoes from distant parts may still be out, or on their way in, when the next pulse starts. The time between pulses, or the pulse rate, must be set to accommodate the thickest part that might be examined. This thickness is one-half the distance between pulses. Remember, the sound is making a round trip, so the maximum thickness that can be examined is only one-half of the distance that the sound can travel. Table 25–6 shows the maximum part thickness that can be imaged at various pulse rates. At the commonly used rate of 1000 pulses/sec, a 75-cm thick part can be examined. At a rate of 10,000, the thickest

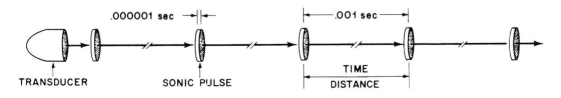

Figure 25–23   Multiple sonic pulses

part is 7.5 cm, which is satisfactory for ophthalmology but not for abdominal imaging.

IMAGING PRINCIPLES

The sonographic image is influenced by the size and shape of both the object and the transducer. The same principle applies to x-ray imaging. The effect of the x-ray focal spot size is made readily apparent if a pinhole is placed half way between the target and film, the resultant image being a picture of the focal spot, not the pinhole. At shorter object-film distances, or with larger objects, the effect is much less dramatic, and we call it penumbra or edge gradient, but the effect is there just the same. Transducers are much larger than focal spots so transducer images are more evident. Figure 25–24 shows a B-mode scan of five equally spaced wire rods imaged with a focused transducer. (Focused transducers will be described later in this section.) The wires are small in diameter relative to the sound beam. As the beam moves from left-to-right, echoes begin when the leading edge of the beam reaches

a wire and continue until the beam has passed beyond all of the wires. The resulting images are a picture of the sound beam, not the wire. Since beam width varies with depth, image width also varies with depth, being closest to the shape of the wire when the beam is narrowest. The wire is the sonographer's pinhole.

Resolution

When we talk about resolution with the A-mode, we are only concerned with the ability of the beam to separate two objects at different depths. However, in the B-mode, we must also be concerned with horizontal, or lateral, resolution, i.e. the ability to separate two objects located side-by-side. We will refer to these as depth and lateral resolution. Neither is accurately defined, at least not by x-ray imaging standards, so our discussion will be in general principles and not in line pairs per mm.

Depth (Axial) Resolution

Depth resolution is the ability of the beam to separate two objects lying in

Figure 25–24　"Imaging" the sonic beam

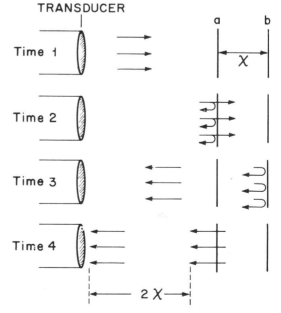

Figure 25–25　Depth (axial) resolution

tandem along the axis of the beam. Figure 25–25 shows a time-sequence of an ultrasonic pulse resolving two surfaces, **a** and **b,** separated by **x** distance. At times 2 and 3, portions of the beam are reflected from surfaces **a** and **b** respectively. The reflected pulses are completely separated and each produces its own signal. The separation of their leading edges is 2x, or twice the original separation, since the second echo had to travel back-and-forth across the distance x. The length of the sonic pulse, called the spatial pulse length,[7] equals the wavelength of the sound times the number of wavelengths in the pulse. The number of wavelengths will depend upon the Q-factor of the transducer. For example, at a frequency of 1.5 MHz, the wavelength of the sound in water is 1 mm (λ = 1,500,000 cycles/sec ÷ 1,500,000 mm/sec). If each sonic pulse consists of 3 wavelengths, the spatial pulse length will be 3 mm. Two objects will be resolved, i.e. recognized as being separate, if the spatial pulse length is less than one-half the separation. Figure 25–26 shows two objects

Figure 25–27   Reverberation images

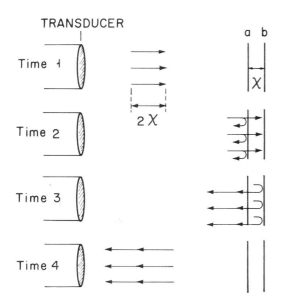

Figure 25–26   Unsatisfactory, or unsuccessful depth resolution

separated by exactly one-half a spatial pulse length. At time 2, the pulse splits, but the first reflected pulse does not clear surface **a** before the pulse returns from surface **b.** The transducer only sees one pulse so the two surfaces are not resolved.

Reverberation Echoes. When we discussed tomography, we described phantom images as images that appear to the eye, but have no physical existence. A similar image, called a reverberation image, occurs in sonography. Figure 25–27 shows how these spurious images are produced. The critical event occurs at time 4 when the returning echoes from **b** reflect off the back surface of **a** and initiate a third echo (time 5) which the transducer interprets as another object. Thus three surfaces are displayed, the third being a reverberation image. Time 6 shows the beginning of a fourth image and with a geometric configuration such as the one shown in the illustration, the number of reverberation images is limited only by the penetrating power of the beam and sensitivity of the detector.

The transducer itself may act as a reflecting surface and produce a reverberation artifact, especially in ophthalmologic sonography. The artifact is recognized by manually changing the distance between the transducer and the globe of the eye. The factitial image moves in synchrony with the transducer.

Lateral (Horizontal) Resolution

Lateral resolution is the ability to separate two objects lying side-by-side. Figure 25–28 shows two objects separated by a narrow space. In order to recognize the objects as discrete entities, the beam must be narrower than the space separating the objects. In A, the beam is too wide so that even when it straddles the space, echoes return from both objects, the display interprets an edge, and the space goes un-

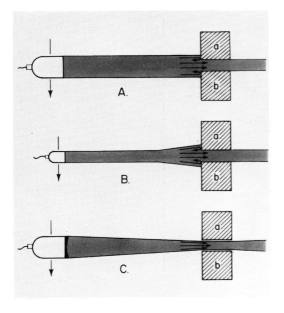

Figure 25–28 Lateral (horizontal) resolution

recognized. An obvious way to narrow the beam, and improve resolution is with a smaller transducer. This works well in some clinical situations, for example, in ophthalmology where small diameter high frequency transducers are used to produce superb resolution. However, the advantages of small transducers are lost in the much thicker abdomen. The Fresnel zone is too short, even at high frequencies, to reach deep structures. Figure 25–28B shows the problem diagrammatically. The beam is well into the Fraunhofer zone at the object plane, and may actually be wider than the beam from a larger transducer.

Focused Transducers. The solution to the above imaging problem is a focused transducer like the one shown in Figure 25–28C. Focused transducers restrict beam width and improve lateral resolution. However, they are designed to focus at a specific depth, or depth range, so they must be selected to optimally display the depth of interest. In the illustration the beam is focused at the proper depth so that it is able to pass through the space between objects **a** and **b,** thus permitting them to appear as separate entities.

Sonic beams can be focused with either a curved piezoelectric crystal or an acoustic lens. Lens material, usually made from polystyrene or an epoxy resin,[8] propagates sound at a greater velocity than body tissues, so the sound is refracted, or bent, toward a point in space. Knowing the radius of curvature of the lens and velocities of sound in the lens material and body tissues, the exact focal point can be calculated. **A close approximation of the focal length is the diameter of curvature of the lens** as shown in Figure 25–29. Focusing moves the transition point between the near and far zones from its anticipated position at x' back toward the transducer to a new position at x'_f. The beam is maximally restricted and of greatest intensity at the focal point, but the point is not sharply defined. Like an optical lens, an acoustic lens has a focal zone, a

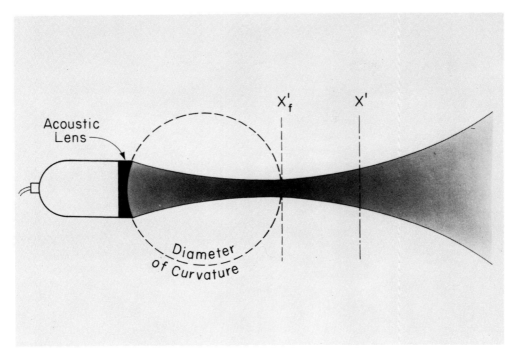

Figure 25–29   Focused transducer

distance over which the focal properties are fairly well maintained. The focal zone is shortest with a large diameter, short focal length lens. Focused transducers are classified as short, medium and long,[8] depending on the depth at which they focus as follows:

    short   .... 4–6 cm
    medium .... 6–8 cm
    long   .... 8–11 cm .

Tomographic Thickness. The expression tomographic thickness is only meaningful with B-mode scanning. It refers to the thickness of the slice that is in sharp focus or to the thickness that the sonic beam "sees." It is closely akin to lateral resolution. We described a B-mode scanner as a saber cutting a gash through the body. Two sabers would be more accurate: two sabers side-by-side separated by the width of the beam and cutting out a slice of tissue. The thinner the slice, the more accurately the images will depict a plane.

The final image is a composite of all objects in the slice. The thickness and shape of the tomographic slice are the same as those of the sonic beam. A cylindrical beam (unfocused) produces a pancake-like slice with parallel sides in the Fresnel zone and a flared-out bottom in the Fraunhofer zone. Slices from focused transducers flare out at both the top and bottom and are narrowest in the center. The top flare is limited by the width of the transducer but the bottom flare increases with increasing depth.

Imaging Curved Surfaces

Curved surfaces are difficult to image with an echo system, and unfortunately most body surfaces are curved. The problem is shown diagrammatically in Figure 25–30, where an attempt is made to image the top of a sphere with a linear scan motion. As the probe moves across the sphere, beam alignment is optimum only

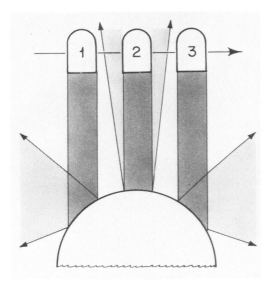

Figure 25–30 Unsatisfactory scan motion for imaging curved objects

at position 2. The reflected echoes from positions 1 and 3 never reach the transducer, so only the central portion of the sphere is imaged and the sides are left open.

The perfect imaging motion for a sphere, or any curved surface, is an arc whose center of curvature is located at the same point as that of the surface being imaged. Such an arrangement is shown in Figure 25–31. The transducer remains perpendicular to the tangent of the sphere at all times as it rotates through a 180° arc. The returning echoes all travel the same distance so they are equally attenuated and the image is a perfect duplication of the object. Obviously, this ideal mode is impossible in clinical work since there are no true spherical structures in the body and even if there were, we would not be able to locate their centers. However, a fair approximation of this system is achieved with cross-

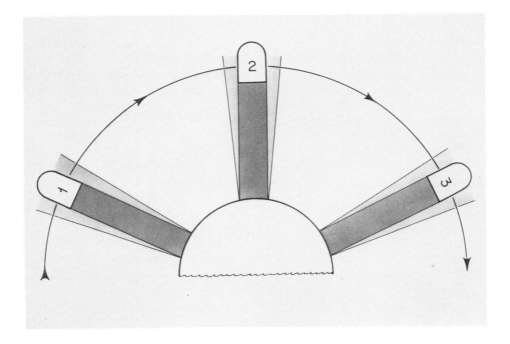

Figure 25–31   Optimum scan motion for imaging curved objects

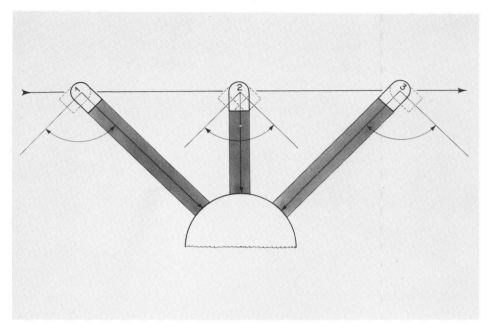

Figure 25–32   Alternative method for imaging curved objects

sectional scanning by sweeping the transducer around 180° of the body surface. Cross-sectional images, especially since the advent of the gray scale, are of excellent quality.

Figure 25–32 shows a third method for imaging curved surfaces, one using a compound scanning motion. The transducer moves slowly from left-to-right and at the same time oscillates back-and-forth through a 90° arc. During at least a part of the scan the beam strikes a large portion of the curved surface at right angles. This method cannot be used for contact scanning, but it works well with the part immersed in a water bath.

Permanent Records of Sonic Images

After the desired image is displayed on the T.V. monitor or cathode ray tube, a permanent record is made for later review. The simplest and most widely used method is probably a polaroid picture of the display tube. Two other methods are gaining in popularity—transparencies, similar to x-ray film, and videotape or disc recorders. The transparencies may be made with either roll film using a 70-mm or larger format camera, or with multiple exposures on a large cut film. Recently, videodisc recorders have become more economical and are being used for ultrasonic display.

DOPPLER TECHNIQUES

The Doppler effect is a change in the perceived frequency of sound emitted by a moving source. The effect was first described by Christian Doppler in 1843. The cause of the frequency change is shown schematically in Figure 25–33. In A, a vibrating source (P) produces a series of concentric waves, all moving out from the center, the oldest in the most peripheral location (time 1) and newest at the center (time 6). The velocity of sound in the particular medium and the frequency of the oscillator determine the wavelength

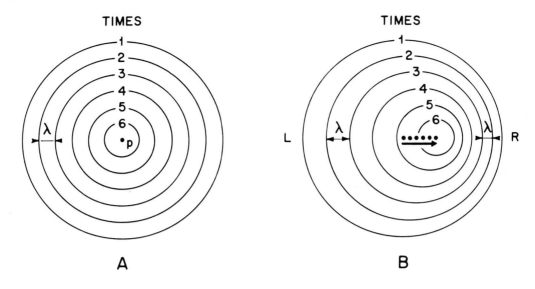

Figure 25–33   The Doppler shift

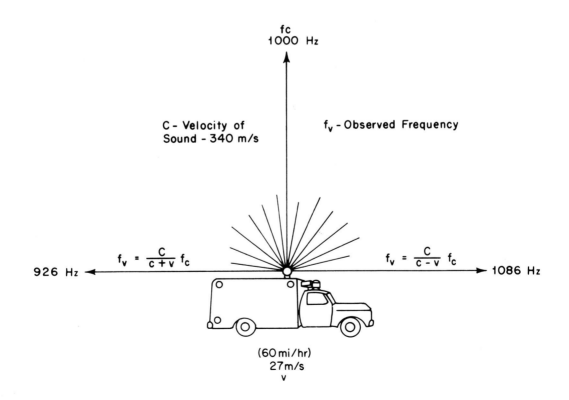

Figure 25–34   Magnitude of the Doppler shift

(λ), or distance between crests. In B, the sound source is moving to the right as it vibrates. It sends out a wave crest and then runs after the crest in one direction and away in the opposite direction. The sound usually moves faster than the source, so the source never catches the crest. However, source motion does change the gap between crests, increasing the frequency and decreasing the wavelength to the right and decreasing the frequency and increasing the wavelength to the left. Sound velocity is not affected by source motion so the sound moves at the same velocity in all directions. The wavelength change is caused by the source motion changing the spacing between crests.

The magnitude of the Doppler shift is shown in Figure 25–34. An ambulance moving 27 m/sec (60 miles/hr) is blowing its siren at a frequency of 1000 Hz. The frequency ahead of the siren is 1086 Hz, while the frequency behind is 926 Hz. A pedestrian would hear a frequency shift of 160 Hz as the ambulance passed. The only person hearing the true frequency of 1000 Hz are passengers in the vehicle.

In contrast to the other ultrasonic modes that we have discussed, all of which are visual, most of the current medical applications of the Doppler effect employ an audio-mode. Doppler techniques are used to study motion, primarily that of the circulatory system. Two transducers are used in the audio-mode, one as a transmitter, and the other as a receiver. Both operate continuously. Pulsed Doppler devices incorporating features of both pulsed sonography and continuous wave Doppler are in various stages of development. They offer considerable promise for the future, but we will not attempt to describe them since the instrumentation is still largely experimental.

Continuous Wave Doppler

The continuous wave Doppler mode employs two piezoelectric elements, both contained in a single head as shown in

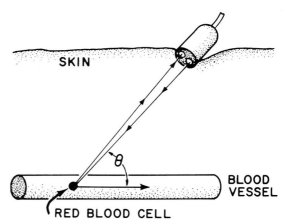

Figure 25–35 Audio-mode Doppler transducer

Figure 25–35. One crystal transmits a continuous sonic signal at a known frequency, usually between 3 and 8 MHz. The other crystal receives the returning echoes and records their frequency. The frequency of the initial signal is algebraically subtracted from that of the returning echoes. The difference, the **Doppler shift,** usually falls within the frequency range detectable by the human ear and, after amplification, this Doppler shift is the audio signal. Returning echoes originate from the cellular elements of the blood, particularly the red blood cell. The Doppler beam is used to detect the motion of the blood within the vessel rather than the motion of the vessel wall.

In contrast to pulsed sonography, where the intensity of returning echoes is greatest when the beam is perpendicular to a reflecting surface, the Doppler shift is greatest when the beam strikes a vessel at a sharp angle. Figure 25–35 shows a vector of red blood cell motion towards the transducer even though the transducer is not in the direct path of flow. The smaller the angle between the sonic beam and the flow direction (θ), the greater the vector of motion towards the transducer and the greater the Doppler shift. Theoretically, motion cannot be detected when the transducer is perpendicular to the direction of blood flow, but this theoretical situation does not occur in actual practice because of divergence of the beam, i.e. some part of the beam is always off of the perpendicular. The frequency change of back scattered echoes can be calculated with the Doppler shift equation:

$$\triangle f = \frac{2\,f\,v}{c}\cos\theta$$

$\triangle f$ = frequency change (Doppler shift–Hz)
f = frequency of initial beam (Hz)
v = velocity of blood (m/s)
c = velocity of sound (1540 m/s)
θ = angle between sound beam and direction of blood flow (Figure 25–35)

The vector of blood cell motion towards the transducer is represented by $\cos\theta$ in the equation. If the angle is increased, there is a smaller vector of motion towards the transducer and consequently $\cos\theta$ is smaller. If the number of degrees in the angle is decreased, the $\cos\theta$ is larger, and it approaches 1 as the transducer looks directly into the blood stream. With this equation as a foundation, the velocity of blood flow can be calculated if the angle θ is known. For example, if a Doppler device is constructed with a fixed angle of 60° (cos 60° is 0.5), and a frequency of 3.08 MHz (3,080,000 Hz), substituting in the Doppler shift equation, converts a measured frequency shift into a blood flow velocity.

$$\triangle f = \frac{2\,f\,v\cos\theta}{c}\;\text{or}\;v = \frac{\triangle f\,c}{2\,f\cos\theta}$$

$$v = \frac{\triangle f \cdot 1540}{2\cdot 3,080,000\cdot 0.5}$$

$$v = .0005\,\triangle f$$

If the measured frequency shift is 1000 Hz, then the velocity of blood flow is:

$$v = .0005 \times 1000 = 0.5\;\text{m/s}$$

At frequencies between 3 MHz and 8 MHz, the Doppler shift falls in the audible range for most physiologic motions. An experienced listener can learn a great deal about the status of the circulatory system with a Doppler device. It can be used to detect blood flow, or its absence, in both arteries and veins, to identify vascular constrictions with their associated eddy currents and venturi jets, and to detect fetal heart motion earlier than any other method.

SUMMARY

Ultrasound is sound with a frequency greater than 20,000 cycles/sec (Hertz abr. Hz). Medical sonography employs frequencies between 1 megaHertz (MHz) and 20 MHz. These high frequencies are produced by subjecting a special ceramic material, a piezoelectric crystal, to a short voltage spike. The crystals may be made of quartz, but more commonly they are a synthetic ceramic of barium titanate or lead zirconate titanate. The electric field, created by the voltage spike, realigns crystalline elements (dipoles) in the ceramic, thereby suddenly changing the crystal's thickness. The sudden change in thickness starts a series of vibrations which produce sound waves.

The piezoelectric crystal is housed in the front of a transducer, a plastic box that protects the crystal from mechanical trauma and provides sonic and electrical insulation. Thin silver or gold electrodes are plated onto the surface of the crystal and the outside electrode is grounded to protect the patient from electrical shock. A backing block dampens vibrations between voltage spikes, so the transducer can be used to generate multiple short pulses of sound. Each transducer vibrates at its own natural frequency, called the resonant frequency, when struck with a short voltage spike. If a clinical situation dictates a different frequency, another transducer must be selected, one designed with the appropriate frequency. Piezoelectric crystals can be damaged by heat. Above a critical temperature, called the Curie temperature, a crystal loses its piezoelectric properties and becomes a worthless piece of ceramic. The Q-factor is a measure of both the purity of tone (narrowness of frequency range) and of the ring down-time, i.e. the time that it takes a transducer to stop vibrating.

An ultrasonic beam is a series of longitudinal waves transmitting energy. They travel through average body tissue at a velocity of 1540 m/sec. Their velocity is independent of frequency. The velocity of sound depends upon the density and compressibility of the conducting medium, and is equal to the frequency times the wavelength. As a sound beam passes through the body, the beam is attenuated, or reduced in intensity, by a combination of diffusion, reflection, refraction and absorption. The sonic beam is fairly coherent with parallel sides in the near, or Fresnel zone. Beyond a certain critical distance, the transition point, the beam reaches the far, or Fraunhofer zone, and begins to flare out and disperse. The length of the near zone is proportional to the square of the diameter of the transducer and inversely proportional to the wavelength of the sound. The beam is rapidly attenuated by dispersion in the far zone. Reflection occurs at tissue interfaces. The incident and reflected angles are equal. The amount of reflection depends upon the difference in the acoustic impedance of the two surfaces and the angle of incidence of the beam. Acoustic impedance is the product of the density and velocity of sound in the conducting medium. Reflection is greatest with a large difference between the acoustic impedances of the two media and with a small incident angle. Reflection is least, and transmission greatest at an incident angle of 90°.

When the velocity of sound changes as it passes from one medium to another, the frequency remains constant but the wavelength changes. If the wavefront strikes the second medium at an angle, the sound is refracted, or bent. The degree of refraction depends upon the angle of incidence and difference in the velocity of sound in the two media. Absorption, which is the conversion of sound into heat, depends upon the frequency of the sound and both the viscosity and relaxation time of the conducting medium. Absorption is directly proportional to frequency, i.e. increasing from 1 to 2 MHz doubles absorption and halves the penetrating power of the beam. Therefore, high frequency sound cannot be used to examine thick parts.

A longitudinal wave is propagated by multiple particles (molecules) oscillating back-and-forth to produce bands of compression and rarefaction in the conducting medium. When these bands are back-scattered to the piezoelectric crystal as echoes, they change the crystal's thickness which produces an electrical signal. This signal forms the basis of the ultrasonic image. The sound is transmitted in short bursts, or pulses, usually 1000/sec. The pulses are short, about one millionth of a second. Between pulses, the transducer acts as a receiver, recording returning echoes. The time delay between the initiation of a pulse and the return of an echo is converted into depth in all imaging modes. The images can be displayed in several modes. The A-mode displays a one-dimensional static image showing echoes as spikes projecting from a baseline. The baseline identifies the central axis of the beam. The TM-mode is similar to the A-mode, except that the echoes are recorded as dots instead of spikes, and the TM-mode is used to study moving parts. Motion is recorded on a strip chart recorder or by sweeping the dots across an oscilloscope during a timed exposure.

The B-mode is a two-dimensional display of the image produced by moving a transducer either longitudinally or in cross section. The transducer is like the handle of a saber with the sound beam as the blade. Multiple controls are provided to augment weaker echoes. The most important is the time gain compensator which logarithmically enhances echoes from selected depths after an adjustable delay.

Depth resolution, the ability to separate

two objects in tandem, depends upon the spatial pulse length which is the number of waves in a pulse times their length. Depth resolution is best with transducers that have a short spatial pulse length. Lateral resolution, the ability to separate two objects lying side-by-side, depends upon the width of the sonic beam. The beam can be narrowed with an acoustic lens which bends the sound toward a focal point.

The Doppler effect is a change in the perceived frequency of a sound emitted by a moving source. Doppler devices are used to study motion, primarily that of blood. This is accomplished by continuously transmitting a sound beam through one transducer while a second transducer records returning echoes. The difference between the two frequencies usually falls in the audible range for most physiologic motions. After amplification the difference becomes an audio signal.

REFERENCES

1. Baker, D. W.: *Diagnostic Ultrasound* (Edited by King, D. L.). St. Louis: The C. V. Mosby Co., 1974.
2. ———: Ultrasonic instruments. Seminars Roentgenol. 10, 265, 1975.
3. Buddemeyer, E. U.: The physics of diagnostic ultrasound. Radiol. Clin. N. Amer., 13, 391, 1975.
4. Feigenbaum, H.: *Echocardiography*. 2nd Ed. Philadelphia: Lea & Febiger, 1976.
5. Felix, W. R., Jr., Sigel, B., and Popky, G. L.: Doppler ultrasound in the diagnosis of peripheral vascular disease. Seminars Radiol. *10*, 315, 1975.
6. Hileman, R.: Shades of gray. Sonix *1*, 30, 1975.
7. Kremkau, F. W.: The physical principles of ultrasound. Seminars Roentgenol. *10*, 259, 1975.
8. Leo, F. P., and Rao, G. U. V.: The technology of diagnostic ultrasound. Radiol. Clin. N. Amer. 3, 403, 1975.
9. McDicken, W. N.: *Diagnostic Ultrasonics: Principles and Use of Instruments*. New York: John Wiley and Sons, Inc., 1976.
10. Sample, W. F., Po, J. B., Gray, R. K., and Cahill, P. J.: Gray-scale ultrasonography. Applied Radiol. *4*, 63, 1975.
11. Sanders, R. C.: Foreword to a symposium on B-scan ultrasound. Radiol. Clin. N. Amer. *13*, 389, 1975.
12. Taylor, K. J. W., Carpenter, D. A., and McCready, V. R.: Gray-scale echography in the diagnosis of intrahepatic disease. J. Clin. Ultrasound, *1*, 284, 1973.
13. Wells, P. N. T.: *The Physical Principles of Ultrasonic Diagnosis*. London: Academic Press, Inc., 1969.

CHAPTER **26**

Protection

HISTORICAL REVIEW

Many of the somatic dangers of radiation became evident a few months after x rays were discovered. Roentgen announced his discovery in December of 1895. In 1896, 23 cases of radiodermatitis were reported in the world literature.[1] Between 1911 and 1914, three review articles identified 54 cancer deaths and 198 cases of radiation-induced malignancy. The first American radiation fatality occurred in 1904 when Thomas Edison's assistant, Clarence M. Dally, died of cancer. A few far-sighted individuals cried out for radiation controls, but their pleas were largely ignored. Catastrophes continued until the whole medical community became alarmed. Finally, in 1921, the first official action was taken when the British X-ray and Radium Protection Committee was founded to investigate methods for reducing exposures. However, their efforts were severely hampered, since they did not have a satisfactory unit of radiation measurement. The crude units of the time, the erythema dose and "slight film fogging" proved completely inadequate. In 1928, the Second International Congress of Radiology (ICR) appointed a committee to define the roentgen (R) as a unit of exposure. The committee did not finish its assignment until 1937, but the roentgen became the accepted unit of measurement even though it was not accurately defined.

The first dose limiting recommendation was made by a group of American scientists, the Advisory Committee on X-ray and Radium Protection, in 1931, 46 years after Roentgen's discovery. The recommendation was 0.2 R per day. The name of the committee has been changed several times, and it is now called the National Council on Radiation Protection and Measurements (NCRP). It is a private organization of scientists, experts in various aspects of radiation, operating under a congressional charter without legal status. The NCRP publishes its recommendations in periodic handbooks. These handbooks are purely advisory, but most state and federal laws are based on NCRP recommendations. Since the first recommendation of 50 R per year (0.2 R per work day) made in 1931, the maximum permissible dose (MPD) has been lowered on three separate occasions as shown in Table 26–1.

Table 26–1. Historical Review of Maximum Permissible Dose (MPD) Recommendations of the National Council on Radiation Protection and Measurements (NCRP)

DATE	ANNUAL MPD (rems)
1931	50
1936	30
1948	15
1958	5

The MPD is now only 1/10 of its initial level. Recommended exposures have been lowered because of a growing concern over the increasing use of diagnostic radiation and apprehension about the mounting evidence that small doses can cause leukemia and carcinoma.

BIOLOGIC EFFECTS OF RADIATION

All ionizing radiation is harmful! This is the premise that mandates a radiation protection policy. The harmful effects fall into two broad categories: (1) somatic, those harmful to the person being irradiated; and (2) genetic, those harmful to future generations. We are not qualified to discuss the biologic effects of radiation in any detail, so our description will be quite superficial. The interested reader should read one of the texts listed at the end of this chapter.[2-4] **One important point must be emphasized—the data are not available to indicate if there is a threshold below which no harmful effect will occur.** Without this knowledge, we cannot say that there is a safe dose. Therefore, a recommendation that 5 rem per year is the maximum permissible dose really means "that, in light of present knowledge, this dose is not expected to cause appreciable bodily injury to a person at any time during his lifetime."[5] **In actual practice, radiation levels should be kept at the lowest practicable level, and we should not think of permissible doses as perfectly safe.**

The most important somatic effect of radiation is carcinogenesis, and leukemia is the most common neoplasia. The exact risk is unknown. Hall[2] makes the statement that "the 20-year risk from leukemia plus all other radiation-induced neoplastic diseases is 6 cases per 100,000 individuals exposed per rem." He admits that this estimate is made on limited data and involves many tenuous assumptions. Nevertheless, most experts agree that low doses of radiation can cause neoplasms. Usually there is a long latent period rang-

ing from 5 to 20 years for leukemia and from 10 to 30 years for other tumors.

The genetic effects of radiation are more frightening than the somatic ones because they may not manifest themselves for several generations. Each new mutant constitutes a potential burden to society, and the burden must be kept at the lowest level consistent with good medical practice. Because of the fear of these genetic effects, dose limits are placed on exposures to large segments of the population, as opposed to maximum permissible doses. This emphasizes the need to restrict exposures. The **genetically significant dose (GSD)** is defined as the dose which, if received by every member of the population, would be expected to produce the same total genetic injury as the actual doses received by the various individuals. For example, if the world population consisted of 1000 individuals and each received a radiation dose of 0.1 rem, the genetic effect would be the same as if 10 individuals received 10 rems and the other 990 received nothing:

$$1000 \times 0.1 = (10 \times 10) + (990 \times 0)$$

The concept implies that the effect of large exposures to a few individuals is greatly diluted by the total population and thus has little overall genetic impact. Radiation workers may receive relatively large exposures without significantly changing the population's genetically significant dose.

RADIATION UNITS

Before discussing maximum permissible dose (MPD) recommendations, we are going to digress and define three units of radiation measurement: the roentgen, the rad and the rem.

1. **The roentgen (R)** is defined as a unit of **radiation exposure** which will liberate a charge of 2.58×10^{-4} coulombs per kilogram of air.[6] This definition is relatively meaningless to most radiologists, since the coulomb is not part of our daily vocabulary. In more familiar terms, a roentgen is the approximate exposure to the body

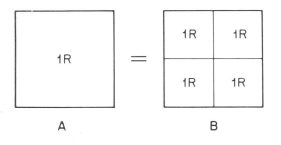

Figure 26-1   The exposures in A and B are identical

surface for an AP film of the abdomen for a patient of average thickness. As a measure of exposure, the roentgen is independent of area, or field size. This independence is shown diagrammatically in Figure 26-1. When a large square (A) is exposed to 1 R, each increment of the square receives 1 R. If the square is divided into multiple smaller squares (B), each of these squares receives 1 R of exposure. It would be improper to add the exposures of the smaller squares and say the total was 4 R, since no area has received that much exposure. This is a familiar concept in other areas of our daily lives. For example, rainfall is measured in inches without regard to area. A 1-inch rain produces a 1-inch deep layer of water in a drinking glass or a washtub, provided they both have flat bottoms and perpendicular sides. Roentgen exposures are exactly the same.

2. The **rad** is the unit of **absorbed dose.** One rad is equal to the radiation necessary to deposit energy of 100 ergs in 1 gm of irradiated material (100 ergs/gm). It is independent of the composition of the radiated material and energy of the beam. However, the number of rads deposited per R of exposure varies both with energy of the beam and the composition of the absorber as shown in Table 26-2. The energy deposited in soft tissue per roentgen is approximately 95 ergs/gm in the diagnostic energy range. It may be five times as much in bone at low energies and actually a little less than 95 ergs/gm at 1

MeV. As a general rule, the absorbed dose is proportional to the degree of attenuation.

3. The **rem** is a unit of **dose equivalent.** It is equal to the absorbed dose multiplied by a **quality factor (QF).**

Rem = Rads × Quality Factor

The rem is a measure of the biologic effectiveness of irradiation. Some practical quality factors are shown in Table 26-3. These are only approximations; the actual numbers depend upon the energy of the beam. Since the quality factor for x rays is one, the rad and rem are equal. In fact, at diagnostic energy levels the rad, rem and roentgen may all be considered equal, since the energy deposited in soft tissues by one roentgen of exposure is only 5% more than a rad.

1 roentgen ≃ 1 rad = 1 rem

Table 26-2. Approximate Absorbed Dose (Rads) per Roentgen of Exposure

TISSUE	RADS PER ROENTGEN OF EXPOSURE	
	50 kVp	1 MeV
Soft tissue	0.95	0.95
Bone	5.0	0.90

Table 26-3. Quality Factors for Various Kinds of Radiation[7]

TYPE RADIATION	QUALITY FACTORS
X-rays	1
Gamma-rays	1
Beta Particles	1
Protons	5
Neutrons:	
Slow	3
Fast	10
Alpha Particles	20

X rays and beta particles have the same quality factor. This is logical since the beta particle is a moving electron and the end product of x-ray attenuation is also a moving electron. They are used as the standard and assigned a quality factor of 1. Larger particles deposit more energy per unit length of travel. The amount of energy deposited per unit length of travel, expressed in keV per micron, is called the **linear energy transfer (LET).** If an electron and proton start with the same energy, the proton will be attenuated more quickly. Because of the proton's large size, it encounters more "friction" as it passes between atoms. Having started with the same amount of energy as the electron, the proton deposits more energy per unit length of travel, so it is a higher LET radiation. The amount of biologic damage is determined by the linear energy transfer of the radiation. A tissue absorbing 100 rads of proton radiation sustains 5 times as much biologic damage as a tissue absorbing the same quantity of x rays. Thus, protons have a quality factor of five. For radiation protection purposes the quality factor is multiplied by the absorbed dose in rads to determine the dose equivalent in rems.

The **relative biologic effectiveness (RBE)** is another expression that is used to compare the effectiveness of several types of radiation. It must be determined for each type of radiation and biologic system, and by convention, is reserved for laboratory investigation.

CURRENT POPULATION EXPOSURES

Mankind has been exposed to radiation since the beginning of time. Initially, the exposure all came from natural sources, but over the past few decades, exposures from man-made sources have gradually increased. Annual exposures in the United States from the various kinds of radiation are summarized in Table 26–4. These are approximations and serve only as a general

Table 26–4. Current Radiation Exposure in the USA from Various Sources[5]

SOURCE OF RADIATION	ANNUAL DOSE (mrem)
1. Natural Radiation (average 125)	
a. External (average 100)	
1.) Cosmic	30–70
2.) Gamma	30–130
b. Internal	25
2. Medical procedures	50–70
3. Applied in human research	–
4. Occupational	1
5. Man-made environmental	4
Total	140–300

guide. They may vary by a factor of 10 under some circumstances.

Natural Radiation

Natural radiation exposure arises from external and internal sources. The external sources are cosmic and gamma radiation. Exposure from cosmic radiation varies slightly with latitude and considerably with altitude. It ranges at sea level from 30 mrem/year in Florida to 35 mrem/year in Alaska, and up to 70 mrem/year at an altitude of 1 mile. Gamma ray exposures are a little lower inside buildings than on the outside. The exposure comes primarily from radionuclides in the rock and building materials. In the United States, gamma ray exposures average about 60 mrem outside and 55 mrem inside of a building. The total exposure from external sources averages about 100 mrem/year.

Internal exposure comes from radionuclides in food, water and air, and it is estimated at about 25 mrem/year. The principal contributors are radium and thorium (and their decay products), radiopotassium (^{40}K), and radiocarbon (^{14}C).

The total natural radiation dose in the United States is estimated at 125 mrem and may range up to 400 mrem/year. No deleterious effect has been validated in persons receiving the higher exposure, but we cannot derive great consolation from this fact since no satisfactory epidemiological study has ever been undertaken.

Man-made Radiation

Exposure to man-made radiation sources contributes less to population exposure than natural sources, but the man-made contribution is constantly rising and it is cause for concern. At present, the major contributor to the genetically significant dose (GSD) is medical radiation for diagnostic and therapeutic procedures, which is estimated at between 50 and 75 mrem/year. Other man-made sources, i.e. radiation used in research, occupational exposure, and man-made environmental radiation make only a minor contribution. Occupational exposures may be as high as 5000 mrem/year (although they are usually much less), but the total number of exposed persons is relatively small and the contribution to the GSD is estimated at only 1%.

Man-made environmental radiation includes effluents from atomic facilities and fallout from nuclear explosions. Fallout from weapons testing is the major contributor at the present time. The radionuclides of principal concern are iodine (^{131}I), strontium (^{89,90}Sr)., cesium (^{137}Cs) and cerium (^{144}Ce). Consumer products contribute little because of tight controls. Exposure comes primarily from some television receivers and luminous watches, clocks and signs. Fortunately, shoe-fitting fluoroscopes are gone. The average national increment from man-made environmental radiation is estimated to be about 4% of the exposure from natural radiation.

DOSE LIMITING RECOMMENDATIONS

"The principal objective of radiation protection is to ensure that the dose received by an individual (other than the patient) does not exceed the applicable maximum permissible value. A secondary objective is to prevent damage or impairment of function of radiation-sensitive film or equipment."[6] To accomplish the principal objective, we must know maximum permissible values and understand the tools that we have to reduce exposures to these levels. We will discuss permissible exposures and dose limits next and deal with methods later.

For the purpose of regulating radiation

Table 26–5. Dose Limiting Recommendations[5]

CATEGORY OF INDIVIDUAL	MAXIMUM PERMISSIBLE DOSE (rem)	
	Annual	Quarterly
1. Occupationally exposed		
Whole body (gonads, lens, and bone marrow)	5	3
Hands	75	25
Forearms	30	10
Other organs	15	5
Fetus (entire gestation)	0.5	–
	DOSE LIMITS (rem)	
2. Occasionally exposed	0.5	–
3. General population		
Genetic	0.17	–
Somatic	0.17	–

exposures, individuals are divided into two categories: (1) the occupationally exposed and (2) the occasionally exposed. The recommendations affecting radiation protection policy deal only with these two categories. A third category, or group, is the population at large. Different exposure recommendations are made for each of these three groups as shown in Table 26–5. Briefly summarized, **the maximum permissible dose for an occupationally exposed individual is 5 rem/year; the dose limit for the occasionally exposed is 1/10 as much, or 0.5 rem/year; and the dose limit for the population is 1/3 of the occasional level, or 0.17 rem/year.** These recommendations apply to radiation incurred under occupational conditions and exclude exposure from the following:

1. Background radiation
2. Medical-dental procedures (diagnostic x rays)
3. Man-made devices outside the occupational environment (T.V. sets, luminous dial watches, etc.)

Occupationally Exposed

The occupationally exposed individual accepts some risk. He takes this slight risk for some tangible benefit, usually gainful employment. As a general rule, he is somewhat knowledgeable of the risks involved, and his numbers are relatively small so his exposure does not contribute appreciably to the genetically significant dose. For this reason, his maximal permissible dose is larger than that of the other groups. By law, no one under 18 may be employed in an occupationally exposed position.

The MPD for the whole body and other critical organs (the gonads, red bone marrow, and lens) shall not exceed 5 rems in any one year, or 3 rems in one-quarter or an accumulated dose of 5 rems times the age in years minus 18.

Maximum permissible accumulative dose =
(N − 18) × 5 rems

For example, if a technologist is 30 years of age, his permissible accumulative dose would be: (30 − 18) × 5 = 60 rems. This is the maximum permissible accumulation that he is allowed to receive up to the age of 30. If a radiation worker accidentally receives a dose exceeding his maximum permissible accumulative dose, he must avoid any further exposure until his accumulative dose falls below that recommended by the formula. The MPD for the skin, hands, forearms and other organs is higher as shown in Table 26–5. Fetal exposures are restricted to only 1/10 of the whole body dose, or 0.5 rems during the entire 9 months of gestation.

Occupationally exposed individuals work in a controlled area, which is an area under the supervision of an individual responsible for radiation protection. Exposures in controlled areas must be kept at a level that would allow a radiation worker to stay in the area during his entire working day without exceeding his MPD. The customary time interval that is used to calculate exposures for controlled areas is 1 week. Dividing the 5 rems maximum permissible annual dose by a 50-week work year gives a maximum permissible weekly exposure of 0.1 roentgen. Notice that we have changed units from rems to roentgens, but this is permissible since the two are almost equal in the diagnostic energy range. If exposures in the entire controlled area are kept below 0.1 R/week, then a radiation worker is free to move about the area in safety.

Occasionally (Non-Occupationally) Exposed

The non-occupationally exposed individual is in a different situation than the radiation worker. Usually the occasionally exposed individual has no knowledge of the risks involved, receives no compensation for taking a risk, and most important, has no freedom to decide if he will accept the risk. When a member of the general population, for example a visitor, enters a radiation area, he becomes an occasionally exposed individual. The radiation is thrust upon him, frequently without his knowledge. Also, the population size of the occasionally exposed is not controlled, so large numbers of individuals could be involved which would have a greater impact upon the genetically significant dose. For all of these reasons, the dose limits for the occasionally exposed is 0.5 rem/year, or 1/10 of the MPD for the occupationally exposed.

Areas occupied by occasionally exposed persons are designated as uncontrolled areas. The area may be a corridor, waiting room, elevator, parking lot, etc. If the area is exposed to radiation, and non-radiation workers have access to it, its radiation restrictions are more stringent than controlled areas. Exposures must be kept at a level consistent with the continuous occupancy by an occasionally exposed individual without exceeding his dose limit of 0.5 rem/year, or 0.01 R/week.

In summary, the occupationally exposed individual has a maximum permissible dose of 5 rem/year and occupies a controlled area with a permissible weekly exposure of 0.1 R. The occasionally exposed individual has a dose limit of 0.5 rem/year and occupies an uncontrolled area with a permissible weekly exposure of 0.01 R.

PROTECTIVE BARRIERS

Three methods can be used to control radiation exposure levels: distance, time and barriers. Distance is obviously an effective method since beam intensity is governed by the inverse square law. Exposures can be controlled with time in a variety of ways: (1) by limiting the time that the generator is turned on; (2) limiting the time that the beam is directed at a certain area; or (3) limiting the time that the area is occupied. All of these factors are taken into consideration in planning a new installation. However, when they prove inadequate, the only alternative is a protective barrier, usually lead or concrete. Barriers are designated as either primary or secondary depending on whether they protect from primary radiation (the useful beam) or stray radiation (a combination of leakage and scatter radiation).

Primary Barriers

Figure 26–2 diagrammatically summarizes the factors that must be considered in determining primary barrier requirements for a radiographic installation. The number of factors seems imposing, but the total concept is quite simple. Our first task is to evaluate the exposure to the area in question. Once we know the exposure, we can use either half-value layers or tables to determine barrier requirements. Five factors must be evaluated in exposure calculations. The five are shown along the central axis of the illustration and include the following:

1. Workload (W) in mA · min/wk
2. Roentgens per mA · min at 1 meter ($\bar{E}$)

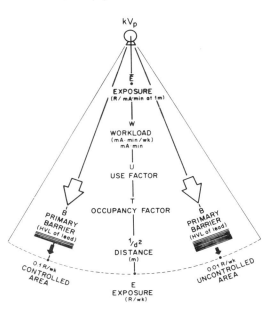

Figure 26–2 Summary of factors involved in primary barrier determinations

3. Use factor (U)
4. Occupancy factor (T)
5. Distance (d) in meters

We will go through the list one step at a time, but first note that no mention is made of attentuation by the patient. Even though patient attenuation may be 90%, it is completely ignored in calculating barrier requirements. The x-ray energy that is used for protection calculations is the maximum voltage (kVp) of the generator, even though the machine will frequently be operated at lower potentials. No distinction is made between single and three-phase generators.

Step 1. The **workload (W)** is the quantity of x rays generated per week. It is the product of tube current in mA and time in minutes of exposure per week (mA · min/wk). For example, if a 125-kVp chest room is being designed to handle 12 patients/hour, the workload is calculated by multiplying the mAs per exposure times the number of exposures per week and then dividing by 60 to convert seconds into minutes. At 125 kVp, we will estimate 2 mAs for a PA, and 8 mAs for a lateral film, i.e. 10 mAs/patient.

$$\frac{mAs}{pt} \times \frac{pts}{hrs} \times \frac{hrs}{wk} = mAs/wk$$

$$10 \times 12 \times 40 = 4800 \; mAs/wk$$

To convert mAs to mA · min, we simply divide by 60:

$$4800 \div 60 = 80 \; mA \cdot min/wk$$

The recommended workload of the NCRP can be used when more specific information is not available. Their recommendations are given in Table 26–6. The recommendation for our 125 kVp chest room is 400 mA · min/wk, which is 5 times the 80 mA · min/wk that we calculated. The NCRP recommendations provide a generous margin for error which is the goal of radiation protection policies. Notice in the table that the workload diminishes as energy increases. The workload for a radiographic room is 1000 mA ·

Table 26–6. Recommended Workloads for Radiographic and Fluoroscopic Installations[6]

MAXIMUM ENERGY (kVp)	WORKLOAD (mA · min/wk)	
	RADIOGRAPHIC ROOM	FLUOROSCOPIC ROOM
100	1000	1500
125	400	600
150	200	300

min/wk at 100 kVp and only 200 mA · min/wk at 150 kVp. The recommended workload is diminished because less mAs is required to expose a film at the higher kVp. Patient handling limits the number of procedures that can be accomplished in a day. Therefore, the recommended workloads in Table 26–6 are all considered equal. This may not seem logical, but it makes good sense. A room can only handle a certain number of patients a day. It takes approximately the same number of milliroentgens to expose a film at 100 kVp as it does at 150 kVp. When the kVp is raised, the mAs can be lowered and the net mR output stays about the same.

Step 2. Since the recommendations regarding maximal permissible dose are all given in roentgens, we must have a way of converting workload into roentgens. The customary way of expressing exposures is in terms of **roentgens/mA · min at a distance of 1 m** from the x-ray source. Table

Table 26–7. X-Ray Output in Roentgens per mA · Minute at 1 Meter (Ē) for Various Energies[7]

PEAK KILOVOLTAGE (kVp)	Ē (R/mA · min at 1 m)
50	0.15
70	0.40
100	0.90
125	1.4
150	2.0

26–7 shows the number of R/mA · min at 1 m for various x-ray energies. This exposure is multiplied by the workload to determine the total roentgen output per week. For example, at a maximum energy of 100 kVp with a workload of 1000 mA · min/wk, Table 26–7 shows an exposure of 0.9 R/mA · min at 1 m. This is a weekly exposure of (1000 mA · min/wk × 0.9 R/mA · min) 900 R/wk at 1 m. The inverse square law is used to determine the exposure at other distances. Note that the exposure per mA · min increases with increasing kVp, and this compensates for the lower workload recommendation described in the previous section.

Step 3. The **use factor (U),** which should really be called the **beam direction factor,** is the fraction of time that the beam is directed at a particular barrier. If it is anticipated that the beam will only be directed at a wall 10% of the time, then the use factor is 0.1. If a wall holds a fixed film changer for chest radiography, where the direction of the beam cannot be changed, then the use factor for that particular wall is 1.0; all other walls are secondary barriers. When specific information is not available, recommended use factors can be obtained from Table 26–8. The use factor for ceilings is always zero since the beam is rarely directed at the ceiling. **The use factor for secondary barriers is always 1,** since the entire room is exposed to stray radiation whenever the x-ray beam is turned on.

Table 26–8. Use Factors for Diagnostic Exposure Rooms[6]

	USEFUL BEAM (Primary Barrier)	STRAY RADIATION* (Secondary Barrier)
Floor	1	1
Walls	1/16	1
Ceiling	0	1

*Stray radiation is the sum of leakage and scatter radiation.

Table 26–9. Occupancy Factors (T) for Non-occupationally Exposed Persons[6]

Full Occupancy (T = 1)
Areas that will be occupied by the same individuals for their full work day such as offices, laboratories, nurses stations, etc.

Partial Occupancy (T = 1/4)
Corridors, restrooms, elevators using operators, etc.

Occasional Occupancy (T = 1/16)
Waiting rooms, stairways, unattended elevators, janitor closets, outside areas used for pedestrian and vehicular traffic, etc.

Step 4. The **occupancy factor (T)** is the fraction that the workload should be decreased to correct for the degree of occupancy of the area in question. It has the same basis as the use factor and is expressed as a fraction which represents the amount of time that the area will be occupied. If the floor of an exposure room is in the basement of a hospital, and no subbasement will ever be constructed, then the floor's occupancy factor is 0, and it is neither a primary nor secondary barrier. Table 26–9 shows recommended occupancy factors for various areas when more specific information is not available. If the area in question is **a controlled area,** i.e. within the x-ray department, it **is assigned an occupancy factor of one.** A radiation worker may spend only a small amount of time in any particular area, but wherever he goes in the department, he will be in a position of potential exposure, so all areas are assumed to be continuously occupied. Therefore, the occupancy factors in the table are only for areas occupied by non-occupationally exposed individuals.

Step 5. Distance (d) is one of the most effective means of radiation protection since exposures change inversely with the square of the distance (the inverse square law). Distances are measured in meters to be consistent with the roentgen output/mA min which is given in the table for a distance of 1 m. If an exposure is 2 R at 1 meter, then at 4 m it will be:

$$2 \text{ R} \times \frac{1}{4^2} = 0.13 \text{ R}$$

It is usually assumed that an individual will be at least 1 foot from a barrier for distance measurements. Some radiation is absorbed in air, but with energies over 50 kVp and distances less than 100 feet, the amount is negligible, and it is ignored.

The product of the factors described in steps 1 through 5 gives the "effective" weekly exposure to any particular point. The term effective is used here to emphasize that the actual exposure may be different, depending upon the occupancy factor.

$$E = \bar{E} \cdot W \cdot U \cdot T \cdot 1/d^2$$

E = weekly exposure reaching the point in question (R/wk)
$\bar{E}$ = R/mA · min at 1 m
W = workload (mA · min/wk)
U = use factor (no units)
T = occupancy factor (no units)
d = distance (in meters from the x-ray tube to the point in question)

The categories of protected areas were discussed earlier under dose limiting recommendations. Two types of areas require protection, those having occupationally exposed individuals and those occupied by persons only occasionally exposed. The recommendations are 5 rem/year for the occupationally exposed and 0.5 rem/year for the occasionally exposed. Dividing by a 50-week work year, the weekly maximum permissible exposures are 0.1 R for occupationally occupied and only 0.01 R for occasionally occupied areas. After an area has been assigned to a category, its weekly exposure must be kept below recommended levels. If the total exposure (E) at the point in question is less than 0.1 R/wk for a controlled area, or 0.01 R/wk for an uncontrolled area, no barrier is required. If E is greater than these maximal permis-

sible exposures, then a protective barrier is required. Its thickness is discussed next.

Methods for Calculating Primary Barrier Thicknesses

Having determined the amount of radiation reaching the area in question, we must reduce this exposure to an acceptable level which depends upon the category of the area. This is accomplished by interposing a barrier of either lead or concrete. Two methods are commonly used to calculate barrier requirements for diagnostic installations: (1) half-value layers (HVL) and (2) precalculated shielding requirement tables. A third method, employing attenuation curves, is commonly used for therapy installations. The attenuation curves are difficult to read at diagnostic exposure levels and they are rarely used by physicists, so we will not bother describing the method.

Half-Value Layers (HVL)

The first method for calculating barrier requirements, and the simplest to understand, is with half-value layers (HVL). The concept of HVL was first used in radiation therapy to express the quality of an x-ray beam. **The half-value layer is the thickness of a specific substance which, when introduced into the path of a beam of radiation, reduces the exposure rate by one-half.** A beam with a half-value layer of 0.2 mm of lead is more penetrating than a beam with a half-value layer of 0.1 mm of

Table 26–10. Half Value Layer (HVL) Thicknesses of Lead and Concrete for Various X-Ray Energies[6]

PEAK KILOVOLTAGE (kVp)	LEAD (mm)	CONCRETE (inches)
50	0.05	0.17
70	0.15	0.33
100	0.24	0.6
125	0.27	0.8
150	0.29	0.88

lead. HVL's in millimeters of lead and inches of concrete are given in Table 26–10. Barrier thickness is calculated by repetitively halving the exposure until it reaches a permissible level, and then multiplying the number of halves times the half-value layer of the beam. For example, if the actual exposure at some point is 3.2 R/wk, and the permissible exposure 0.1 R/wk, the required number of HVL's is determined as follows:

$$3.2 \div 2 = 1.6$$
$$1.6 \div 2 = 0.8$$
$$0.8 \div 2 = 0.4$$
$$0.4 \div 2 = 0.2$$
$$0.2 \div 2 = 0.1$$

Five HVL's reduces 3.2 R/wk down to 0.1 R/wk. If the half-value layer of the beam was 0.25 mm of lead, the barrier would be:

$$0.25 \times 5 = 1.25 \text{ mm of lead}$$

A problem arises in using half-value layers with heterochromatic radiation. Remember, filtration changes the quality of a diagnostic beam as it passes through a barrier. The beam increases in mean energy, or is hardened, so if we use its initial HVL, we could underestimate barrier requirements. Table 26–11 explains how this

problem arises. We start with a 150 kVp heterochromatic beam with a mean energy of 50 keV, a HVL of 0.29 mm of lead and a hypothetical 100 R/wk from the beam. These are the characteristics of the beam as it emerges from the x-ray tube. It has already been filtered by both inherent and added filtration. To reduce the intensity to 50 R, we place 0.29 mm (1 HVL) of lead at point A. The 0.29 mm of lead further filters the radiation, increases its mean energy from 50 to 57 keV, and therefore increases its HVL. Now we must place 0.32 mm of lead at point B to reduce intensity by one-half. In the example given, it is assumed that there is no intensity loss from inverse square. As we continue adding newly determined HVL's to reduce intensity to 12.5 R at point P in the table, we change the mean energy from 50 to 66 keV and the HVL of the beam from 0.29 to 0.35 mm of lead, 0.06 mm more than its initial thickness. Summing the three HVL's placed at points A, B and C shows that 0.95 mm of lead is required to reduce the intensity at point P to 12.5 R. If we had assumed that three of the original HVL's would have accomplished this objective, we would have underestimated the barrier,

Table 26–11. Filtration Changes the Quality of a Diagnostic X-ray Beam (table described in text)

		0.29 mm Pb	+	0.32 mm Pb	+	0.34 mm Pb	=	0.95 mm Pb
		A		B		C		P
Peak Energy (kVp)	150		150		150			150
Mean Energy (keV)	50		57		63			66
HVL (mm Lead)	0.29		0.32		0.34			0.35
R in Beam*	100		50		25			12.5

*Assumes no reduction in intensity from the inverse square law; i.e., the distances between points A, B, and C is zero.

since 0.29 × 3 is only 0.87, which is 0.08 mm less than that actually required. However, the error is not significant if the original HVL is for an already hardened beam. The numbers given in Table 26–11 are for such a beam. In other words, the radiation has been passed through numerous half-value layers and the last one is used to express beam quality.

Precalculated Shielding Requirement Tables

Most physicists use precalculated tables like Table 26–12 to determine barrier requirements for diagnostic installations. The tables are easy to use because the inverse square effect and barrier thicknesses are precalculated. All one needs do is determine the effective workload by multiplying the actual workload (W) by the use factor (U) and occupancy factor (T). The effective workload is still in mA · min/wk, since the use and occupancy factors have no units. Knowing the kVp and

distance, the table indicates primary and secondary barrier requirements in both lead and concrete. For example, to determine the barrier requirements at 10 feet for a busy 100 kVp radiographic room with a workload of 1000 mA · min/wk with the use and occupancy factors both 0.25, we would multiply the workload times the use and occupancy factors.

$$W \cdot U \cdot T = mA \cdot min/wk$$
$$1000 \cdot 0.25 \cdot 0.25 = 62.5$$

We then go to the table and find 62.5 mA · min/wk in the 100 kVp column. Moving to the right to a distance of 10 feet, we find primary barrier requirements of 0.5 mm of lead for a controlled and 1.25 mm for an uncontrolled area. Under the same column we can find barrier requirements in concrete and also secondary barrier thicknesses. All of this is accomplished with little mathematical manipulation, which explains the popularity of the tables.

Table 26–12. Shielding Requirements for Radiographic Installations[6]

WUT* in mA · min/week			DISTANCE IN FEET FROM SOURCE (X-RAY TUBE TARGET) TO OCCUPIED AREA									
100 kVP	125 kVp	150 kVp										
1,000	400	200	5	7	10	14	20	28	40			
500	200	100		5	7	10	14	20	28	40		
250	100	50			5	7	10	14	20	28	40	
125	50	25				5	7	10	14	20	28	40
62.5	25	12.5					5	7	10	14	20	28

TYPE OF AREA	MATERIAL	PRIMARY PROTECTIVE BARRIER THICKNESS									
Controlled	Lead, mm	1.9	1.65	1.4	1.2	1.0	0.75	0.5	0.3	0	0
Noncontrolled	Lead, mm	2.65	2.4	2.2	1.95	1.7	1.5	1.25	1.0	0.8	0.5
Controlled	Concrete, inch	5.9	5.2	4.6	4.0	3.3	2.7	2.1	1.6	1.0	0.4
Noncontrolled	Concrete, inch	8.0	7.3	6.7	6.0	5.4	4.8	4.1	3.5	2.9	2.2

		SECONDARY PROTECTIVE BARRIER THICKNESS									
Controlled	Lead, mm	0.55	0.4	0.2	0.1	0	0	0	0	0	0
Noncontrolled	Lead, mm	1.2	1.0	0.8	0.6	0.45	0.25	0.1	0	0	0
Controlled	Concrete, inch	1.9	1.4	0.8	0.2	0	0	0	0	0	0
Noncontrolled	Concrete, inch	3.8	3.2	2.6	2.1	1.5	1.0	0.4	0	0	0

*W—workload in mA · min/week, U—use factor, T—occupancy factor.

SECONDARY BARRIERS

Secondary barriers provide protection from scatter and leakage radiation, which we will lump together and call stray radiation. As a general rule, **no secondary barrier is required for areas protected by a primary barrier,** i.e. the primary serves as both a primary and secondary barrier. All of the factors that played a role in calculating barriers for the useful beam will have to be reconsidered in determining secondary barriers except the use factor. The use factor is really a beam direction factor, and since stray radiation goes in all directions, the use factor is always one.

Protection From Scatter Radiation

To determine primary barrier thickness, we make numerous estimates and allow a generous margin for error. Secondary barrier calculations are even less precise. The two most important factors, the intensity and the energy of the scatter radiation, are both unknown. Therefore, before we can go any further, we must make two assumptions.

1. **The energy of the scatter radiation is assumed to be equal to that of the primary** (provided the primary is less than 500 kVp). This assumption is reasonably accurate, especially below 100 kVp where little energy is lost in Compton's scattering, and where the secondary beam is hardened (its mean energy increased) by passing through the patient. If the assumption errs, it errs on the side of conservatism.

2. **The intensity of 90° scatter radiation, relative to the primary beam, is reduced by a factor of 1000 at a distance of 1 meter for a field size of 400 sq cm.** The 1 m distance is measured from the center of the beam on the patient's surface. When radiation can be forced to scatter more than once, for example with a maze, its intensity is reduced to inconsequential levels, well below permissible exposures, so we will not concern outselves with multiple scatterings.

Field size is one of the factors that controls scatter radiation, so it is not surprising that it plays a role in determining secondary barrier requirements. The other two factors that control scattering, peak kilovoltage and patient thickness, are ignored. Field size is measured at the patient's surface. A correction factor is used for fields other than 400 sq cm.

$$\text{Correction factor} = \frac{F}{400}$$

F = actual field size (cm²)
400 = control field size (cm²)

The correction factor has no units, since both F and 400 are in square centimeters, and they cancel each other. For fields smaller than 400 sq cm, the correction factor is less than one; for larger fields, it is greater than one. For example, with 200 sq cm, the correction factor is:

$$\text{Correction factor} = \frac{200}{400} = 0.5$$

The roentgen output of the x-ray tube (exposure in R/mA · min at 1 m, i.e. $\bar{E}$), workload (W), and occupancy factor (T), are the same as they were for the primary barrier calculations. Inverse square attenuation is also the same except that the distance is measured from the center of the patient rather than from the center of the x-ray tube. The use factor is dropped since it is always one. A correction factor is added for field size, and the total exposure is divided by 1000 for right angle scattering.

$E_s = \bar{E} \cdot W \cdot T \cdot 1/d^2 \cdot 1/1000 \cdot F/400$
E_s = weekly exposure from scatter radiation (R/wk)
$\bar{E}$ = R/mA · min at 1 m
W = workload (mA · min/wk)
T = occupancy factor (no units)
d = distance (in meters from the center of the beam on the patient's surface)
F = actual field size (cm²)

The weekly exposure is then handled in the same manner that it was for primary barrier calculations. Exposures are reduced to permissible levels by one of the two previously described methods, i.e. half-value layers or precalculated tables.

Protection From Leakage Radiation

Leakage radiation is radiation that passes through the lead shielding in the tube housing when the beam is turned on. By law, the **maximum permissible leakage exposure 1 meter from a diagnostic x-ray tube is 0.1 R/hour** with the tube operating continuously at its maximum kVp and mA. This does not mean the maximum mA that the tube is capable of generating, rather it means the maximum mA at which the tube can be run continuously without overheating. The tube may be rated at 150 kVp and 1000 mA, but it cannot be operated continuously at this level. At 150 kVp, its maximum mA will probably be around 500, and it will only tolerate that for a few milliseconds. The maximum mA at which the tube can be run continuously must be determined from anode heat cooling charts. Figure 26–3 shows a cooling chart for a Dynamax "69" tube. The maximum continuous mA is the maximum amount of heat per second (1400 heat units in this case), divided by the peak voltage, which may be from 100 to 150 kVp. At 150 kVp, the maximum continuous mA would be:

$$1400 \div 150 = 9.3 \text{ mA}$$

The Dynamax "69" is a large tube. Smaller tubes have maximum continuous loads of 3 to 5 mA. The manufacturer must build the housing to limit exposure to 0.1 R/hour at 1 meter with the tube operating at peak potential, and the highest mA that does not exceed the housing's ability to dissipate heat.

In calculating exposures from primary and scatter radiation, we could look up the roentgen output at 1 meter ($\bar{E}$) for each mA of workload. Both the exposure and workload involve the primary beam. For leakage radiation, we need a comparable unit of exposure, i.e. R/mA · min at 1 m, but the "mA · min" refers to the useful beam and the "R at 1 meter" to the leakage

ANODE THERMAL CHARACTERISTICS

Figure 26–3   Anode thermal characteristics of a Machlett Dynamax "69" x-ray tube radiation. Leakage occurs whenever the x-ray beam is "on". It is completely independent of the useful beam itself and will occur even if the collimator shutter is completely closed. As long as x rays are being generated within the tube housing, leakage radiation occurs.

Figure 26–4 shows the relationship between the workload of the primary beam and the permissible leakage level of 0.1 R/hour. In the illustration, 5 mA is given as the maximum continuous current that the tube can tolerate. If the tube runs at this level for only 1 second, the exposure is 5 mAs, which is the unit technicians use to describe radiographic techniques. However, to be consistent with our previous methods, we will continue using the unit mA · min, which is the number of mA times the "on" time in minutes. Thus, in 1 minute of continuous operation, the output will be 5 mA · min. The leakage exposure is 0.1 R/hour at a distance of 1 meter from the x-ray tube. To convert to R/min, we simply divide by 60:

$$0.1 \text{ R/hr} \div 60 \text{ min/hr} = 0.00167 \text{ R/min}$$

This is the leakage exposure that results from the tube being "on" for 1 minute. The workload of the primary beam for the same minute was 5 mA · min. To determine the leakage exposure at 1 meter for each mA · min of workload, we must divide by 5:

$$\frac{0.00167 \text{ R/min}}{5 \text{ mA} \cdot \text{min/min}} = 0.00033 \text{ R/mA} \cdot \text{min at 1 m } (\bar{E}_L)$$

Now that we have determined the exposure in R/mA · min at 1 m ($\bar{E}_L$), it is a simple task to calculate the exposure at some other point. We multiply the number of R/mA · min times the workload, occupancy factor, and inverse square of distance as we did for primary and scatter exposure calculations.

$E_L = \bar{E}_L \cdot W \cdot T \cdot 1/d^2$
E_L = weekly exposure from leakage radiation (R/wk)
$\bar{E}_L$ = leakage exposure at 1 m per mA · min of workload (R/mA · min)
W = workload (mA · min/wk)
T = occupancy factor (no units)
d = distance from x-ray tube (meters)

The customary method for reducing leakage exposures to permissible levels is with half-value layers of barrier. Leakage radiation is already heavily filtered by the lead in the tube housing, so the half-value method is quite accurate.

There is one last "rule of thumb" regarding radiation protection. If the difference between the barrier requirements for scatter and leakage radiation is greater than three half-value layers, use the large one and ignore the smaller one; if less than three half-value layers, add one half-value layer to the larger and ignore the smaller. However, for diagnostic installations, this rule is relatively meaningless. Leakage exposures are almost always within the permissible range without any barrier. Even more important, the walls of diagnostic rooms are almost always planned as primary barriers and they provide ample protection from stray radiation.

EXAMPLE

Figure 26–5 shows a general radiographic room with an upright Bucky mounted on the wall protecting area C. The generator, a three phase unit, is rated

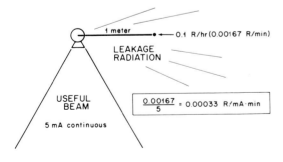

Figure 26–4 Maximum permissible leakage exposure at 1 meter in R/mA · min with a maximum continuous exposure of 5 mA

3 meters

PATHOLOGY LAB
(BASEMENT)

(B)

(A)

2 meters •

RADIOLOGIST'S
OFFICE

(C)

• 4 meters

REST
ROOM

Figure 26–5   Floor plan of the general radiographic room described in the example

at 125 kVp and 600 mA. We will calculate barrier requirements for areas A, B and C, where A is a radiologist's office, B is the floor above a basement pathology laboratory and C is a restroom. The distances from the points in question to the x-ray tube are given in the illustration, and notice that the points are 1 foot from the wall which is the NCRP recommendation.[6] We will assume that the x-ray tube is never directed at area A.

Since we do not know how many patients will be done in an 8-hour shift, we will accept the NCRP recommendation for a busy general radiographic room of 400 mA · min/wk for a 125 kVp installation. Then we need not concern ourselves with the generator's mA capacity, and of course, single and three phase units are treated the same. We can look up the occupancy factors, use factors, and roentgen output at 1 m in the appropriate tables. Since the beam is never directed at area A, its use factor as a primary barrier is 0, and it will only require a secondary barrier. In actual practice, it would be better to provide a primary barrier for

area A so that the room's function could be changed at a later date without the need for additional protection. We will return to area A when we discuss secondary barriers. The use factor for point B, the pathology laboratory, is 1 since it is a floor, and the use factor for a floor is always 1 (Table 26–8). The table shows a use factor of 1/16 for walls, but a large number of upright chest examinations are anticipated, so we will use a use factor of 1/4 and not follow the NCRP recommendations. The occupancy factors are 1/4 for the restroom and 1 for the pathology laboratory. We will calculate primary barriers first, and in this example we will use both methods to determine barrier thickness.

Primary Barriers

Precalculated Tables

We will start with the table method, since it requires the least mathematics. To use the method, we must find the product of the workload (W), use factor (U) and occupancy factor (T):

	W · U · T = mA · min/wk
Point B:	400 · 1 · 1 = 400
Point C:	400 · ¼ · ¼ = 25

We can look up barrier requirements for points B and C in Table 26–12, but we have a bit of a problem, since the distances in the table are given in feet and our distances are in meters. One meter equals 39.37 inches, or approximately 3.25 feet. Converting from meters to feet, we get:

Point B: 3 × 3.25 = 10 ft.
Point C: 4 × 3.25 = 13 ft.

To look up the barrier thickness for point B in Table 26–12, we find 125 kVp and 400 mA · min/wk at a distance of 10 feet. Both the pathology laboratory and restroom are uncontrolled areas. The primary barrier thickness is 2.2 mm of sheet lead, or 6.7 inches of concrete, for an uncontrolled area. Since B is in a basement, we would simply make sure that the concrete floor is at least 6.7 inches thick. Point C is done in a similar manner, but 13 feet is not shown in the table so we have to extrapolate between 10 and 14 feet. At 25 mA · min/wk, a lead thickness between 1.25 and 1.0 mm, say 1.20 mm, would be needed for an uncontrolled area. No secondary barrier would be required for these walls, since the primary would provide ample protection from stray radiation.

Half-Value Layers

To use HVL's, we must calculate the potential exposure at the points in question. The roentgen output at 1 m ($\bar{E}$) is 1.4 R/mA · min (Table 26–7).

	E = $\bar{E}$ · W · U · T · 1/d³
Point B:	E = 1.4 · 400 · 1 · 1 · ⅓² = 62
Point C:	E = 1.4 · 400 · ¼ · ¼ · ¼² = 0.154

The pathology laboratory and restroom are both uncontrolled areas with maximum permissible exposure levels of 0.01 R/wk. The exposures to both points are excessive, i.e. above permissible levels, so our next step is to determine the number of HVL's required to reduce them to permissible levels.

Point B:	Exposure — HVL's
	62 R/wk — 0
	31 — 1
	15.5 — 2
	7.75 — 3
	3.88 — 4
	1.94 — 5
	0.97 — 6
	0.48 — 7
	0.24 — 8
	0.12 — 9
	0.06 — 10
	0.03 — 11
	0.015 — 12
	0.01 — approx 12.6 HVL's
	0.007 — 13

If the number of half-value layers does not come out evenly, we can extrapolate as we did above, but it is simpler to use the whole number that reduces exposures below the permissible level, i.e. 13 in this case, a practice that errs on the side of conservatism. Table 26–10 shows the HVL for 125 kVp to be 0.27 mm for lead and 0.8 inches for concrete. Multiplying these values by the 12.6 HVL's required to attenuate the beam to permissible levels:

Lead: 0.27 × 12.6 = 3.4 mm
Concrete: 0.8 × 12.6 = 10 inches

Since B is the floor, we would probably use the 10 inches of concrete. Following the same procedure for point C:

Point C:	Exposure — HVL's
	0.14 R/wk — 0
	0.07 — 1
	0.35 — 2
	0.17 — 3
	0.10 — approx 3.3 HVL's
	0.085 — 4

Lead: 0.27 × 3.3 = 0.89 mm
Concrete: 0.8 × 3.3 = 2.6 inches

The barrier thicknesses are different for the two methods (i.e. tables and HVL's), but this is not important since our purpose is to explain principles. Also, the differences emphasize the fact that radiation protection is not a precise science.

Secondary Barriers

Wall A protects a radiologist's office and will require a secondary barrier. It is a controlled area with a maximum permissible exposure of 0.1 R/wk, and since it is a controlled area, its occupancy factor is 1. For convenience, we will calculate the exposures for both leakage and scatter radiation at a distance of 2 meters as shown in Figure 26–5.

Precalculated Tables

Table 26–12 gives both primary and secondary barrier requirements. We simply multiply the workload (W), use (U) and occupancy (T) factors (WUT) and find the barrier thickness for the appropriate distance.

$$W \cdot U \cdot T = mA \cdot min/wk$$
$$400 \cdot 1 \cdot 1 = 400\ mA \cdot min/wk$$

Converting the distance of 2 meters into feet, we get a little over 6 feet. At 125 kVp, the secondary barrier thickness for a controlled area (Table 26–12) is 0.55 mm of lead for 5 feet and 0.40 mm for 7 feet. We will need a thickness between these two, say 0.5 mm, and this would handle both the leakage and scatter radiation. In other words, we would be finished. But we will go on to make the calculations for scatter and leakage radiation separately using half-value layers.

HVL Method for Scatter Radiation

The workload will be the same as it was for the primary barrier, i.e. 400 mA · min/wk at 125 kVp. The occupancy factor is 1 since it is a controlled area. The exposure is 0.14 R/mA · min (Table 26–7). This exposure is at 1 meter, which we will assume is the patient's surface. This is a reasonably accurate assumption since most films are taken from 40 inches. We will estimate an average field size of 14 × 14 inch (196 sq inch). There are approximately 6.5 sq cm per sq inch (2.54 × 2.54 cm), so our field will be 1270 sq cm (6.5 cm/sq inch × 196 sq inch). We will also assume one right angle scattering.

$$E_S = \bar{E} \cdot W \cdot T \cdot 1/d^2 \cdot 1/1000 \cdot F/400$$
$$E_S = 1.4 \cdot 400 \cdot 1 \cdot 1/2^2 \cdot 1/1000 \cdot 1270/400$$
$$E_s = 0.45\ R/wk$$

Using the HVL method to reduce this exposure to the permissible level of 0.1 R/wk:

The HVL at 125 kVp (Table 26–10) is 0.27 mm of lead and 0.8 inch of concrete.

Point A: Exposure — HVL's
           0.45 R/wk — 0
           0.225   — 1
           0.113   — 2
           0.10   — 2.3 HVL's
           0.056   — 3

Lead: 0.27 × 2.3 = 0.62 mm
Concrete: 0.8 × 2.3 = 1.8 inches

HVL Method for Leakage Radiation

We will assume that 6 mA is the maximum continuous exposure the tube will tolerate without overheating. To determine the R/mA · min ($\bar{E}_L$), we divide the 0.1 R/hour permissible leakage exposure by 60 min/hour and 6 mA · min/min:

$$(0.1 \div 60) \div 6 = 0.00028\ R/mA \cdot min$$

The weekly leakage exposure at point A will be:

$$E_L = \bar{E}_L \cdot W \cdot T \cdot 1/d^2$$
$$E_L = 0.00028 \cdot 400 \cdot 1 \cdot \tfrac{1}{2}^2 = 0.028\ R/wk$$

An exposure of 0.028 R/wk is less than the permissible level for a controlled area, so no barrier is required for leakage radiation. The total secondary barrier would be the 0.62 mm of lead required for scatter radiation.

SHIELDING REQUIREMENTS FOR RADIOGRAPHIC FILM

A secondary objective of radiation protection is "to prevent damage or impairment of function of radio-sensitive film or equipment."[6] We will limit our discussion to x-ray film. "An exposure of 1 milliroentgen (mR) over a portion of a film may produce undesirable shadows."[6] For protection purposes, an exposure of 0.2 mR is considered safe. This is the maximum permissible exposure that the film should receive during its entire storage life. We (radiologists) think more of our films than we do of ourselves. The maximum permissible exposure for film is only 0.2 mR as compared to 100 mR/week for ourselves, 500 times as much, and this assumes that the film will only be stored for one week.

Protective barrier calculations for film are exactly the same as those for controlled and uncontrolled areas with one exception. The permissible exposure for the film varies with storage life. For one week of storage, the customary time interval for protection calculations, the permissible level is 0.2 mR. For monthly storage (4 weeks), the film is only permitted a weekly exposure of 0.05 mR (0.2 mR ÷ 4 weeks). The number of HVL's of lead and concrete must be sufficient to bring exposures to the appropriate level. Barrier thicknesses can also be determined from a table[6] similar to Table 26–12.

SUMMARY

Man has lived with, and tolerated, natural radiation since the beginning of time. However, evidence is gathering that small doses of radiation can cause both mutations and neoplasms. No one knows just how much radiation is tolerable, but it is clear that the genetically significant dose has been increasing from man-made sources. The National Council on Radiation Protection's recommendations are designed to protect both the general public and radiation worker. Many of the recommendations have been turned into laws. The most important recommendations are those involving maximum permissible doses, which are currently 5 rem/year for a radiation worker and 0.5 rem/year for the occasionally exposed individual. These levels are broken down into weekly permissible exposures of 0.1 R/wk for controlled areas occupied by radiation workers and 0.01 R/wk for uncontrolled areas occupied by the occasionally exposed individuals. Three modalities are available to reduce radiation exposures: time, distance and barriers. Time plays its role in three ways: (1) in the amount of time that the machine is turned "on" at a particular mA, expressed as mA · min/wk, and called the workload; (2) in the amount of time the beam is directed at a particular area, called the use factor; and (3) in the amount of time that an area is occupied, the occupancy factor. Distance attenuates the beam via the familiar inverse square law. If time and distance fail to bring exposures to permissible levels, then the third method, a barrier, is required. Barriers are usually constructed of either sheet lead or concrete depending on which is cheaper.

Protection must be provided against three kinds of radiation: (1) the primary, or useful beam, (2) scatter radiation and (3) leakage radiation. The latter two, together, are called stray radiation. If the useful beam can be directed at a wall, the wall must be a primary barrier. If the useful beam cannot be directed at a wall, it is a secondary barrier and need only protect from stray radiation. Primary barriers serve a dual function as both primary and secondary barriers.

The exposure from the primary beam can be calculated by multiplying the workload, use factor, occupancy factor, and inverse square of the distance times an R output at 1 meter for each mA of workload. If this exposure, which is expressed in R/wk, exceeds permissible levels, then a barrier is required. Barrier thicknesses can be calculated in two ways: (1) with precalculated tables or (2) with HVL's of lead or concrete. A secondary barrier protects against stray radiation and it is only required when the useful beam cannot be directed at a particular wall. Secondary barriers protect against scatter and leakage radiation. For scatter radiation, the exposure is assumed to be attenuated by a factor of 1000, i.e. reduced to 0.001 at a distance of 1 meter for each right angle scattering, and it is also assumed that its quality does not change. A correction factor is added for field size and the use factor is always 1, since scatter and leakage radiation go in all directions. Otherwise, the calculation is the same as it is for the primary beam. The R output at 1 meter for each mA · min of workload is multiplied by the workload, occupancy factor and inverse square of the distance, a conversion factor for field size and 1/1000 for a right angle scattering.

The exposure from leakage is based upon the law that the maximum radiation level at 1 meter is 0.1 R/hour, or 0.00167 R/min. This exposure must be converted to R/mA · min. The maximum operating mA for continuous exposure at maximum kVp is determined from anode heat rating charts and it is usually about 5 mA. The conversion to R/mA · min is accomplished by dividing the 0.00167 R/min by the maximum continuous mA. This exposure at 1 meter is multiplied by the occupancy factor and inverse square of distance to determine the leakage exposure at the point in question. If the barrier requirements for scatter and leakage differ by more than three half-value layers, the larger suffices; if less than three half-value layers, add one half-value layer to the larger.

REFERENCES

1. Buschong, S. C.: *The Development of Radiation Protection in Diagnostic Radiology.* Cleveland: CRC Press, 1973.
2. Hall, E. J.: *Radiobiology for the Radiologist.* Hagerstown: Harper & Row, 1973.
3. Dalrymple, G. V., Gaulden, M. E., Kollmorgen, G. M., and Vogel, H. G., Jr.: *Medical Radiation Biology.* Philadelphia: W. B. Saunders Co., 1973.
4. Pizzarello, D. J., and Witcofski, R. L.: *Basic Radiation Biology.* 2nd Ed., Philadelphia: Lea & Febiger, 1975.
5. *Basic Radiation Protection Criteria.* National Council on Radiation Protection and Measurements: Washington, D.C.: NCRP Report No. 39, 1971.
6. *Medical X-ray and Gamma-ray Protection for Energies up to 10 MeV–Structural Shielding Design and Evaluation.* National Council on Radiation Protection and Measurements: Washington, D.C.: NCRP Report No. 34, 1970.
7. Schultz, R. J.: *Primer of Radiation Protection.* 2nd Ed., New York: GAF Corporation, X-ray Products, 1969.

Index

Page numbers in *italics* refer to figures;
page numbers followed by t refer to tables.